Teaching Medical Professionalism

Supporting the Development
of a Professional Identity

Second Edition

Teaching Medical Professionalism

Supporting the Development of a Professional Identity

Second Edition

Edited by

Richard L. Cruess
Professor of Surgery and Core Faculty Member in the Centre for Medical Education, Faculty of Medicine, at McGill University in Montreal, Canada

Sylvia R. Cruess
Professor of Medicine and Core Faculty Member in the Centre for Medical Education, Faculty of Medicine, at McGill University, Montreal, Canada

Yvonne Steinert
Professor of Family Medicine and Director of the Centre for Medical Education, Faculty of Medicine, at McGill University, Montreal, Canada

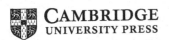

CAMBRIDGE
UNIVERSITY PRESS

University Printing House, Cambridge CB2 8BS, United Kingdom

Cambridge University Press is part of the University of Cambridge.

It furthers the University's mission by disseminating knowledge in the pursuit of education, learning and research at the highest international levels of excellence.

www.cambridge.org
Information on this title: www.cambridge.org/9781107495241

© Cambridge University Press (2009) 2016

First published 2009
Second edition 2016

A catalogue record for this publication is available from the British Library

Library of Congress Cataloguing in Publication data
Cruess, Richard L., editor. | Cruess, Sylvia R. (Sylvia Robinson), 1930– , editor. | Steinert, Yvonne, 1950– , editor.
Teaching medical professionalism : supporting the development of a professional identity / edited by Richard L. Cruess, Sylvia R. Cruess, Yvonne Steinert.
Second edition. | Cambridge ; New York : Cambridge University Press, 2016. | Includes bibliographical references and index.
LCCN 2015042974 | ISBN 9781107495241 (paperback)
| MESH: Professional Competence. | Education, Medical. | Physician's Role. | Physicians – psychology. | Self Concept. | Students, Medical – psychology.
LCC R737 | NLM W 21 | DDC 610–dc23
LC record available at http://lccn.loc.gov/2015042974

ISBN 978-1-107-49524-1 Paperback

....

Contents

Contributors

Louise Arnold, PhD
Professor Emerita and Former Dean of Education, University of Missouri-Kansas City School of Medicine, Kansas City, Missouri, USA

J. Donald Boudreau, MD
Associate Professor of Medicine, Core Faculty Member, Centre for Medical Education, Faculty of Medicine, McGill University, Montreal, Quebec, Canada

Era Buck, PhD
Senior Medical Educator, Assistant Professor, Department of Family Medicine, Office of Educational Development, University of Texas Medical Branch, Galveston, Texas, USA

Richard L. Cruess, MD
Professor of Surgery, Core Faculty Member, Centre for Medical Education, Former Dean of Medicine, Faculty of Medicine, McGill University, Montreal, Quebec, Canada

Sylvia R. Cruess, MD
Professor of Medicine, Core Faculty Member, Centre for Medical Education, Former Director of Professional Services, Royal Victoria Hospital, Faculty of Medicine, McGill University, Montreal, Quebec, Canada

Janet de Groot, MD MSc
Associate Dean, Office of Equity and Professionalism, Associate Professor of Psychiatry and Oncology, Cumming School of Medicine, University of Calgary, Calgary, Alberta, Canada

Mark J. DiCorcia, OTR PhD
Associate Professor of Clinical Biomedical Science, Assistant Dean of Academic Affairs, Charles E. Schmidt College of Medicine, Florida Atlantic University, Boca Raton, USA

Elizabeth Gaufberg, MD MPH
Jean and Harvey Picker Director, Arnold P. Gold Foundation Research Institute, Associate Professor of Medicine and Psychiatry, Harvard Medical School, Boston, Massachusetts, USA

Frederic William Hafferty, PhD
Professor of Medical Education, Division of General Internal Medicine, College of Medicine, Program in Professionalism & Values, Mayo Clinic, Rochester, Minnesota, USA

Brian D. Hodges, MD PhD
Vice President Education, University Health Network, Professor of Psychiatry, Richard and Elizabeth Currie Chair in Health Professions Education Research, University of Toronto, Toronto, Ontario, Canada

Mark D. Holden, MD
Professor and Director, Division of General Internal Medicine, University of Texas Medical Branch, Galveston, Texas, USA

Thomas A. Hutchinson, MB
Professor of Medicine, Director, McGill Programs in Whole Person Care, Faculty of Medicine, McGill University, Montreal, Quebec, Canada

Sir Donald Irvine, CBE MD FRCGP FMedSci
Former President, UK General Medical Council, London, UK

Koshila Kumar, PhD
Lecturer (Clinical Educator Development), Flinders University Rural Clinical School, Adelaide, Australia

Lee A. Learman, MD PhD
Professor of Clinical Biomedical Science, Senior Associate Dean for Graduate Medical Education and Academic Affairs, Charles E. Schmidt College of Medicine, Florida Atlantic University, Boca Raton, USA

Jocelyn Lockyer, PhD
Professor, Department of Community Health
Sciences, Senior Associate Dean of Education,
Cumming School of Medicine, University of Calgary,
Calgary, Alberta, Canada

John Luk, MD
Assistant Dean for Interprofessional Integration,
Assistant Professor of Medicine, Dell Medical School,
University of Texas at Austin, Austin, Texas, USA

Karen V. Mann, PhD
Professor Emeritus, Division of Medical Education,
Dalhousie University, Halifax, Nova Scotia, Canada

Lynn V. Monrouxe, PhD CPsychol FAcadMEd
Professor and Director of the Chang Gung Medical
Education Research Centre, Chang Gung Memorial
Hospital, Linkou, Taiwan

John J. Norcini, PhD
President and Chief Executive Officer, Foundation for
Advancement of International Medical Education
and Research (FAIMER), Philadelphia, Pennsylvania,
USA

Jennifer Quaintance, PhD
Director of Medical Education Support Services,
Associate Research Professor, Department of
Biomedical and Health Informatics, University of
Missouri-Kansas City School of Medicine, Kansas
City, Missouri, USA

**Christopher Roberts, MB ChB FRACGP
MMedSci PhD**
Associate Professor in Primary Care and Medical
Education, Sydney Medical School – Northern
Hornsby Ku-Ring-Gai Hospital, Hornsby, Australia

Judy A. Shea, PhD
Professor of Medicine, Associate Dean of Medical
Education Research, University of Pennsylvania,
Philadelphia, Pennsylvania, USA

Ivan Silver, MD
Professor, Department of Psychiatry, Vice President,
Education, Centre for Addiction and Mental Health,
University of Toronto, Toronto, Ontario,
Canada

Mark Smilovitch, MD
Associate Professor, Division of Cardiology, Faculty
Member, McGill Programs in Whole Person Care,
Faculty of Medicine, McGill University, Montreal,
Quebec, Canada

Linda Snell, MD MHPE FRCPC MACP
Professor of Medicine, Core Faculty Member, Centre
for Medical Education, Faculty of Medicine, McGill
University, Montreal, Quebec, Canada

Yvonne Steinert, PhD
Professor of Family Medicine, Director, Centre
for Medical Education, Richard and Sylvia
Cruess Chair in Medical Education, Faculty of
Medicine, McGill University, Montreal, Quebec,
Canada

Robert Sternszus, MD
Assistant Professor of Pediatrics, Core Faculty
Member, Centre for Medical Education, Faculty of
Medicine, McGill University, Montreal, Quebec,
Canada

Christine Sullivan, MD FACEP
Associate Dean for Graduate Medical Education,
Associate Professor of Emergency Medicine,
University of Missouri-Kansas City School of
Medicine, Kansas City, Missouri, USA

William M. Sullivan, PhD
New American Colleges and Universities,
San Francisco, California, USA

Jill E. Thistlethwaite, MBBS PhD
Adjunct Professor, School of Communications,
University of Technology, Ultimo, Australia

Foreword

This is a report from a movement. It presents ideas, evidence, and guidance for those interested in using the most recent advances in knowledge about learning and human development to enhance medical education's ability to form competent, caring, and publicly responsible physicians. Like all genuine social movements, this new approach is emerging from experience and experiment, in this case by the medical educators involved in articulating a new way of understanding their mission. For that reason, it is an optimist book. The voices are those of many of the leaders, theorists, and experienced practitioners of the new approach who have found in it a promising way to confront the challenges of a new era in medicine.

Though it is not formally a manifesto, this book makes a strong case that professional identity formation needs to become the central focus in educating tomorrow's physicians. In a time when medicine in general, and medical education in particular, finds itself under great stress, the book provides a way in which the profession can respond constructively through a new focus on the professional identity of physicians. The book is also not a how-to manual. But it does provide a thorough review of the learning science and social scientific insights that underlie the changes in training that it calls for, while vividly exemplifying these new educational practices in functioning programs. Neither is this a policy document, though it ought to provide persuasive evidence to support bold proposals to implement the vision of medical education that the book sets out, one that can sustain physicians' commitment to high standards of practice over an entire career.

Since the publication of the first edition of *Teaching Medical Professionalism* in 2009, medical education in the United States and Canada has seen an upsurge in efforts to ensure that physicians at all stages of their training encounter a learning environment that embodies the practice of medicine at its best. "Professionalism" is the term that is often used to encapsulate the complex but utterly essential features of such high-performance practice that is grounded in continuing improvement, focused on the needs of patients, and guided by a sense of social responsibility shared between the profession and the public it is meant to serve. The point of focusing attention on professionalism in medical education, however, is not simply aspirational. It is to effect positive developmental growth in the thinking, skills, and dispositions of future physicians as they move from beginners toward growing competence as professionals.

Through years of careful experimentation and the sharing of insight and experience, the authors gathered in this volume have come to recognize the need to take a further step to deepen medical professionalism, both in understanding and in practice. Teaching medical professionalism has always involved more than simply teaching skills or imparting knowledge. But there has been little consensus about how to describe and understand that "something further." Now, with this volume, the authors propose that the goal of teaching professionalism be named in a clearer and more encompassing way. They call it the formation or "development of professional identity." This is the unifying theme of this book and the topic that all the contributors address from their various perspectives.

From concepts to evidence and then to cases

The volume is organized to first clarify what the development of professional identity is, in both its cognitive base and the theories and research that support it. Next, the import and implications of these concepts – which turn out to be quite wide-ranging – are explored in a section entitled "Principles." Then, as befits a book intended to be useful in spreading and supporting a growing movement, the fourth section provides an arresting group of case studies of how attention to professional identity formation changes and enhances medical education. This section includes illuminating descriptions of learning from mistakes as well as accounts of programmatic success. The fifth section looks to the future.

Much of the value of the book lies in this sequence. Moving from conceptual exploration to empirical evidence, to application of theory, and then to actual case studies, enables the reader to grasp something of the excitement the authors have experienced in their collective intellectual journey. Perhaps most saliently, the volume's organization makes it easy to grasp how much the contemporary learning sciences have contributed to a better understanding of how professionalism actually can be decisive for a developing physician's identity. This knowledge about how identity is formed is further illuminated by new research on how learning environments, ultimately meaning the whole situation of the learner, including relationships with faculty, peers, other professionals, and patients, can be better understood and more effectively managed to support the development of competent practitioners. To grasp the book's breadth of approach, it is worthwhile to attend a bit more closely to how the authors identify the problems they are addressing as well as the assumptions on which their responses are based.

The current moment in medicine as problem and as opportunity

In medicine, as in all professions, identity is closely tied to education. It is in the years of training that extend from medical school through residency and fellowships that physicians learn the craft of modern healing. It is also then that they achieve a sense of themselves as members of the distinct society that comprises medicine as a profession, with its social roles, nomenclature, specific understandings, distinctive practices, and characteristic deportments. Moreover, in medicine, this education is closely linked with the care of patients. While intensively dependent upon the advancing frontiers of biological science and pharmacological as well as technological invention, medicine is ultimately an evolving tradition of practice.

Because medicine is a way of life as well as a body of knowledge and technique, its expertise can only be learned, as the skills of practice can only be transmitted through sustained, face-to-face relationships between mentors and students. In today's healthcare environment, the number and kind of such

educational relationships is expanding. They now routinely include relations among peers and between physicians and nurses and other healthcare professionals working in teams. However, the fundamental reality remains that medicine is an intensely human and social art of healing as well as a highly organized profession. And this fact makes medicine always vulnerable to disruption and loss when the social and economic conditions that support a given organization of the profession begin to change, especially when, as recently, they change rapidly.[1]

The large upsurge in interest in professionalism over the past two decades can best be understood as medicine's response to major changes that, for many in the profession, have threatened to harm the transmission of what they see as essential values. These threatening changes are well-known. One might be called the "Technocratic Illusion." This is the utopian program of turning medicine into an application of bioengineering that would eliminate all ambiguity and uncertainty from clinical practice. Without disparaging the value of new technology or evidence-based care, it is important to note what is left out by the technocratic vision, namely the uncertainties inherent in clinical judgment, as well as any public discussion of the ends, as well as the means, of providing healthcare. The second threat might be called the "Economistic Chimera." This refers to the supposed gains in efficiency promised by the massive commercialization of medicine. These trends undermine the profession's relationship with the public by restructuring practice with little regard to the values intrinsic to medicine. These disruptive changes are common across subspecialties but their effects seem especially acute in medical education. And while in the current jargon of business, "disruption" has become a desirable state, disruption less often plays a positive role in the therapeutic realm.

At least that is the judgment of the influential historian of medical education, Kenneth M. Ludmerer. In his most recent book, *Let Me Heal*, Ludmerer analyzes the shift from what he calls the "educational era" that saw the establishment of the teaching hospital and the residency system as pacesetting innovations in American medical education, to today's medical centers governed by the imperative of "maximum throughput" of patients.[1] Ludmerer underlines the negative implications of this change for the crucial transmission of medical learning and identity through the residency system. The problem is that the push to maximize hospital (and physician) revenue distorts the organizational culture required for successful medical education. It leaves less and less time, attention, and resources to support the sustained teaching relationships on which becoming a good doctor depends. The seriousness of these problems, and their negative effects on developing professional identity, were also analyzed in *Educating Physicians*, the 2010 study of medical education by the Carnegie Foundation for the Advancement of Teaching.[2]

Professionalism as supporting the evolving identity of physicians

In this difficult context, it is clear that it can no longer be presumed that the values of medicine will survive, let alone be effectively transmitted, unless they are consciously fostered in ways that can be effective under changing conditions. Professionalism entails attributes of organizational culture as well as those of individuals. Both must be renewed by being adapted to new circumstances. As a living culture, medicine depends upon intensive, sustained, personal contact. This contact can be augmented and mediated electronically, but, at basis, it is bodily and spatially rooted. The professionalism movement has brought to the foreground these human features of the medical landscape that current trends often inadvertently push to the periphery of attention.

Consider the important issue of student motivation. Studies of student motivation in college and elsewhere underscore the highly contextual nature of motivation for learning. Far from being an inherent and invariant trait of individuals, motivation turns out to be highly malleable, varying significantly over time even for the same individuals. To motivate learning, it turns out that the key is the student's perception that the educator actually cares about whether and how well the student learns. Among colleagues, something similar operates, so that professional performance improves when practitioners understand themselves to be members of a community committed to high standards of professional performance. Recognizing the interrelationship between individual motivation and the quality of relationships prevailing within a specific organizational setting expands the horizon within which medical educators can consider their goals and practices. It also opens the potential for a stronger sense of agency on the part of the educators themselves to improve the organizational culture in which they live.

Professionalism as an educational movement: the key elements

How does the turn to the development of professional identity develop these insights? How might it help to turn present threats to medical education into opportunities for significant improvement? This is to ask how professionalism can succeed as a social movement within the healthcare environment. Like all successful educational movements, it needs to do three things. First, it must provide a catalytic reframing of the issues and articulate overarching goals for change in a convincing way. Second, the movement's participants have to elaborate clear principles that embody what is possible thanks to this new framing of the situation. And, third, the movement has to inspire and nurture core groups of participants who can develop exemplary centers of practice that demonstrate the potentials of the new way of seeing things.

At the heart of all successful social movements, the educational as well as the political kind, lies a reframing of the situation that elicits agreement and mobilizes energy from individuals who until then had experienced the deficiencies of their situation as purely private problems. Such reframing can transform individual acquiescence in a bad situation into collective efforts at improvement. Over the last half-century, a series of social movements – civil rights, women's rights, and marriage equality, to name a few of the most prominent – have reshaped laws and institutions that deeply affect daily life. Each of these movements reframed what had been suffered as merely private difficulties as common problems to be solved. Like a catalytic agent, the new framing of the situation that these movements provided generated bonds among formerly unaffiliated individuals and groups, weaving trust and connection based upon a new sense of sharing common goals. By so doing, the new, shared understanding generated hope and the confidence that made sustained action toward improvement possible.

Something similar has operated at moments of major change in medical education and practice. The Flexner Report, for example, framed the problem of early twentieth-century North American medicine as inadequate training in science, especially clinical science, and proposed the new model medical school with teaching hospital as the exemplary way to overcome these deficiencies. Once taken up by the medical profession, the result was the establishment of an enduring pattern of preparing physicians that has virtually defined the profession for a century.

Reframing the focus of medical education as developing professional identity

The increased attention to professionalism in medical education embodies a deepened understanding that the development of competent and engaged physicians requires more than the acquiring of knowledge and skills by learners. Especially under the conditions sketched above, educating doctors for the healthcare needs of today and tomorrow demands a wholesale reframing of what teaching and learning are about. In doing this, the professionalism movement has brought about a very important shift in perspective. Professionalism has expanded the goals of medical training. By locating the acquisition of knowledge and skills within a larger process of gradual induction into the community of medical practice, it has emphasized the goal of educating physicians who identify with the values and purposes of the profession. It has therefore raised to awareness the necessarily ethical, as well as intellectual and technical, dimensions of medical practice. Articulating these aims has, in turn, focused new attention to the role of physicians as members of a profession with public ethical responsibility as defined by medicine's contract with society at large.

The professionalism movement has therefore called increased attention to the profession's need to ensure that its members develop the identity that the public expects and the ideals of medicine demand. As a result, the question of how best to support the formation of professional identity has assumed greater prominence as a focus of pedagogical research and experimentation. And, as the process of forming a professional identity has become an object of attention and scrutiny, the notion of knowledge presumed by discussions of medical education has itself begun to shift. From an older view that thought of knowledge and skill as being acquired by the learner, often imagined in isolation from contexts of social interaction and apart from institutional norms and expectations, a new view has emerged. Instead, learning is now increasingly understood as an interactive process of social participation.

This shift in perspective significantly strengthens the agenda of the professionalism movement. Indeed, the shift to a participatory understanding of learning gives new depth and clarity to the reframing of medical education as the development of professional identity. The perspective of participation highlights the contexts of learning and, importantly, the changing social position and personal stance of the learner across the process of becoming a doctor. Effective learning of medicine, in this view, means moving from a stance of observer on the outside or periphery of the practice through graduated stages toward becoming a skilled participant at the center of the action. Seen as growing participation in the profession's community of expert practice, developing competence becomes inseparable from the formation of a sense of identity committed to the profession's mission and standards.

Convergence on the idea of social learning

A striking feature of this second edition of *Teaching Medical Professionalism* is the convergence among the authors of the chapters toward a common focus of attention on the process of social learning. This serves as the fundamental notion underlying the framing of medical education as professional identity development. Within this new framework of understanding, developing a professional identity is a process that is at once a transformation of an individual's identity, in which the individual is ultimately the key actor, and a passage through shared environments. These learning environments are shaped by particular organizational cultures that embody, to notably different degrees, the norms of the profession and which can either support or undermine the efforts to make professionalism prevail as the overarching value.

The key concept is that learning to practice medicine is always, implicitly or explicitly, also a process of learning to *be* a physician. Before the professionalism movement called attention to this fact, medical education typically carried out much of its formative work tacitly. As noted, this made the whole process easily vulnerable to disruption. The chapters gathered here provide several theoretical perspectives on learning and psychosocial development that make articulation of medicine's implicit goals more powerful.

These perspectives derive from social research and the learning sciences.

One approach proceeds from the inside out. It is derived from cognitive psychology, particularly the "constructivist" idea of learning that underlies much of current research on human development. This approach calls attention to the active role of the learner. Rather than the proverbial "blank slate," the learner is understood as always actively trying to make sense of what is encountered, trying to weave newly acquired knowledge and performance skills into the individual's existing fabric of understandings of the world and the self in the world. An important implication of this viewpoint for medical educators is the value to them of grasping the sense their students are making of their experience, which may be quite different from what the educators intend, and engaging with their students' understanding to advance their development.

The other approach proceeds from the outside in. It derives from social psychology and sociology, especially the theory of socialization. The underlying metaphor here is learning as bringing new entrants into an ongoing team effort to achieve shared goals. This viewpoint highlights the fact that learners always occupy roles in relation to others in social groups – roles that strongly affect both the cognitive and the emotive stance of the learner. There is ample evidence of how strongly social role and position can influence the learner's stance toward her experience, including the way the learner comes to feel about her own capacity to understand the world and her legitimacy in occupying a particular social role. These insights are crucial to making medicine a more welcoming environment in a diverse society. This perspective also emphasizes the importance for motivation and learning of role models and mentors in medical education. Its attention to social context illuminates the way different, even conflicting, expectations and norms can be embodied in the culture of an organization, with the result that the implicit but unacknowledged norms can become more formative of professional identity than the organizations' formal, stated values, as in the idea of the "hidden curriculum."

The key point of convergence between the two approaches, with their respective research literatures, lies in the idea of learning as a function of participation. The metaphor of learning as participation spans the psychological and the social while emphasizing the agency of both the learner and the community of educators. The very movement from periphery toward the center depends upon a synergy between the movements from the inside out and the outside in. On the one hand, the literature makes it clear that active sense-making is a key contributor to identity development, and that this process can be analyzed and its components intentionally strengthened through pedagogical interventions. On the other hand, it is equally clear that students' sense of agency is best engaged toward positive identification with professional values when educators and learners both become more aware of the often unseen power of organizational cultures. As educators themselves become more aware of these influences, they become better able to intentionally foster a more reflective and proactive stance on the part of learners toward their own development.

Principles and implications: three illustrations

The chapters in Part I and Part II explain these concepts and the research literatures from which they derive. From this enhanced theoretical base, the authors of chapters in the subsequent sections go on to explore the implications of the approach for a number of topics important for the success of the professionalism movement. Later chapters take up, for example, what is known about how to reliably assess progress toward the development of professional identity; the means available for remediating lapses in professional behavior; and the most effective ways to implement programs of faculty development in support of identity formation. There is also discussion of how licensing and accrediting bodies might play more constructive roles in advancing the formation of professional identity.

In addition, three other topics can illustrate the power of the book's framing concepts: the emerging conception of professional education environments as "developmental networks"; strategies for fostering continuity in learning and identity development across major moments of transition; and attention to new forms of practice, especially interprofessional educational experiences.

Developmental networks

The synergy between fostering students' own meaning-making, and explicitly modeling professionalism and providing mentoring relationships, has given rise in the literature to the idea of professional schools as evolving "developmental networks." At the center of this idea lies the notion that a strong professional identity requires that students develop a proactive stance toward their own learning and career choices. However, it is not assumed that this should happen in isolation from efforts to design and foster educational environments built around explicit criteria of professionalism.

One of the points of convergence among educational researchers concerned with formation of identity is the importance of developing habits of self-reflection among students. This is entirely consistent with the metaphor of learning as participation. Reflection in that perspective names the process by which the learner develops greater awareness of her own capacities and ways of thinking and responding to experiences. Well-designed learning spaces and experiences – those that provide explicit modeling of what is to be learned, opportunity for the learners to practice this, and the provision of feedback on their performance – make the objectives of learning clear and assessable. Clear learning objectives, in turn, enable learners to orient their efforts and to become aware of their progress, as well as to relate their new experience to their ongoing sense of who they are.

Practices of reflection are quite varied and can take different forms at different points in the educational journey, ranging from the directed to the spontaneous. Reflection can be carried out privately or in small groups, with or without feedback from instructors or preceptors. The evidence is increasingly strong that in all its forms, reflection can be a powerful tool. Carried on in a context explicitly structured around the norms of professionalism, reflection proves an important aid toward becoming a self-directed learner, an essential quality for a successful later life as a physician.

What is perhaps most striking in the examples the book provides is the value of formally cultivating reflective practices among educators themselves. By becoming more aware of their own progress and difficulties, reflection helps educators recognize the need for change and further learning. But most importantly, it encourages greater empathy with students' struggles toward a well-integrated professional identity, promoting the kind of mutual engagement that is optimal for professional and personal development.

Attention to continuity at transition points

Medical education is marked by major transitions between different environments for learning – transitions that require students and more advanced practitioners alike to navigate large discontinuities in the roles they occupy, as well as in the cognitive and emotive stance they are expected to assume. Entering medical school, the first experience of the dissection lab, the first encounter with death in a clinical context: all these provoke tension, uncertainty, and reflection about one's sense of purpose and one's fit with the world of medicine. Similar moments of discontinuity appear in the transition from predominantly classroom-based to clinical education, in gradually assuming responsibility for patient care and entry into residency. Such moments continue into the years of practice.

The literature on role modeling and mentorship presented in many chapters gives important resources for making sure that continuity of purpose and identity remains strong across these disorienting moments. Programs intending to foster identity development can draw upon a growing base of experience and research for tested methods of making it through the transitions with an enhanced, rather than wounded, sense of agency and meaning. Today's fuller understanding of how identity matures can help students with what for many is a highly challenging transition: the cognitive and emotive shock attendant upon realizing that medical practice will frustrate expectations of certainty. Developing a new resiliency in the face of having to take responsibility in the face of endemic ambiguity and uncertainty, one of the most important professional virtues, can be greatly aided when the student is able to reflect on this experience in a supportive context and with awareness that this too is a necessary transition.

Attention to changing forms of practice: interprofessional learning experiences

The rapid changes in the contexts and forms of medical practice make this an issue that is likely to loom ever larger for future medical students and residents. With its discussion of interprofessional education in the health fields, the book provides an illuminating example of how recent research in learning and socialization theory can assist in designing and testing new learning experiences to help students who will work in healthcare teams that are, like the settings in which they function, organized quite differently than has been typical. Learning from, with, and about allied healthcare professionals, including nurses but also pharmacists and technicians, is an area fraught with the possibility of missteps. So, it is important that experiments in this area proceed with as much knowledgeable guidance as possible.

Research is already identifying promising strategies for fostering forms of "cohesive practice" involving multiple professions. For example, longitudinal integrated clinical placements that enable medical and nursing students to train and work together in carefully designed settings seem to promote trust and collaboration that result in good patient outcomes. However, what is still to be determined is how such experiences can and ought to contribute to the physicians' and nurses' developing sense of identity. The issues such experiments raise echo some of those described above, especially the problem of coping with dissonance among points of view and social roles in ways that build a genuinely interprofessional sense of participation in the enterprise of healthcare provision.

"Rounds" of professional identity formation: learning from cases

For readers seeking a fuller sense of what is entailed in the shift toward professional identity formation as an overarching goal of medical education, the most inspiring section of the book is likely to be the fourth. This section presents a set of well-developed cases that describe the experiences of several institutions that have made large-scale attempts to implement the ideas set out earlier in the volume. Since reasoning and learning by cases is the classic method by which medicine advances, it is fitting that a book seeking to advance a movement of reform in medical education should conclude with the presentation and discussion of such cases.

Four chapters present stories of three institutions that have engaged in reform addressing diverse aspects of medical formation. The University of Texas Medical Branch has implemented a new undergraduate curriculum based on professional identity formation. McGill University's Faculty of Medicine

has reshaped its undergraduate program on professionalism to now center on professional identity formation, while the same institution has also introduced identity formation into its residency programs. Colleagues at Indiana University have described ways to alter the learning environment so that it can support professional identity formation.

With more than a decade of experience, McGill's four-year, longitudinal, undergraduate Physicianship Program provides an illuminating example of the possibilities opened up by making professional identity development the common focus of a whole educational program. At its center are an interconnected set of practices and roles that emphasize the students' biographical coherence. This represents a departure from the inherited pattern of medical schools, which, like most other professional schools, have often distanced the beginner from previous ways of thinking and earlier identities. The idea behind this boot-camp or ordeal-like approach seems to have been a belief that the old, lay self had first to be decommissioned before a new, fully professional identity, with its attendant new way of thinking about self and world, could be constructed in its place. The student's role in this process was largely reactive, allowing herself to be reshaped by new authorities.

Instead, the Physicianship Program draws on the theories of social learning to support students as they negotiate actively their movement from the periphery of the medical community toward deeper participation. To accomplish this, the program deliberately asks students to articulate and draw upon their earlier motivations and predispositions toward a medical career. The program provides concepts, common experiences, reflection, and active guidance to enable students to weave together a narrative that links their past lives and significant communities, with their present efforts to understand and enter the new community of medicine. The program aspires to give students the understanding and confidence necessary to look toward a future identity as a professional, a purpose that can enable them to create continuities across the difficult points of transition they must navigate.

When they enter medical school, McGill's students are placed in small learning communities of six peers who, together with two volunteer upperclass students, meet three times each semester, throughout the four undergraduate years. These groups are led by selected members of the clinical faculty who have become Osler Fellows, named after the famous clinician. The fellows act as mentors to the group, having themselves already spent a year in similar groups of faculty engaged in the program. Known as Physician Apprenticeship, the learning communities take up different topics each year, appropriate to the group members' progress through the medical curriculum. They begin with discussions of their own goals in relation to definitions of modern roles of healer and professional and conclude in the fourth year with deliberative sessions that explore basic tensions endemic to the physician's identity as preparation for residency and the further transitions to come.

It is worth noting how many of the emphases and pedagogical approaches discussed in the earlier chapters of the volume show up as important practices in the cases presented. McGill's Physicianship Program is not an outlier in this regard. Practices of reflection, for instance, appear in a myriad of forms. Every program has developed ways to make the modeling of professional virtues and judgment a conspicuous feature of daily life for all involved. Perhaps most significantly, all the programs have worked out, including through trial and error, methods of fostering, not only continuity in medical learning but biographical coherence as well. This enables students to more intentionally and reliably develop as physicians who will embody the best values of medicine.

These cases, then, illustrate how the ideas promoted in this volume look in practice. They invite the reader to enter imaginatively into the atmosphere of a set of ongoing educational experiments that are helping to advance the agenda of professional identity formation. And so, they lead back to the proposal that begins the book: that learning medicine for our time is best reframed as the development of a professional identity centered on the central values of the community of physicians. The ideas as well as the examples presented in this book are all works in various stages of progress. The important point, however, is that this experiment is now ongoing and gathering momentum. As an educational movement, it is serious, increasingly well-grounded in evidence, and spreading. Perhaps most valuable of all, it is inspiring.

William M. Sullivan

References

1. Ludmerer, KM. *Let Me Heal: The Opportunity to Preserve Excellence in American Medicine.* Oxford, UK: Oxford University Press; 2015.

2. Cooke, M, Irby, DM, O'Brien, BC. *Educating Physicians: A Call for Reform of Medical School and Residency.* San Francisco, CA: Jossey-Bass; 2010.

Introduction

Richard L. Cruess, Sylvia R. Cruess, and Yvonne Steinert

When the first edition of *Teaching Medical Professionalism*[1] was published, considerable experience on teaching and assessing professionalism had been developed in medicine's educational establishments. The book was therefore based upon a body of knowledge that existed, and the authors formed their recommendations upon their own experiences and that of others working in the field. The emphasis has recently shifted from teaching professionalism to supporting professional identity formation,[2–4] despite a lack of literature outlining how professional identity formation can be supported throughout the continuum of medical education. It is our hope that this book can partially fill the void, as it brings together educators and researchers who have focused on the subject of professional identity formation in medicine.

The idea that physicians actually have a professional identity is not new. In 1957, Merton published one of the first studies of the sociology of medical education.[5] In the introduction to the book, Merton stated (p. 5) that medical education has a dual purpose: "to shape the novice into the effective practitioner of medicine, to give him the best available knowledge and skills, and to provide him with a professional identity so that he comes to think, act, and feel like a physician."[5] Through the ages, great emphasis has been placed on ensuring that medical graduates possess the requisite knowledge and skills, using increasingly sophisticated methods of teaching and assessment.[6]

Until recently, it was assumed that medical students and residents would acquire their professional identities by patterning their behavior after respected role models.[7] The desired identities were encompassed in the concept of professionalism, and physicians were expected to behave like professionals. While there were frequent references in the literature to professionalism, it was not addressed explicitly, being mainly taught in the informal curriculum.

There is agreement that this historic system functioned reasonably well, as long as a homogeneous medical profession that was largely male and made up of members of the dominant social group served a comparably homogeneous population.[7] There was also general agreement between medicine and society on shared values. The world changed after World War II. As the medical profession and the society that it served became wonderfully diverse, passing on the traditional values cherished by both the profession and society became more difficult. This was occurring as medicine and systems of healthcare delivery became more complex. The day of the solo practitioner treating a paying patient is a part of history, along with a type of professionalism that has been termed "nostalgic."[8] As the practice of medicine was transformed after World War II from a cottage industry into an activity that consumes a significant percentage of the gross national product of every country, medicine's adherence to its traditional value systems was questioned.[9,10] Individual physicians and the profession were thought to place their own interests ahead of the interests of patients and of society, and the profession was accused of a lack of rigor in setting and maintaining standards. There was a loss of public trust in individual physicians and in the profession. There was general agreement in both society and within the medical profession that medicine's professionalism was threatened.[6]

The medical profession did react, motivated in part by a desire to maintain medicine's privileged position in society.[11] Nevertheless, the response did include attempts at more rigorous and open self-regulation and a major effort on the part of the educational establishment to ensure that each physician entering practice would understand the nature of professionalism and the importance of meeting medicine's professional obligations.[7,12] What has been termed "the professionalism project"[13] began in the

Teaching Medical Professionalism, 2nd Edition, ed. Richard L. Cruess, Sylvia R. Cruess and Yvonne Steinert.
Published by Cambridge University Press. © Cambridge University Press 2016.

1980s and 1990s. The objective was to teach professionalism explicitly, thus transferring it from the informal to the formal curriculum. As the movement grew, definitions of professionalism emerged,[14] and methods of teaching[15] and assessing[16] professionalism were developed. Faculty development programs also supported these activities.[17] Finally, the importance of professionalism in the medical curriculum at both the undergraduate and postgraduate levels was established when accrediting bodies throughout the world required that it be taught and assessed.

Until now, the educational objective has been teaching professionalism, with the implication that it is incumbent upon students to learn it, along with other aspects of the formal curriculum. The literature on teaching professionalism does contain frequent references to the desirability of medical students and residents acquiring a professional identity. However, as was true of the words *profession* and *professionalism* prior to the 1980s, the concept remained aspirational in nature and was rarely defined. This situation has changed dramatically during the past decade. An extensive literature exists in developmental psychology and other academic fields that describes how each human being proceeds through developmental stages from birth and throughout adult life, emerging with a unique identity or identities.[18] Individuals with backgrounds in both medicine and the social sciences have examined the nature of professional identity in medicine, provided definitions of it and of identity formation, and have explored the nature of the process of socialization through which professional identities are formed.[4] There is now an extensive literature, easily accessible to medical educators on the subject.

As this literature appeared, there began to be questions on the assumptions underlying programs devoted to teaching professionalism. It was assumed that if practitioners understand the nature of contemporary professionalism and the obligations that they must fulfill in order to meet societal expectations, they would consistently exhibit professional behaviors. Hafferty[19] wondered if this is sufficient. He asked, "Does it really matter what one believes as long as one acts professionally?" (p. 54) He answered his own question[19] by stating that "the fundamental uncertainties that underscore clinical decision making and the ambiguities that permeate medical practice, require a professional presence that is best grounded in what one is rather than what one does." (p. 54) The Carnegie Foundation report on the future of medical education broke new ground when it recommended that professional identity formation in medicine represent a foundational element to medical education.[2] Subsequent to this influential report, others have supported this approach, agreeing with Merton et al. that professional identity formation is a fundamental aspect of medical education.[2,4]

When assisting learners at all levels of medical education to develop their own professional identities becomes the educational objective, the emphasis shifts from faculty members teaching professionalism to a new paradigm in which students are actively engaged in the development of their own professional identities. The role of faculty is to assist students in understanding the process of identity formation and of socialization, and to engage them in monitoring their own journey from layperson to professional.

We believe that the true aim of medical education throughout the ages has always been the creation of a professional identity in emerging physicians. If this transformational change is accepted, a new approach to education based upon the duality proposed by Merton[5] is required in which knowledge, skills, and professional identity are given equal attention.

Concurrent with an interest in identity formation has been the growing acceptance of the concept of communities of practice as being applicable to both medicine and medical education.[20] Medical students voluntarily wish to join the community of practice that is medicine, and, in the process of joining, they acquire the identity of members of the group. In acquiring this identity, they must also accept the norms of the community of practice.

If the objective of medical education becomes supporting professional identity formation, there are major implications for curricular design. New educational objectives must be established; definitions of professionalism, professional identity, and socialization currently available must be incorporated into the curriculum; and methods of engaging and supporting students and residents as they develop their identities must be developed. Faculty development is essential, and methods of assessing progress toward a professional identity must be created.

Much has already been accomplished. The experience gained in teaching professionalism is invaluable and can serve as the basis for instituting programs to support professional identity formation. The norms of the community of practice, of great importance to the professional identity of physicians,[4,20] are encompassed in the word *professionalism*. Programs that have been devoted to teaching professionalism can use these norms as they move toward supporting professional identity formation.

The aim of this book is to assist those who wish to institute programs devoted to professional identity formation. The content of many chapters is truly new and innovative and built on past achievements. The authors have examined the foundational aspects of medical education through the lens of identity formation. In many instances, this reorients what has been done in the past without requiring great changes. In others, it provides new insights that can guide us in the future. As an example, examining remediation or continuing professional development through the lens of identity formation can engender hope for real progress in areas that have proved difficult in the past.

The book provides guidance on what must be taught, the cognitive base of professionalism, the theoretical basis of identity, and the nature of the process of socialization. It describes the educational theory and strategies for supporting professional identity formation. It also analyzes those educational methods most relevant to identity formation, role modeling and mentoring, and experiential learning and reflection. General principles for establishing programs on professional identity formation are provided, along with information relevant to including professionalism in identity formation. Assessment and remediation are reinterpreted in terms of identity formation, methods of reorienting faculty development are outlined, and the important role of licensing and certifying bodies is discussed. A section of the book contains case studies from institutions that have begun the transformation from teaching professionalism to supporting professional identity formation at the undergraduate and postgraduate levels. A case study on changing the learning environment so that it is supportive of identity formation is also present. In the final section of the book, the evolving nature of professional identities is recognized in an attempt to look forward to the possible identities of the future.

It is hoped that this book will be of assistance to those responsible for designing and implementing programs of instruction on professionalism and professional identity formation. It should also be of interest to both teachers and learners. While aimed specifically at the medical community, it should be noted that the terms *profession*, *professional*, and *professionalism* are generic and applicable to other occupations, both within and outside the healthcare field. All healthcare professionals have professional identities that are formed through socialization. The authors hope that the chapters in this book will be of assistance to those responsible for educating other members of the healthcare team, with whom future physicians will most certainly interact. Those who read the book from cover to cover can obtain a comprehensive background for program development and teaching in the field of medical professionalism. However, each chapter can stand alone and be used by readers with specific areas of interest.

The authors who have contributed to this work are true experts in the field and have been pioneers in addressing professional identity formation. The editors would like to thank each and every one for their support, their extraordinary creativity and innovation, and their commitment to the project. We are also grateful to the students, residents, and faculty members of McGill University for their enthusiastic participation in our work. Finally, we thank our colleagues at the Centre for Medical Education for their intellectual engagement, honest feedback, and creative suggestions as we have tested our concepts and beliefs with them. We are also grateful to Melissa Como for her assistance in preparing this volume.

William Sullivan[21] has written that "recognizing the formative nature of medical education gives medical educators an opportunity to become more self-aware and intentional about how future physicians actually develop." (p. xi) It is our hope that by intentionally and explicitly addressing professional identity formation during the continuum of medical education, we will move toward our aspirational goal of ensuring that each graduating medical student or resident "thinks, feels, and acts like a physician."

References

1. Cruess, RL, Cruess, SR, Steinert, Y, eds. *Teaching Medical Professionalism*. New York, NY: Cambridge University Press; 2009.

2. Cooke, M, Irby, DM, O'Brien, BC. *Educating Physicians: A Call for Reform of Medical School and Residency*. San Francisco, CA: Jossey-Bass; 2010.

3. Jarvis-Selinger, S, Pratt, DD, Regehr, G. Competency is not enough: integrating identity formation into the medical education discourse. *Acad Med*. 2012; 87(9):1185–90.

4. Cruess, RL, Cruess, SR, Boudreau, JD, Snell, L, Steinert, Y. Reframing medical education to support professional identity formation. *Acad Med.* 2014; **89**(11):1446–51.

5. Merton, RK, Some preliminaries to a sociology of medical education. Preface. In Merton, RK, Reader, LG, Kendall, PL, eds. *The Student Physician: Introductory Studies in the Sociology of Medical Education.* Cambridge, MA: Harvard University Press; 1957:vii–ix.

6. Bonner, TN. *Becoming a Physician: Medical Education in Great Britain, France, Germany, and the United States, 1750–1945.* New York, NY: Oxford University Press; 1995.

7. Cruess, RL, Cruess, SR. Teaching medicine as a profession in the service of healing. *Acad Med.* 1997; **72**(11):941–52.

8. Hafferty, FW, Castellani, B. A sociological framing of medicine's modern-day professionalism movement. *Med Educ.* 2009; **43**(9):826–28.

9. Starr, P. *The Social Transformation of American Medicine.* New York, NY: Basic Books; 1982.

10. Freidson, E. *Professionalism: The Third Logic.* Cambridge, UK: Polity; 2001.

11. Martimianakis, MA, Maniate, JM, Hodges, BD. Sociological interpretations of professionalism. *Med Educ.* 2009; **43**(9):829–37.

12. Cohen, JJ. Professionalism in medical education, an American perspective: from evidence to accountability. *Med Educ.* 2006; **40**(7):607–17.

13. Wear, D, Kuczewski, MG. The professionalism movement: can we pause? *Am J Bioeth.* 2004; **4**(2):1–10.

14. Birden, H, Glass, N, Wilson, I, Harrison, M, Usherwood, T, Nass, D. Defining professionalism in medical education: a systematic review. *Med Teach.* 2014; **36**(1):47–61.

15. Birden, H, Glass, N, Wilson, I, Harrison, M, Usherwood, T, Nass, D. Teaching professionalism in medical education: a Best Evidence Medical Education (BEME) systematic review. *Med Teach.* 2013; **35**(7): e1252–e1266.

16. Hodges, BD, Ginsburg, S, Cruess, R, Cruess, S, Delport, R, Hafferty, F, Ho, MJ, Holmboe, E, Holtman, M, Ohbu, S, Rees, C, Ten Cate, O, Tsugawa, Y, Van Mook, W, Wass, V, Wilkinson, T, Wade, W. Assessment of professionalism: recommendations from the Ottawa 2010 Conference. *Med Teach.* 2011; **33**(5):354–63.

17. Steinert, Y, Cruess, RL, Cruess, SR, Boudreau, JD, Fuks, A. Faculty development as an instrument of change: a case study on teaching professionalism. *Acad Med.* 2007; **82**(11):1057–64.

18. Monrouxe, LV. Identities, self and medical education. In Walsh, K, ed. *Oxford Textbook of Medical Education.* Oxford, UK: Oxford University Press; 2013:113–23.

19. Hafferty, FW. Professionalism and the socialization of medical students. In Cruess, RL, Cruess, SR, Steinert, Y, eds. *Teaching Medical Professionalism.* New York, NY: Cambridge University Press; 2009:53–73.

20. Lave, J, Wenger, E. *Situated Learning: Legitimate Peripheral Participation.* Cambridge, UK: Cambridge University Press; 1991.

21. Sullivan, WM. Introduction. In Cruess, RL, Cruess, SR, Steinert, Y, eds. *Teaching Medical Professionalism.* New York, NY: Cambridge University Press; 2009: ix–xvi.

Professionalism and professional identity formation: the cognitive base

Richard L. Cruess and Sylvia R. Cruess

The task of medical education is to "shape the novice into the effective practitioner of medicine, to give him the best available knowledge and skills, and to provide him with a professional identity so that he *comes to think, act, and feel like a physician.*"[1] (p. 5)

During the past few decades, it has become apparent that the issue of the professionalism of individual physicians and of the medical profession must be addressed explicitly at all levels of medical education. For this reason, the subjects of professionalism and professional identity are being addressed directly throughout the continuum of medical education.[2–10] As is true of any significant topic that must be learned, there is a defined body of knowledge called the cognitive base that serves as the basis of the teaching, learning, and assessment of the subject. The purpose of this chapter is to outline the cognitive base that should underpin educational activities designed to support learners in medicine as they become professionals and acquire their professional identities.

As physicians, patients, and members of the general public have come to believe that medicine's professionalism is under threat, virtually all have concluded that any action to address the issue must include major initiatives throughout medical education aimed at ensuring that physicians both understand the nature of contemporary medical professionalism and live according to its precepts – that they come to "think, act, and feel like a physician."[1–6] As a result, there is now a substantial literature describing how this can best be accomplished, with a recent shift in emphasis toward supporting professional identity formation.[7–10]

For centuries, professionalism as a subject was not addressed directly. There were no courses on professionalism and it was not included in the standard medical curriculum. This is not because it was deemed unimportant. The Hippocratic Oath, subsequent codes of ethics, and a host of writers addressed the values and beliefs of the medical profession, often linking them to the word "professionalism." However, it was assumed that these values and beliefs that are the foundation of the profession would be automatically acquired during the educational process as students "acquire the complex ensemble of analytic thinking, skillful practice, and wise judgment."[5] The learning of professionalism depended heavily upon the use of role models, that is, situations in which students, residents, and, indeed, practicing physicians patterned their behavior on "individuals admired for their ways of being and acting as professionals."[11] While this method remains essential and powerful, by itself it is no longer deemed adequate.[3,4,6,12]

At first, general agreement developed among educators that professionalism must be taught and evaluated as a specific topic at both the undergraduate and postgraduate levels. In recent years, certifying and accrediting bodies have required this.[13–16] As a result, a substantial literature emerged defining medical professionalism and its relation to medicine's social contract. The difficult issue of how best to assess professionalism was also addressed.[17,18] While disagreements continued to exist over the nature of professionalism and how best to communicate it, there was agreement that what had been largely implicit in medical education must be made explicit.[18] The intent of the first edition of this book was to present the theoretical basis for teaching and assessing professionalism and to outline the means by which this could be accomplished, based on the knowledge and best practices of the time.

The commonly stated educational objective was to ensure that learners at all levels understood the

Teaching Medical Professionalism, 2nd Edition, ed. Richard L. Cruess, Sylvia R. Cruess and Yvonne Steinert.
Published by Cambridge University Press. © Cambridge University Press 2016.

cognitive base of professionalism, internalized the value system of the medical profession, and consistently demonstrated the behaviors expected of a professional.[19] While the idea of professional identity was occasionally invoked, assisting students to develop a professional identity was not a stated goal, in part due to a lack of understanding of the process of identity formation within the medical profession. This is no longer true. There is now an extensive and rich literature devoted to professional identity formation in medicine that has contributed to our understanding of the nature of medical professional identity and the process of socialization through which this identity is formed.[20–47] Accompanying the emergence of this literature has been the belief by many that the real objective of teaching professionalism has always been to assist students as they develop their own professional identities. Teaching and assessing professionalism have thus represented a means to an end rather than ends in themselves. As a result, there have been calls to reframe medical education around professional identity formation,[7,9,10] an approach that we strongly support.

This does not mean that past efforts devoted to the teaching and assessment of professionalism are without value and can be discarded. The attributes of the professional represent the norms to which learners aspire. The programs devoted to the teaching and assessment of professionalism can be modified to support the educational objective of assisting learners as they develop their own professional identity or identities, particularly as both lean so heavily on reflection as a formative element.

This chapter will propose that medicine represents a community of practice (or practices) that students and residents wish to join. As they join the community, they acquire the professional identity expected of members of the community. They must learn and adhere to the values and norms of the community to acquire this identity. Understanding the values and norms requires a definition of profession or professionalism, the reasons for the existence of professions, knowledge of the attributes of a member of the profession, and the relationship of professionalism to medicine's social contract with society. This material, along with an understanding of the concepts of professional identity formation and socialization, constitute the cognitive base to be communicated to those wishing to enter the profession of medicine.

Medicine as a community of practice

Social learning theory has been invoked to both understand and guide medical education (see Chapter 5). The concepts of communities of practice and situated learning developed by Lave and Wenger[48] have been particularly helpful because they appear to reflect the reality of both medical education and practice. The concept is presented schematically in Figure 1.1.

Lave and Wenger[48] and Wenger[49] propose that social interaction between individuals promotes learning, and that a community of practice is created when those who wish to share a common body of knowledge engage in activities whose aim is to become knowledgeable and skilled in a defined field.

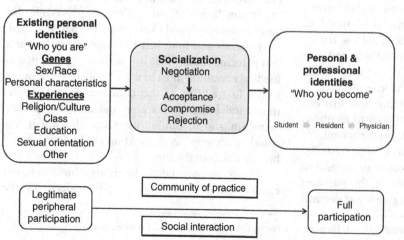

Figure 1.1. A schematic representation of professional identity formation and socialization, indicating that individuals enter the process of socialization with partially developed identities and emerge with both personal and professional identities (upper portion). The process of socialization in medicine results in an individual moving from legitimate peripheral participation in a community of practice to full participation, primarily through social interaction (lower portion).[46] Reprinted with permission by *Academic Medicine* © 2015.

The result is the acquisition of both a body of knowledge and skills and a set of acceptable behaviors – a way of "being." The learning, which is both explicit and tacit, takes place within the defined domain and thus is "situated." As a consequence, the individual moves from "legitimate peripheral participation" to full participation in the community. An important aspect of full participation, according to these authors, is the acquisition of the identity associated with the community. This activity is voluntary – the individual wishes to join the community and over time accepts its values and norms. The movement from peripheral participation to the center is not linear, but occurs in stages, proceeding from observation to imitation to carrying out uncomplicated tasks and culminating in more complex activities. This description applies to the transformation of a medical student from a member of the lay public to a professional. The sense of belonging that accompanies the development of a professional identity is an important component of a community of practice. It translates into the collegiality of the profession.[50] Finally, the profession exerts a compelling social influence on its members, as compliance with professional norms and values eventually emerges from within the individual.[51,52]

The health of the community depends upon the voluntary engagement of its members and on the presence of leadership. According to Wenger et al.[53] (p. 11), "one of the primary tasks of a community of practice is to establish the common baseline and standardize what is well-understood." These standards represent the norms of medicine's community of practice. While there certainly are values that have persisted through the ages, such as caring and compassion, some norms change over time as the social contract between medicine and society evolves, altering the expectations of patients, society, and physicians.[54] Each individual wishing to join the community must adhere to the majority of these norms. Failure to do so can inhibit progress to full membership or elicit sanctions or exclusion from the community.[24,51]

In the past, the identity of physicians has been exclusionary because the profession was dominated by white males of the dominant religion.[22,24,26,31] The hierarchical organization of the profession tended to perpetuate the existing power relationships, making change difficult. Even though progress has been made, with the community becoming more representative of the society it serves, minority and class distinctions still exist, making entry challenging for many.[22,24,31,37] In addition, and without question, tension arises between the imperative to impose norms and standards in an effort to homogenize values and the desire of individuals to maintain important aspects of their own identity as they join the community of practice.[26,37]

The description of communities of practice presented by Wenger et al.[51] (p. 38) seems to describe the practice of medicine: "a set of socially defined ways of doing things in a specific domain: a set of common approaches and shared standards that create the basis for action, communication, problem solving, performance, and accountability." This is an accurate description of the practice of medicine.

Profession, professionalism, professional identity, and professional identity formation

In dealing with the interconnected concepts of profession, professionalism, professional identity, and professional identity formation, words and definitions become important. This is particularly relevant because the literature frequently states that professionalism is difficult to define, often accompanied by the admonition that it cannot be taught, learned, or assessed without such a definition.[18,55] We have long believed that the definitions, most of which deal with the word "professionalism," enjoy many more commonalities than differences. What is unquestionably true, and widely accepted, is that each institution involved in teaching professionalism or promoting the development of professional identities must have a set of institutional definitions accepted by all within the institution.[2,3,18] What is taught, learned, and assessed should spring from these definitions. What cannot be explicitly defined cannot be taught, learned, or assessed.[18]

If medical education is to be reframed around the concept of professional identity formation, the definitions of identity, professional identity, and professional identity formation become foundational elements of any educational program. The definitions of the words "profession" and "professionalism" become important descriptors of the desired identity associated with medicine as a community of practice. They should both represent the historical value systems of medicine as a healing art and reflect their contemporary state.

Chapters 3 and 4 present in-depth analyses of the nature of professional identity, professional identity formation, and socialization. In this chapter, we will use material drawn from these chapters so that it can serve as the basis of educational programs to support professional identity formation.

Professional identity

The Oxford English Dictionary definition of identity is the following: "a set of characteristics or a description that distinguishes a person or thing from others."[56] While this definition is certainly accurate, it is too broad to be useful as the basis of a program in medical education. With our colleagues in the Faculty of Medicine at McGill University, we have therefore developed a definition of medical professional identity. A physician's professional identity is "a representation of self, achieved in stages over time, during which the characteristics, values, and norms of the medical profession are internalized, resulting in an individual thinking, acting, and feeling like a physician."[9]

Conceptually, professional identity formation must be congruent with the processes through which all human beings develop a personal identity.[51] Psychological theory proposes that individuals proceed through life continuously organizing their experiences into a meaningful whole that incorporates their personal, private, public, and professional "selves."[51,52,57-61] As they pass through each stage, from infancy to childhood, adolescence, and beyond, individuals gain experience and become capable of constructing an increasingly complex persona.

Medical students enter medical school with clearly established identities that have been formed since birth (see Chapter 3). Developmental psychologists have contributed a rich literature that documents the various developmental stages through which humankind pass. Piaget and Inhelder,[57] Kohlberg,[58] Erikson,[59] Kegan,[60] Marcia,[61] and others have contributed to our understanding of the process. Kegan's framework[60] has proved particularly helpful and it has been applied to professional identity formation in medicine, dentistry, and the military. Two points are of particular significance to medical educators. First, the identities of individuals beginning their medical studies, while containing elements and characteristics

that will remain with them throughout their lives, are still not fully formed and can and will be influenced by multiple factors, including the educational process.[57-61] Second, the process of choosing an occupation has a significant impact on identity formation. Becoming competent in a chosen field has a stabilizing influence on one's identity.[59] Thus, learners at both the undergraduate and the postgraduate levels of medical education are in a transformative phase of their development. Educational programs can either support students through this journey or divert them from it.

Figure 1.1 presents a schematic representation of the process.[46] Students enter with identities that have resulted from the impact of both internal and external factors.[51,60,61] Individuals possess personal characteristics that are genetically determined – physical characteristics, gender, race, and a host of others. However, the sum total of their experiences in life has an enormous and lasting impact – religion, culture, socioeconomic class, level of education, sexual orientation, and many others.

During their educational experiences, learners in medicine become exposed to the norms of the community of practice and, if they wish to acquire the identity of a physician, they must adapt to these norms.[25,38] This involves a series of negotiations, most of which are internal to the self. An individual can accept all or some of the norms or can attempt to compromise by making accommodations to any given norm or practice. Finally, he or she can reject some norms. The recent emphasis on lifestyle represents an instance of a generation rejecting patterns of practice that were widely accepted in the past.[62,63] When significant numbers of learners wish to compromise or reject some of the accepted norms of the community, the negotiations are no longer internal – they take place within the larger community. It is important that this be understood, because the environment within which the majority of these negotiations take place is the educational community.

Learners emerge from the process of socialization with an altered identity that contains the core of who they were when they entered medical school and who they have become.[1,26,64,65] Transitions are important.[39,43,64,65] Entering medical school represents a transition, as does beginning residency and practice. Medical students have been shown to have a distinct identity that is different from that of a resident, and practitioners have their own distinct identities.[64,65]

Without question, there is tension in all phases of development that arises as individuals attempt to retain elements of who they are, as they are consciously and unconsciously being altered into who they are to become.[28,29,59]

It is important to emphasize that when the educational goal becomes the formation of a professional identity, the nature of that identity must be clearly delineated. Daniels[66] and others[67,68] have suggested that there is a socially negotiated ideal of the "good physician," and that, at any given point in time, a physician's behavior is both guided and constrained by this ideal. While there is some latitude in the expectations of both physicians and society due to individual, national, and cultural differences and specialty choices, certain core values such as caring, compassion, commitment, confidentiality, honesty, and integrity are universally accepted.[2,4] In joining the profession, an individual must accept these values and has a limited ability to pick and choose among the obligations resulting from them. The concept is not immutable and is being constantly renegotiated as "conditions inside and outside medicine change."[54,66] What it means to be a professional establishes the norms of the identity of an individual who wishes to join medicine's community of practice. Thus, the definitions of profession and professionalism, as well as the attributes of the professional, can provide a guide to assist learners who are attempting to "integrate their various statuses and roles, as well as their diverse experiences, into a coherent image of self."[8]

Professional identity formation

Jarvis-Selinger et al.[8] have described the process of professional identity formation as "an adaptive developmental process that happens simultaneously at two levels: (1) at the level of the individual, which involves the psychological development of the person and (2) at the collective level, which involves the socialization of the person into appropriate roles and forms of participation in the community's work." (p.1185) Thus, the journey from layperson to professional is internal to the self but is influenced by many external factors, both within the community of practice and external to it.

Profession and professionalism – defining the norms

As we have come to believe that medicine is a community of practice, the word "profession" has come to represent and define this community. A member of the community can be described as a professional, and professionalism will outline the behaviors expected of a professional. The attributes ascribed to a professional become descriptive of the professional identity to which individuals aspire. Thus, the efforts of the past few years, whose aim was to make the teaching of professionalism more explicit, can bear fruit when professional identity formation becomes an educational objective. The norms of the community of practice are contained in these definitions and descriptions and can be readily adapted to support professional identity formation.[9]

Although there is general agreement on the salient features of professionalism,[4,69] it has proved difficult to develop universally accepted definitions of "profession" and the words "professional" and "professionalism," which are derived from it. In part, this stems from the frequent use of the words as if they are interchangeable, which they are not. However, another cause is the difference in the background and approach of those studying all professions, including medicine.[69–71] The largest independent body of literature referring to the professions is found in the social sciences. Sociologists have been studying and writing about the professions for more than a century, and medicine has figured prominently in this literature. While there are certainly different approaches within the field of sociology, the primary interest is in the organization of society (and of work within society) and the role of the professions in this organization.[70] While sociologists recognize the importance of the doctor–patient relationship, they are primarily interested in the interface between the medical profession and the society which it serves.

To members of the medical profession, the definition must convey something more than the organization of society, important as this may be. Physicians require something that can assist in defining their own professional identity and establishing the ideology of the profession,[5,8,30,71] thus helping to establish the ideals to which they aspire and the norms to which they must adhere. Those responsible for teaching professionalism must address aspects relating to the relationship of physicians with both patients and society, as there are clearly expressed concerns about the performance of individual practitioners and of the profession in both areas.[5,72,73] These concerns relate to issues of morality, conflicts of interest, the state of the doctor–patient relationship, self-regulation, and to the impact of the healthcare system on the practice of medicine.[2–5,72,74] For this reason, we believe that any definition of medical professionalism must encompass the approaches found in both the medical and the sociological literature.

The literature contains many definitions of profession, professionalism, and medical professionalism. Most are similar and present common concepts because they generally begin with the assumption that the physician is a virtuous person and that the practice of medicine is a moral endeavor.[4,69–71] Profession, derived from the word "profess," is the etymological root of the frequently used terms professional and professionalism.[56]

It seems to us preferable to start with a definition of the root word "profession." We will provide two definitions, either of which can easily serve to communicate the norms of medicine's community of practice and hence of the desired professional identity.

Those preferring a short definition that stresses broad categories generally include descriptions of professions as containing common elements, work based on command of a complex body of knowledge, autonomy (sometimes linked to self-regulation), and a service orientation. We would suggest the following, developed by Starr in his seminal book, *The Social Transformation of American Medicine*[74] (p. 15):

> Profession: "An occupation that regulates itself through systematic, required training and collegial discipline; that has a base in technical specialized knowledge; and that has a service rather than profit orientation, enshrined in its code of ethics."[74]

It must be stressed that if this definition is to be used as a part of the cognitive base, the attributes of the profession that are outlined below must also be taught and should be linked to one of the broad themes included in the definition.

For those who prefer a more complete definition, the following is offered. It is based on the Oxford English Dictionary's,[56] to which have been added elements drawn from the medical and social sciences literature, which are felt to be fundamental parts of contemporary professionalism. Its disadvantage is its length and complexity, but it does contain the major elements that the literature indicates should be included. In addition, it indicates that professional status is granted by society, with the important implication that society can alter the terms should it wish to do so.

> Profession: "An occupation whose core element is work based upon the mastery of a complex body of knowledge and skills. It is a vocation in which knowledge of some department of science or learning or the practice of an art founded upon it is used in the service of others. Its members are governed by codes of ethics and profess a commitment to competence, integrity and morality, altruism, and the promotion of the public good within their domain. These commitments form the basis of a social contract between a profession and society, which in return grants the profession a monopoly over the use of its knowledge base, the right to considerable autonomy in practice and the privilege of self-regulation. Professions and their members are accountable to those served, to the profession, and to society."[75]

It should be pointed out that there are other examples of long and short definitions of "profession," "professionalism," and "medical professionalism" that are both acceptable and operationally useful.[69] The *International Charter on Medical Professionalism* explicitly outlines the nature of professionalism, stressing the obligations of a medical professional in contemporary society,[76] as does Swick's *Towards a Normative Definition of Medical Professionalism*.[77] Both are comprehensive and can serve effectively as the basis of a program on professionalism and professional identity formation.

Professionalism

Professionalism is a term used to describe the behavior of a professional. The Royal College of Physicians of London definition, "a set of values, behaviors and relationships that underpins the trust the public has in doctors,"[78] is commonly used. When the emphasis was on teaching and learning professionalism, it was particularly useful, because the assessment of professionalism leaned heavily on the assessment of observable behaviors – "what one does."[17] If professional identity formation becomes the educational objective, "what one is" becomes much more significant in terms of both pedagogical approaches and assessment methods.[9,10] Behaviors will continue to have an important place in the educational continuum as they assist in assessing progress toward the acquisition of a professional identity. In addition, unprofessional behavior will always be with us, and it will therefore be necessary to continue to assess behaviors.

While it has been understood for some time that there were differences in how professionalism is expressed in different countries and cultures,[79] experience gained in establishing programs centered around the teaching of professionalism has highlighted our understanding of these differences. The different interpretations of professionalism found in Asian and Middle Eastern countries have been documented,[80,81] and the importance of highlighting these differences is now widely accepted. While the type of professionalism espoused in any country or culture is clearly important within that jurisdiction, it must be understood that other countries and other cultures have their own equally valid interpretations. Documentation is yet to be established, but it is quite clear that a professional identity appropriate for both individual physicians and for a given society will also vary between countries and cultures. Monrouxe indicates this in Chapter 3, where she proposes that there are national differences in the nature of professional identity. Educational programs must recognize this and must not seek to impose an inappropriate identity on students destined for practice in other cultures. Of equal importance, respect must be given to the professionalism and professional identities found in other countries and cultures.

The attributes of a professional identity

Both individuals and society require the services of the healer, a role that has been with us since before the advent of recorded history. As society uses the concept and structures of the professions to organize the delivery of the services of the healer, any consideration of the attributes expected of a physician must recognize this by either separating the two roles (healer and professional) or by including the attributes of both when discussing professionalism.[2,19] In our teaching we have preferred to separate the roles, stating that physicians in their day-to-day activities must simultaneously fulfill the roles of healer and professional (see Chapter 15). Together, the attributes of the healer and the professional represent the desired identity of those wishing to enter the medical profession. They are foundational to the norms of the professional identity of a physician.

The separation of the two roles can be justified in historical terms because their origins and evolution, while parallel, have been different[72,82] (see Figure 1.2).

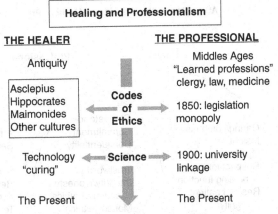

Figure 1.2. The dual roles of healer and professional. The healer and the professional have different origins and have evolved in parallel but separately. As shown on the left, all societies have required the services of healers. The western tradition of healing began in Hellenic Greece and is the part of the self-image of the medical profession. Curing became possible only with the advent of scientific medicine. The modern professions arose in the guilds and universities of medieval Europe and England. They acquired their present form in the middle of the nineteenth century, when licensing laws granted a monopoly over practice to allopathic medicine. When science caused medicine to be more knowledge-based, the profession moved closer to universities. Codes of ethics have always guided the behavior of both the healer and the professional and science empowers both.

The healer has been found in all societies throughout recorded history.[83]

The evolution of the concept in Western society can be traced through Hellenic Greece to the present, with the Hippocratic and Aesculapian traditions being part of the foundation of Western medicine.[2,82,83] Other cultures and religions have their own traditions, but the role of the healer seems to be remarkably constant, almost certainly because it responds to a basic universal human need.

The professions have different origins. The modern professions arose in the guilds and universities of medieval Europe and England.[2,72,74] They acquired their present form in the middle of the nineteenth century, when most Western societies granted them a monopoly over the practice of medicine by establishing licensure. Society used the professions as a means of organizing the delivery of the complex services which it came to require[2,5] – in this case, those of the healer. While the division is obviously somewhat arbitrary, one can postulate that those qualities traditionally associated with the relationship between a doctor and a patient are derived from the role of the healer, while medicine's relationship with society as a

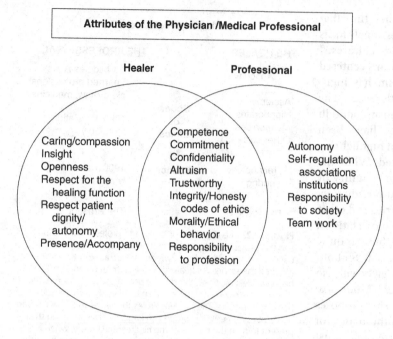

Attributes of the Physician /Medical Professional

Healer   Professional

Caring/compassion
Insight
Openness
Respect for the
  healing function
Respect patient
  dignity/
  autonomy
Presence/Accompany

Competence
Commitment
Confidentiality
Altruism
Trustworthy
Integrity/Honesty
  codes of ethics
Morality/Ethical
  behavior
Responsibility
  to profession

Autonomy
Self-regulation
  associations
  institutions
Responsibility
  to society
Team work

Figure 1.3. The attributes of the healer and the professional. The attributes traditionally associated with the healer are shown in the left-hand circle, and those with the professional on the right. As can be seen, there are attributes unique to each role. Those shared by both are found in the large area of overlap of the circles. This list of attributes is drawn from the literature on healing and professionalism.

whole has evolved from the development of the modern profession.[2]

Figure 1.3 is a diagram of the attributes that constitute the identities of the physician/medical professional, which have been derived from the literature on healing and on professionalism. As can be seen, there are attributes, such as caring and compassion, that have been long recognized as fundamental to the healing function.[4,82,83] On the other hand, there are others associated with being a contemporary professional that historically have not been linked with the traditional healing role, such as autonomy, responsibility to society, or teamwork. In the middle is a group of important shared attributes, each of which is fundamental to the practice of medicine.

The nature of these attributes is well known to the medical profession and it does not seem necessary to give a detailed description of each. Table 1.1 lists them with operational definitions.

It is important to discuss the evolution of medical professionalism because some attributes have changed in their meaning, while others are new to the list. Castellani and Hafferty[71] have warned that we must not practice or teach "nostalgic professionalism," an idealized version that is rooted in the past and does not recognize the emergence of a professionalism or of a professional identity that must cope with the presence of healthcare systems, some of which encourage different forms of professionalism. Others

have concurred in this opinion, calling for a "reborn professionalism,"[72] "civic professionalism,"[5] or redefining the term, stating that many of the traditional aspects are no longer appropriate.[78] In addition, as many have pointed out, students and young physicians are emerging from a society that places great emphasis on lifestyle for whom nostalgic professionalism, with an approach to altruism that they regard as being open-ended, is not acceptable.[63]

The professionalism that is communicated as the contemporary norm of professional identity must recognize these forces and be capable of providing a moral base for the physicians of the future whose task it is to ensure that both the role and the values of the healer survive. It is the services of the healer that society needs and if this need is properly met, it seems likely that a form of professionalism acceptable to both society and medicine will evolve.

Changes in the attributes

Changes in the attributes of the healer

The role of the healer appears to have been relatively constant throughout the ages. Consequently, its attributes appear to have changed little. Caring and compassion, openness, and presence, and the need for the physician to be present for the patient, are timeless

Table 1.1. The attributes of the medical professional or of the dual roles (healer and professional) of the physician

Attributes of the healer

Caring and compassion: a sympathetic consciousness of another's distress together with a desire to alleviate it.

Insight: self-awareness; the ability to recognize and understand the patient's and one's actions, motivations, and emotions.

Openness: willingness to hear, accept, and deal with the views of others without reserve or pretense.

Respect for the healing function: the ability to recognize, elicit, and foster the power to heal inherent in each patient.

Respect for patient dignity and autonomy: the commitment to respect and ensure subjective well-being and sense of worth in others, and to recognize the patient's personal freedom of choice and right to participate fully in his or her care.

Presence/accompany: to be fully present for a patient without distraction and to fully support and accompany the patient throughout care.

Attributes of both the healer and the professional

Competence: to master and keep current the knowledge and skills relevant to medical practice.

Commitment: being obligated or emotionally impelled to act in the best interest of the patient; a pledge given by way of the Hippocratic Oath or its modern equivalent.

Confidentiality: to not divulge patient information without just cause.

Altruism: the unselfish regard for, or devotion to, the welfare of others; placing the needs of the patient before one's self-interest.

Integrity and honesty: firm adherence to a code of moral values; incorruptibility.

Morality and ethical conduct: to act for the public good; conformity to the ideals of right human conduct in dealings with patients, colleagues, and society.

Trustworthiness: worthy of trust, reliable.

Attributes of the professional

Autonomy: the physician's freedom to make independent decisions in the best interest of patients and for the good of society.

Responsibility to the profession: the commitment to maintain the integrity of the moral and collegial nature of the profession and to be accountable for one's conduct to the profession.

Self-regulation: the privilege of setting standards; being accountable for one's actions and conduct in medical practice and for the conduct of one's colleagues.

Responsibility to society: the obligation to use one's expertise for, and to be accountable to, society for those actions, both personal and of the profession, that relate to the public good.

Teamwork: the ability to recognize and respect the expertise of others and work with them in the patient's best interest.

and cross both national and cultural boundaries.[82,83] The concept of respecting patient autonomy is the attribute that has undergone the greatest transformation. The doctor-patient relationship of the past was paternalistic in nature and is no longer acceptable. It is widely recognized that patients must control the direction and details of their own care, with the physician offering expert advice.[84] This fundamental aspect of patient-centered care is now a societal expectation[85] and must be incorporated into the identities of practicing physicians.

Changes in the attributes of the professional

Some attributes ascribed to the professional are either new or have changed significantly. Physician autonomy has been limited in part because of the growth of patient autonomy. However, the most severe intrusions into physician autonomy have resulted from the new levels of accountability expected of contemporary physicians, who are now accountable not only to their patients but also to third-party payers, be they government or corporate, and to society for the health of populations.[86,87] Essentially, physician autonomy and physician accountability are reciprocal. The more that physicians and the medical profession are held accountable, the less autonomous they become. Society is also demanding new levels of accountability. This dimension of medical professionalism, which now represents an important societal expectation, must be communicated as the new reality.[54,88]

Medicine's responsibility to society is not part of the Hippocratic tradition but it is now a major expectation.[54,88] The importance of modern scientific healthcare to society, in the presence of apparently infinite demand for healthcare services, makes responsiveness to societal needs imperative. Contemporary physicians must balance their fiduciary duty to place their patients' interests first, with the knowledge that resources devoted to healthcare are limited and must benefit the largest possible number of individuals. This has been described as representing a conflict between the "social purposes" of medicine and a physician's fiduciary duty to an individual patient.[89] This ongoing conflict leads to considerable tension in the practice of medicine, which must be addressed in teaching programs on professionalism.

Self-regulation, as covered in Chapter 14, is a privilege granted to the medical profession, not because it is good for medicine, but because it was assumed that only the profession was competent to make judgments in an area of great complexity.[72,74] Well-publicized failures in self-regulation on the part of the medical profession have cast doubt upon this assumption,[90–92] and medicine's regulatory powers are being diminished or altered by actions of the state, the courts, and the corporate sector.[93,94] For this reason, the details of self-regulation and the role of the individual physician, and of medicine's associations and regulatory bodies, become an important part of the cognitive base of professional identity formation.

Finally, the necessity to practice in teams of healthcare professionals represents a new requirement.[85,92,94] The historical image of the solo practitioner serving a single patient has not represented reality for some time. Because of the complexity of contemporary healthcare, a major expectation of current society is that physicians will function as members of a healthcare team. This often conflicts with a student's, resident's, or practitioner's image of themselves as an independent and autonomous practitioner. This image must be challenged and, if present, altered in teaching programs. Establishing programs where clinical activities and professionalism may be learned in an interprofessional setting, as outlined in Chapter 10, represents a new and challenging imperative.

Changes in the attributes shared by the healer and the professional

Perhaps the greatest changes, and consequently the greatest challenges, between nostalgic and contemporary professionalism are found in this category.

Historically, physicians were licensed and certified as being competent in their chosen field of medicine, and it was assumed they would remain so for the rest of their professional lives. As outlined in Chapter 19, it has been amply demonstrated that this is not true, and that graduates of the future will be required to demonstrate that they remain competent throughout their careers.[90,95] Furthermore, in those jurisdictions where the profession retains the right to self-regulate, it will remain a professional obligation to accept responsibility for one's own competence, as well as for the competence of one's colleagues.[5,72,74] This concept must be introduced at a very early stage of medical education and be reinforced throughout the continuum if it is to be incorporated into the professional identities of emerging practitioners.

The subject of altruism must also be addressed, as it remains a fundamental societal expectation.[29,30,96,97] Simply put, it is expected that physicians will place the patient's needs above their own, something which is essential if a patient is to trust a physician.[4,8,23,29,96–98] One traditionally important aspect of altruism has been the expectation that a patient's physician will be available when needed. The current generation of graduates comes from a society in which lifestyle is of primary importance, resulting in a questioning of the concept of altruism.[63,99,100] It is of note that there appears to be very little objection to other aspects that are closely linked to altruism, such as commitment, caring, and compassion. The balance between altruism and lifestyle must be addressed in programs aimed at supporting professional identity formation. Denial of the obligation to be altruistic could mean that it is acceptable for a physician to place his or her own interests above that of the patient. Students and residents must understand that altruism is fundamental to patient trust and that, in the absence of trust, healing will be severely impaired. However, with proper planning and with the organization of practice so that someone competent and informed is always available, it should be possible to meet patients' legitimate expectations while maintaining a satisfactory balance between work and personal life. Establishing this system is the responsibility of the physician caring for the patient. Students and residents should be encouraged to consider possible methods of balancing the needs of patients with their own desired lifestyle before they actually enter practice, remembering that they must both place and be seen to place the meeting of their patients' needs above their own.

The final group of attributes that must be stressed because they are under threat is the constellation of honesty, integrity, morality, and ethical behavior. The threats come from a variety of sources including health-care systems that rely on market forces and competition,[72–74,101] and on the presence of a powerful and well-funded pharmaceutical, medical device, and hospital industry.[101–102] They endanger "the ethical foundations of medicine, including the commitment of physicians to put the needs of patients ahead of personal gain, to deal with patients honestly, competently, and compassionately, and to avoid conflicts of interest that could undermine public trust in the altruism of medicine."[102] (p.2668) Students, residents, and practicing physicians must understand that conflicts of interest, which are more present than they have ever been, are not going to disappear, and that professionalism requires that these conflicts be managed in a way that does not diminish physicians' trustworthiness. These issues must be discussed openly in the context of professional identity and individuals must be encouraged to reflect on them in a safe environment before they must actually deal with them in practice.

Professional identity formation and socialization

Chapters 3 and 4 describe in detail how socialization impacts individuals as they develop their own unique professional identities. This section will provide schematic representations of the process of socialization, along with the responses and roles of individuals experiencing the process. The intent is to organize the multiple factors involved, in order to allow medical educators to better understand the process and guide interventions aimed at ensuring that professional identity formation is supported throughout the continuum of medical education.

Socialization is "the process by which a person learns to function within a particular society or group by internalizing its values and norms."[56] It is the principal process through which identities are developed.[25,38] Socialization is different from training. Hafferty puts it well in Chapter 4: "While any occupational training involves learning new knowledge and skills, it is the melding of knowledge and skills with an altered sense of self that differentiates 'training' from 'socialization'."

Figure 1.4 is a representation of the factors that the literature indicates affect individuals as they are transformed from members of the lay public into skilled professionals. Chapters 3 through 7 provide in-depth exploration of the major factors involved.

Role models, mentors, and experiential learning

Role models and mentors and the totality of the clinical and nonclinical experiences of each individual have been shown to be the major factors that assist students, residents, and practicing physicians as they develop their professional identities (see Chapters 6 and 7). Indeed, this is not surprising as it has long been recognized that a fundamental objective of medical education is to bring together students, teachers, and patients to provide learning experiences.

Role models are "individuals admired for their ways of being and acting as professionals"[11] (see chapter 6). Mentors – "experienced and trusted counsellors" – have more prolonged contact with individuals and hence can exert greater influence.[56,103] Their importance is underlined by the fact that they are members of the community of practice to which medical students and residents wish to belong.[8,34,48,104] Consequently, looking, sounding, and behaving like them become aspirational objectives. Both role models and mentors exert their influence through both conscious and unconscious pathways.[104–106] Conscious behavior patterns result from observation, imitation, and practice,[107] a process made more effective by guided reflection.[104,108–110] Of greater importance is the unconscious pathway that leads to the acquisition of tacit knowledge – "that which one knows but cannot tell."[111] In attempting to engage learners in the development of their professional identities, an essential educational objective is to encourage reflection on role modeling and mentoring by shifting the learning to the conscious pathway, making it explicit.[106]

Both clinical and nonclinical experiences also exert a powerful effect on the development of a professional identity. Again, both conscious and unconscious pathways are operative. The literature on identity formation is quite clear – experiences with patients have an enormous impact, and the earlier in the educational experience that they take place, the earlier students begin to feel like physicians.[21,27–30,32] Guided reflection increases the impact of the experiences and increases explicit knowledge.[104,108,110]

Role models, mentors, and experiences are essential to the development of a professional identity. However, if these are not interpreted as being positive

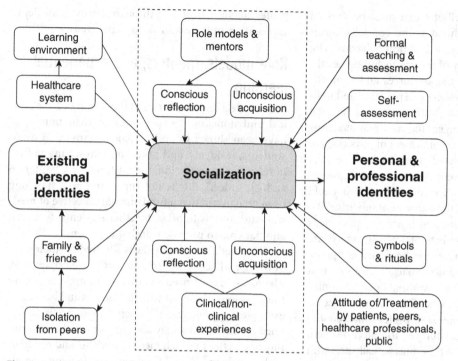

Figure 1.4. A schematic representation of the multiple factors involved in the process of socialization in medicine. The large center box surrounded by the dotted line, which includes role models and mentors, and experiential learning, indicates their importance to this process. The direction of the arrows from existing professional identities to personal and professional identities indicate the dynamic nature of the process.[46] Reprinted with permission by *Academic Medicine* © 2015.

and supportive of the development of a professional self, they can inhibit professional identity development.[33–39] Thus, the organization of the curriculum must ensure that role modeling and mentoring are positive aspects of the process of socialization, and that appropriate clinical experiences take place. Time for guided reflection on both is essential to success.[108–110]

Role models and mentors must become knowledgeable about identity formation and socialization. For this reason, faculty development has been found to be essential to the success of programs aimed at teaching professionalism.[112,113] This becomes even more important as the emphasis shifts to supporting professional identity formation (see Chapter 9).

The teaching milieu

The upper right-hand and left-hand sides of Figure 1.4 address the many factors in the educational environment that impact professional identity formation.

Until recently, professionalism and professional identity formation were not taught explicitly and were therefore addressed indirectly in the informal curriculum.[114] This is no longer true. Accreditation of undergraduate and postgraduate programs has required that they be transferred to the formal curriculum. Thus, much of the content of this chapter – the cognitive base – must be included in the formal curriculum.

As the emphasis switches from teaching professionalism to supporting professional identity formation, self-assessment must come to play a more important role because the presentation of self is so central to one's identity. While self-assessment of knowledge and skills is believed to be unreliable, self-assessment, along with assessment by individual students and residents, is central to determining how each individual charts their own progress toward the development of their professional identity. Tools have been developed to assist individuals as they determine their progress in the journey toward a professional identity.[20,115]

The upper left-hand side of Figure 1.4 is concerned with the nature of the learning environment, a subject that is covered in Chapter 18. The corrosive impact of a negative learning environment on professional behavior and professional identity formation is well documented.[116,117] Viewed through the lens of communities of practice, a healthy and inclusionary environment is welcoming and models appropriate behaviors.[108] On the other hand, an exclusionary, hostile, or negative environment, or one populated by individuals who model unprofessional behavior, can impact identity formation negatively by failing to welcome learners into the community or by communicating unacceptable norms of behavior. These factors, which are generally ascribed to the informal and hidden curriculum, must be addressed specifically, to ensure that they support professional identity formation.[116,117]

The nature of the healthcare system becomes more significant as learners progress through their educational experience. As students spend more time in patient-related activities, they are functioning within the healthcare system with its many pressures.[70,118] Pressures to increase throughput often make it difficult to protect time for active role modeling and the reflection necessary to make learning effective. In addition, the idealism of incoming medical students meets the reality of medical practice.[119] As changing the healthcare system is not a realistic goal, it is important for learners at all levels to reflect on the impact of the healthcare system on their emerging professional identities. The objective is to be aware of the threats posed to the core values of medicine by healthcare systems that sometimes fail to support these values.[5,71]

External factors

The lower-right and left-hand corners of Figure 1.4 include factors external to the learner that can influence professional identity formation.

Symbols and rituals have been used by the medical profession for hundreds of years.[33,36] The Hippocratic Oath, or its modern equivalent, has served to unify the profession around the ideology of service by requiring a public profession of commitment to the ideals of the profession. It is an important indicator that an individual has joined medicine's community of practice. The stethoscope is also an important symbol, and other events during medical education have symbolic importance: the first contact with a cadaver; the first contact with death; the White Coat Ceremony and other rituals. Experiencing them alters the students' sense of self, making them feel as if they are becoming physicians.[20,24,29,32]

How one is treated also has a powerful influence on professional identity formation.[34–36] Certainly, treatment by patients is the most important, but how peers, nurses, and other healthcare professionals as well as the general public treat students can either solidify a developing sense of a "professional" self or inhibit it.[38,39,45]

As illustrated in the lower left-hand corner of Figure 1.4, medical students and residents have, since time immemorial, been isolated from many aspects of their former lives – friends, family, and outside interests.[20,24,29,32] This isolation is shared with their fellow students as they become immersed in the wider healthcare community, sharing a new language and experiences.[43,120] The isolation facilitates the acquisition of the identity of the community, as does the presence of peers undergoing the same experiences. Peer pressure to acquire the identity of the community of practice supports individuals as they join the group.[43,51] While the current generation of students insists on maintaining a balanced lifestyle, the end result appears to be a diminution of their isolation rather than its elimination. Some degree of isolation with like-minded individuals is both desirable and necessary if the process of socialization is to be successful.[25,45,47,51]

Figure 1.5 continues the analysis of socialization. It outlines the roles that learners must play and their common responses to the process of socialization.

The upper portion of Figure 1.5 documents the widely accepted concept that learners in medicine throughout the educational process are continually expected to appear to "think, act, and feel" like a physician before they actually possess the necessary knowledge and skills or the identity of a physician.[21,26,38,47] They therefore, of necessity, play the role, "pretending" to be a physician. In order to fulfill this role, they must learn the language of medicine that is unique to the profession. They must also learn to live with the ambiguity that is inherent to the practice of medicine.[121] The literature on identity formation within medicine stresses that by continually playing a role, an individual gradually grows into the role and the role becomes who that person "is."[8,47] When successful, behaviors spring intuitively from within the individual.

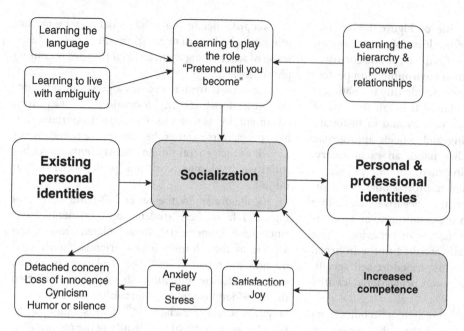

Figure 1.5. A schematic representation of the roles that medical students and residents play during the process of socialization and their potential responses to this process. Medical students and residents who go through the process of socialization must play certain prescribed roles and respond to the process in a variety of predictable ways.[46] Reprinted with permission by *Academic Medicine* © 2015.

Every organization, including medicine, must have a structure and organization that establishes a hierarchy and allocates power to individuals.[26,28,122,123] In order to successfully join the community of practice, it is necessary for learners to learn the hierarchy and power relationships within medicine. To support professional identity formation and learners, each institution must examine its own internal order to be certain that its impact on professional identity formation is positive.

The lower portion of the diagram outlines the responses of individuals to the process of socialization. Of paramount importance is the impact of increasing levels of competence on the sense of self of students, residents, and, indeed, practitioners.[38,42,43,120] As mentioned earlier, successfully mastering the details of any occupation has a powerful stabilizing effect on the identity of all individuals, including of those wishing to become physicians.[51,52]

A very beneficial result of feeling competent is a sense of confidence, satisfaction, and often joy.[36,45] The literature rarely mentions this important aspect, generally emphasizing the stressful nature of medical education. Celebrating increasing levels of competence appears to us to be an important method of diminishing stress.

Anxiety and fear are, without question, present throughout the continuum of medical education and practice, and they do result in well-documented levels of stress.[26,44,124,125] However, developmental psychologists make it clear that stress cannot be avoided if identity change is to take place. Erikson[59] believed that it was necessary to actually repress portions of a previous identity for change to occur and that stress must inevitably result. Monrouxe[28] speaks of identity dissonance that occurs as aspects of the new identity clash with the established identity. The first stress-performance curve was developed in 1910, and it has been known since then that some levels of stress are beneficial to performance up to a point, at which the curve plateaus, performance declines, and, as the level of stress increases, it becomes destructive.[126] It is impossible to eliminate stress from medical education, and it would undoubtedly be more difficult to develop professional identities in the unlikely event that this were to occur. The educational objective should be to ensure that the level of stress remains within the constructive range. In addition, learners should understand and reflect on the very normal reasons for their unease as they develop their professional identities.

Finally, on the lower left side of Figure 1.5 are the responses of learners in medicine to the process of socialization. They of course mimic the responses of any human being to change and stress. Detached concern is well documented in medical students, as is loss of innocence.[24,28,29] Medical students have employed humor – both appropriate and inappropriate – through the ages as a natural defense.[127,128] In addition, they have been shown to utilize silence as a means of withdrawal.[128] Many studies are said to have shown increased levels of cynicism, often linked with loss of innocence,[129] although this is controversial.[40] In fact, there are those who believe that confronting the reality of the practice of medicine is a necessary step in the development of a professional identity.

It must be emphasized that the intent of providing schematic representations of professional identity formation and socialization is two-fold. First, it is hoped that those planning curricula to support professional identity formation can use the diagrams as guides for the design of educational interventions to make socialization more effective. Second, providing schema to students can help them understand their experiences in the continuum of medical education and, of utmost importance, reflect on the impact of these factors and their responses to them. The schema can serve to engage students actively in understanding and taking charge of the development of their own professional identities.

Medicine's social contract with society

The desired professional identity must be related to the needs of both individual patients and society. Societal expectations of the individual physician should be built into the substance of a professional identity. For this reason, the relationship of medicine to society is an important part of the cognitive base of programs devoted to teaching professionalism and supporting professional identity formation. Most observers have utilized the term "social contract" to describe this relationship.

It has long been said that professionalism is the basis of medicine's relationship with society.[5,74,130] This relationship was not analyzed in great detail when both medicine and society appeared to be satisfied with the state of affairs. This is no longer true. One observer has noted that "a better informed community is asking for accountability, transparency, and sound professional standards," whereas the profession feels that its "autonomy is severely restricted by budgets, bureaucracy, guidelines, and peer review."[131] Because of the evident discontent on both sides, the interface between medicine and society has come under scrutiny during recent years. The most accurate and useful descriptor of the relationship is the historical concept of the "social contract."[2,5,77,132] Originally

elaborated over three centuries ago, it has always been based upon reciprocal rights and obligations on the part of the parties to the contract. An advantage of using the term is that it has been a part of the discourse on the organization of society for so long and is therefore widely understood.

A useful definition of social contract is as follows: "The rights and duties of the state and its citizens are reciprocal and the recognition of this reciprocity constitutes a relationship which by analogy can be called a social contract."[133]

Medicine's social contract with society is not an identifiable legal document to which one can refer, although important parts of it are written. The written parts are found in a variety of sources: the laws and rules governing the regulatory framework of medicine, including education, licensure, certification, and revalidation; the legislation establishing the healthcare system of any given country; and legal judgments found in jurisprudence. There are also documents produced by the profession itself, such as the Hippocratic Oath and contemporary codes of ethics, the *International Charter on Medical Professionalism*,[76] and *Good Medical Practice*.[15] However, important aspects of the contract relating to the moral basis of the practice of medicine are unwritten. Caring and compassion, commitment, and altruism are fundamental to the social contract, representing almost existential expectations on the part of individual patients and of society. They cannot be legislated and must arise from within individual physicians. They are important aspects of who the physician "is" and learners must become.[25,29,30,35,36]

Conceptually, medicine's social contract is not complex.[54] Society grants professional status through laws and customs that delegate authority to the professions, including medicine. Medicine is given, and therefore expects, substantial autonomy in practice, a privileged position in society, the right to self-regulation, and substantial financial and nonfinancial rewards. In return, individual physicians and the organizations representing them are expected to fulfill and support the traditional role of the healer, to demonstrate honesty and morality in all of their activities, to put the needs of patients and society above their own (altruism), to ensure the competence of practitioners, and to address the needs of society within their domain. Medicine's principal obligations are based upon public expectations and they form a central core of its professional identity. The profession's conduct is, however, dependent upon society meeting medicine's reasonable expectations.

Table 1.2. An outline of the expectations that society has of medicine and medicine of society based upon the literature

Society's expectations of medicine	Medicine's expectations of society
• To fulfill the role of the healer	• Trust
• Assured competence	• Autonomy
• Access to care	• Self-regulation
• Altruistic service	• Healthcare system
• Morality, integrity, honesty	• Value-laden
• Codes of ethics	• Adequately funded
• Trustworthiness	• Reasonable freedom
• Accountability/ transparency	• Role in public policy
• Respect for patient dignity/autonomy	• Accept some responsibility for health
• Source of objective advice	• Monopoly
• Promotion of the public good	• Lifestyle
	• Rewards
	• Nonfinancial
	• Financial

Implications of the use of the term "social contract"

Understanding societal expectations of medicine and medicine's expectations of society under the contract, and making them explicit, have important implications. Table 1.2 outlines what the literature can tell us about these expectations.[54] As can be seen, they correlate well with the attributes of the professional that are outlined in Figure 1.3. Societal expectations must be foundational to determining the norms of medicine's community of practice. If societal expectations are not met, society will alter the social contract, and the nature of professionalism and of professional identity will change.

If individual practitioners or the profession fail to meet society's expectations, the contract will be changed. On the other hand, if society does not meet the legitimate expectations of the profession, it can be expected that the profession will also respond by attempting to negotiate a more favorable "bargain," and, if that proves impossible, by changing its behavior. As an example, the emphasis on a market-oriented system in the United States has caused the emergence of what has been termed "entrepreneurial professionalism," with unintended consequences.[70,71]

Other advantages to the use of the term "social contract" are that it identifies the parties to the relationship, something which is essential if the complexities of contemporary healthcare are to be fully understood.[54,132] It allows the discussion to be focused on areas of disagreement as well as consensus. Finally, as contracts are subject to negotiation, using this approach can cause both individuals and the profession to negotiate with society in an attempt to create a healthcare system that actually supports the healer role.[54,132,134]

There is also a pedagogic advantage. Presenting professionalism as the basis of a social contract emphasizes its relevance to the practice of medicine and makes the profession's obligations and the reasons for their existence more understandable. Emphasizing the reciprocal nature of medicine's relationship to society can lead to an understanding of the consequences of a failure of medicine or society to meet the reasonable and legitimate expectations of the other.[54]

Conclusion

The Carnegie Foundation report on the future of medical education was unequivocal in one of its major recommendations. It stated that: "professional identity formation – the development of professional values, actions, and aspirations – should be the backbone of medical education."[7] For this to occur, professional identity formation must be acknowledged as a major educational objective throughout the continuum of medical education. This can be facilitated by recognizing that medicine is a community of practice and that entering the profession is a voluntary act. Individuals doing so "are disposed to learn its ways and take its ideology seriously."[89] (p. 336) Learners should understand both identity formation and socialization and become engaged in consciously developing their own medical professional identity. For this to occur, faculty and learners must understand the norms of the community of practice historically encompassed in the words "profession" and "professional." As a consequence, definitions and lists of attributes, as well as an understanding of societal expectations of physicians, become foundational elements in the construction of a professional identity. Finally, it must be recognized that the power of educational programs to influence identity formation either positively or negatively is substantial. It is our task to ensure that educational programs support physicians in training at all levels as they develop their own professional identities.

References

1. Merton, RK. Some preliminaries to a sociology of medical education. In Merton, RK, Reader, LG, Kendall, PL, eds. *The Student Physician: Introductory Studies in the Sociology of Medical Education.* Cambridge, MA: Harvard University Press; 1957:3–79.

2. Cruess, RL, Cruess, SR. Teaching medicine as a profession in the service of healing. *Acad Med.* 1997; 72(11):941–52.

3. Cruess, SR, Cruess, RL. Professionalism must be taught. *BJM.* 1997; 315(7123):1674–77.

4. Inui, TS. *A Flag in the Wind: Educating for Professionalism in Medicine.* Washington, DC: Association of American Medical Colleges; 2003.

5. Sullivan, W. *Work and Integrity: The Crisis and Promise of Professionalism in North America.* Second edition. San Francisco, CA: Jossey-Bass; 2005.

6. Cohen, JJ. Professionalism in medical education, an American perspective: from evidence to accountability. *Med Educ.* 2006; 40(7):607–17.

7. Cooke, M, Irby, DM, O'Brien, BC. *Educating Physicians: A Call for Reform of Medical School and Residency.* San Francisco, CA: Jossey-Bass; 2010.

8. Jarvis-Selinger, S, Pratt, DD, Regehr, G. Competency is not enough: integrating identity formation into the medical education discourse. *Acad Med.* 2012; 87(9):1185–90.

9. Cruess, RL, Cruess, SR, Boudreau, JD, Snell, L, Steinert, Y. Reframing medical education to support professional identity formation. *Acad Med.* 2014; 89(11):1446–51.

10. Holden, MD, Buck, E, Luk, J, Ambriz, F, Boisaubin, EV, Clark, MA, Mihalic, AP, Sadler, JZ, Sapire, KJ, Spike, JP, Vince, A, Dalrymple, JL. Professional identity formation: creating a longitudinal framework through TIME (Transformation In Medical Education). *Acad Med.* 2015; 90(6):761–67.

11. Côté, L, Leclère H. How clinical teachers perceive the doctor-patient relationship and themselves as role models. *Acad Med.* 2000; 75(11):1117–24.

12. Ludmerer, KM. Instilling professionalism in medical education. *JAMA.* 1999; 282(9):881–82.

13. Batalden, P, Leach, D, Swing, S, Dreyfus, H, Dreyfus, S. General competencies and accreditation in graduate medical education. *Health Aff (Millwood).* 2002; 21(5):103–11.

14. Royal College of Physicians and Surgeons of Canada. *CanMEDS 2015.* Ottawa, ON: RCPSC; 2015. [Accessed June 3, 2015.] Available from www.royalcollege.ca/canmeds2015.

15. General Medical Council. *Good Medical Practice.* Fifth edition. London, UK: GMC; 2013.

16. Liaison Committee on Medical Education. *Functions and Structure of a Medical School: Standards for Accreditation of Medical Education Programs Leading to the M.D. Degree.* Washington, DC: Association of American Medical Colleges; 2008. [Accessed June 3, 2015.] Available from http://umsc.org.uic.edu/documents/LCME_standards.pdf.

17. Wilkinson, TJ, Wade, WB, Knock, LD. A blueprint to assess professionalism: results of a systematic review. *Acad Med.* 2009; 84(5):551–58.

18. Hodges, BD, Ginsburg, S, Cruess, R, Cruess, S, Delport, R, Hafferty, F, Ho, MJ, Holmboe, E, Holtman, M, Ohbu, S, Rees, C, Ten Cate, O, Tsugawa, Y, Van Mook, W, Wass, V, Wilkinson, T, Wade, W. Assessment of professionalism: recommendations from the Ottawa 2010 Conference. *Med Teach.* 2011; 33(5):354–63.

19. Cruess, RL, Cruess, SR. Teaching professionalism: general principles. *Med Teach.* 2006; 28(3):205–08.

20. Niemi, PM. Medical students' professional identity: self-reflection during the preclinical years. *Med Educ.* 1997; 31(6):408–15.

21. Niemi, PM, Vainiomäki, PT, Murto-Kangas, M. "My future as a physician" – professional representations and their background among first-day medical students. *Teach Learn Med.* 2003; 15(1): 31–39.

22. Beagan, BL. Everyday classism in medical school: experiencing marginality and resistance. *Med Educ.* 2005; 39(8):777–84.

23. Forsythe, GB. Identity development in professional education. *Acad Med.* 2005; 80(10 Suppl):S112–S117.

24. Bebeau, MJ. Evidence-based character development. In Kenny, N, Shelton, W, eds. *Advances in Bioethics: Volume 10. Lost Virtue: Professional Character Development in Medical Education.* Oxford, UK: Elsevier; 2006:47–86.

25. Hafferty, FW. Professionalism and the socialization of medical students. In Cruess, RL, Cruess, SR, Steinert, Y, eds. *Teaching Medical Professionalism.* New York, NY: Cambridge University Press; 2009:53–70.

26. Lempp, H. Medical-school culture. In Brosnan, C, Turner, BS, eds. *Handbook of the Sociology of Medical Education.* Oxon, UK: Routledge; 2009:71–88.

27. Crossley, J, Vivekananda-Schmidt, P. The development and evaluation of a Professional Self Identity Questionnaire to measure evolving professional self-identity in health and social care students. *Med Teach.* 2009; 31(12):e603–e607.

28. Monrouxe, LV. Identity, identification and medical education: why should we care? *Med Educ.* 2010; 44(1): 40–49.

29. MacLeod, A. Caring, competence and professional identities in medical education. *Adv Health Sci Educ Theory Pract.* 2011; **16**(3):375–94.

30. Monrouxe, LV, Rees, CE, Hu, W. Differences in medical students' explicit discourses of professionalism: acting, representing, becoming. *Med Educ.* 2011; **45**(6):585–602.

31. Weaver, R, Peters, K, Koch, J, Wilson, I. 'Part of the team': professional identity and social exclusivity in medical students. *Med Educ.* 2011; **45**(12):1220–29.

32. White, MT, Borges, NJ, Geiger, S. Perceptions of factors contributing to professional identity development and specialty choice: a survey of third- and fourth-year medical students. *Ann Behav Sci Med Educ.* 2011; **17**(1):18–23.

33. Burford, B. Group processes in medical education: learning from social identity theory. *Med Educ.* 2012; **46**(2):143–152.

34. Goldie, J. The formation of professional identity in medical students: considerations for educators. *Med Teach.* 2012; **34**(9):e641–e648.

35. Helmich, E, Bolhuis, S, Dornan, T, Laan, R, Koopmans, R. Entering medical practice for the very first time: emotional talk, meaning and identity development. *Med Educ.* 2012; **46**(11):1074–86.

36. Helmich, E, Dornan, T. Do you really want to be a doctor? The highs and lows of identity development. *Med Educ.* 2012; **46**(2):132–34.

37. Frost, HD, Regehr, G. "I am a doctor": negotiating the discourses of standardization and diversity in professional identity construction. *Acad Med.* 2013; **88**(10):1570–77.

38. Monrouxe, LV. Identities, self and medical education. In Walsh, K, ed. *Oxford Textbook of Medical Education.* Oxford, UK: Oxford University Press; 2013:113–23.

39. Wilson, I, Cowin, LS, Johnson, M, Young, H. Professional identity in medical students: pedagogical challenges to medical education. *Teach Learn Med.* 2013; **25**(4):369–73.

40. Boudreau, JD, Macdonald, ME, Steinert, Y. Affirming professional identities through an apprenticeship: insights from a four-year longitudinal case study. *Acad Med.* 2014; **89**(7):1038–45.

41. Hill, E, Bowman, K, Stalmeijer, R, Hart, J. You've got to know the rules to play the game: how medical students negotiate the hidden curriculum of surgical careers. *Med Educ.* 2014; **48**(9):884–94.

42. Mavor, KI, McNeill, KG, Anderson, K, Kerr, A, O'Reilly, E, Platow, MJ. Beyond prevalence to process: the role of self and identity in medical student well-being. *Med Educ.* 2014; **48**(4):351–60.

43. McNeill, KG, Kerr, A, Mavor, KI. Identity and norms: the role of group membership in medical student wellbeing. *Perspect Med Educ.* 2014; **3**(2):101–12.

44. Monrouxe, LV, Rees, CE, Endacott, R, Ternan, E. 'Even now it makes me angry': health care students' professionalism dilemma narratives. *Med Educ.* 2014; **48**(5):502–17.

45. Dornan, T, Pearson, E, Carson, P, Helmich, E, Bundy, C. Emotions and identity in the figured world of becoming a doctor. *Med Educ.* 2015; **49**(2):174–85.

46. Cruess, RL, Cruess, SR, Boudreau, JD, Snell, L, Steinert, Y. A schematic representation of the professional identity formation and socialization of medical students and residents: a guide for medical educators. *Acad Med.* 2015; **90**(6):718–25.

47. Sharpless, J, Baldwin, N, Cook, R, Kofman, A, Morley-Fletcher, A, Slotkin, R, Wald, HS. The becoming: students' reflections on the process of professional identity formation in medical education. *Acad Med.* 2015; **90**(6):713–17.

48. Lave, J, Wenger, E. *Situated Learning: Legitimate Peripheral Participation.* Cambridge, UK: Cambridge University Press; 1991.

49. Wenger, E. *Communities of Practice: Learning, Meaning, and Identity.* Cambridge, UK: Cambridge University Press; 1998.

50. Ihara, CK. Collegiality as a professional virtue. In Flores, A, ed. *Professional Ideals.* Belmont, CA: Wadsworth; 1988:56–65.

51. Vignoles, VL, Schwartz, SJ, Luyckx, K. Introduction: toward an integrative view of identity. In Schwartz, SJ, Luyckx, K, Vignoles, VL, eds. *Handbook of Identity Theory and Research.* New York, NY: Springer; 2011:1–27.

52. Skorikov, VB, Vondracek, FW. Occupational identity. In Schwartz, SJ, Luyckx, K, Vignoles, VL, eds. *Handbook of Identity Theory and Research.* New York, NY: Springer; 2011:693–714.

53. Wenger, E, McDermott, R, Snyder, WM. *Cultivating Communities of Practice: A Guide to Managing Knowledge.* Cambridge, MA: Harvard Business Press; 2002.

54. Cruess, RL, Cruess, SR. Expectations and obligations: professionalism and medicine's social contract with society. *Perspect Biol Med.* 2008; **51**(4):579–98.

55. Birden, H, Glass, N, Wilson, I, Harrison, M, Usherwood, T, Nass, D. Defining professionalism in medical education: a systematic review. *Med Teach.* 2014; **36**(1):47–61.

56. *Oxford English Dictionary.* Second edition. Oxford, UK: Clarendon Press; 1989.

57. Piaget, J, Inhelder, B. *The Psychology of the Child.* New York, NY: Basic Books; 1969.

58. Kohlberg, L. *The Psychology of Moral Development: Moral Stages and the Life Cycle*. San Francisco, CA: Harper & Row; 1984.

59. Erikson, EH. *The Life Cycle Completed*. New York, NY: WW Norton; 1982.

60. Kegan, R. *The Evolving Self: Problem and Process in Human Development*. Cambridge, MA: Harvard University Press; 1982.

61. Marcia, JE. Identity in adolescence. In Adelson, J, ed. *Handbook of Adolescent Psychology*. New York, NY: Wiley; 1980:159–87.

62. Hafferty, FW, Castellani, B. A sociological framing of medicine's modern-day professionalism movement. *Med Educ*. 2009; **43**(9):826–28.

63. Ross, S, Lai, K, Walton, JM, Kirwan, P, White, JS. "I have the right to a private life": medical students' views about professionalism in a digital world. *Med Teach*. 2013; **35**(10):826–31.

64. Bosk, C. *Forgive and Remember: Remembering Medical Failure*. Chicago, IL: University of Chicago Press; 1979.

65. Becker, HS, Geer, B, Hughes, EC, Strauss, AL. *Boys in White: Student Culture in Medical School*. Chicago, IL: University of Chicago Press; 1961.

66. Daniels, N. *Just Health: Meeting Health Needs Fairly*. Cambridge, UK: Cambridge University Press; 2008.

67. Cassell, EJ. The changing concept of the ideal physician. *Daedalus*. 1986; **115**(2):185–208.

68. Pellegrino, ED. Character formation and the making of good physicians. In Kenny, N, Shelton, W, eds. *Advances in Bioethics: Vol. 10. Lost Virtue: Professional Character Development in Medical Education*. Oxford, UK: Elsevier; 2006:1–15.

69. Birden, H, Glass, N, Wilson, I, Harrison, M, Usherwood, T, Nass, D. Defining professionalism in medical education: a systematic review. *Med Teach*. 2014; **36**(1):47–61.

70. Hafferty, FW. Definitions of professionalism: a search for meaning and identity. *Clin Orthop Relat Res*. 2006; **449**:193–204.

71. Castellani, B, Hafferty, FW. The complexities of medical professionalism: a preliminary investigation. In Wear, D, Aultman, JM, eds. *Professionalism in Medicine: Critical Perspectives*. New York, NY: Springer; 2006:3–23.

72. Freidson, E. *Professionalism: The Third Logic*. Cambridge, UK: Polity Press; 2001.

73. Fuchs, VR, Cullen, MR. The transformation of U.S. physicians. *JAMA*. 2015; **313**(18):1821–22.

74. Starr, P. *The Social Transformation of American Medicine*. New York, NY: Basic Books; 1982.

75. Cruess, SR, Johnston, S, Cruess, RL. "Profession": a working definition for medical educators. *Teach Learn Med*. 2004; **16**(1):74–76.

76. ABIM Foundation, American Board of Internal Medicine; ACP-ASIM Foundation, American College of Physicians-American Society of Internal Medicine; European Federation of Internal Medicine. Medical professionalism in the new millennium: a physician charter. *Ann Intern Med*. 2002; **136**(3):243–46.

77. Swick, HM. Toward a normative definition of medical professionalism. *Acad Med*. 2000; **75**(6):612–16.

78. Working Party of the Royal College of Physicians. Doctors in society. Medical professionalism in a changing world. *Clin Med (Lond)*. 2005; **5**(6 Suppl 1): S5–S40.

79. Hafferty, FW, McKinlay, JB, eds. *The Changing Medical Profession: An International Perspective*. New York, NY: Oxford University Press; 1993.

80. Ho, MJ, Yu, KH, Hirsh, D, Huang, TS, Yang, PC. Does one size fit all? Building a framework for medical professionalism. *Acad Med*. 2011; **86**(11):1407–14.

81. Al-Eraky, MM, Chandratilake, M. How medical professionalism is conceptualised in Arabian context: a validation study. *Med Teach*. 2012; **34**(Suppl 1):S90–S95.

82. Dixon, DM, Sweeney, KG, Gray, DJ. The physician healer: ancient magic or modern science? *Br J Gen Pract*. 1999; **49**(441):309–12.

83. Kearney, M. *A Place of Healing: Working with Suffering in Living and Dying*. Oxford, UK: Oxford University Press; 2000.

84. Emanuel, EJ, Emanuel, LL. Four models of the physician-patient relationship. *JAMA*. 1992; **267**(16):2221–26.

85. Coulter, A. Patients' views of the good doctor. *BMJ*. 2002; **325**(7366):668–69.

86. Emanuel, EJ, Emanuel, LL. What is accountability in health care? *Ann Intern Med*. 1996; **124**(2):229–39.

87. Broadbent, J, Laughlin, R. "Accounting logic" and controlling professionals: the case of the public sector. In Broadbent, J, Dietrich, M, Roberts, J, eds. *The End of the Professions? The Restructuring of Professional Work*. London, UK: Routledge; 1997:34–49.

88. Gruen, RL, Pearson, SD, Brennan, TA. Physician-citizens – public roles and professional obligations. *JAMA*. 2004; **291**(1):94–98.

89. Bloche, MG. Clinical loyalties and the social purposes of medicine. *JAMA*. 1999; **281**(3):268–74.

90. Irvine, D. *The Doctors' Tale: Professionalism and Public Trust*. Abingdon, UK: Radcliffe Medical Press; 2003.

91. DeAngelis, CD. Medical professionalism. *JAMA*. 2015; **313**(18):1837–38.

92. Cohen, JJ. Tasking the "self" in self-governance of medicine. *JAMA*. 2015; **313**(18):1839–40.

93. Marcovitch, H. Governance and professionalism in medicine: a UK perspective. *JAMA*. 2015; **313**(18):1823–24.

94. Baker, DP, Day, R, Salas, E. Teamwork as an essential component of high-reliability organizations. *Health Serv Res.* 2006; **41** (4 Pt 2):1576–98.

95. Teirstein, PS, Topol, EJ. The role of maintenance of certification programs in governance and professionalism. *JAMA.* 2015; **313**(18):1809–10.

96. Pellegrino, ED. The medical profession as a moral community. *Bull N Y Acad Med.* 1990; **66**(3):221–32.

97. Coulehan, J. Viewpoint: today's professionalism: engaging the mind but not the heart. *Acad Med.* 2005; **80**(10):892–98.

98. McGaghie, WC, Mytko, JJ, Brown, WN, Cameron, JR. Altruism and compassion in the health professions: a search for clarity and precision. *Med Teach.* 2002; **24**(4):374–78.

99. Borges, NJ, Manuel, RS, Elam, CL, Jones, BJ. Comparing millennial and generation X medical students at one medical school. *Acad Med.* 2006; **81**(6):571–76.

100. Watson, DE, Slade, S, Buske, L, Tepper, J. Intergenerational differences in workloads among primary care physicians: a ten-year, population-based study. *Health Aff (Millwood).* 2006; **25**(6):1620–28.

101. Brennan, TA, Rothman, DJ, Blank, L, Blumenthal, D, Chimonas, SC, Cohen, JJ, Goldman, J, Kassirer, JP, Kimball, H, Naughton, J, Smelser, N. Health industry practices that create conflicts of interest: a policy proposal for academic medical centers. *JAMA.* 2006; **295**(4):429–33.

102. Relman, AS. Medical professionalism in a commercialized health care market. *JAMA.* 2007; **298**(22):2668–70.

103. Sambunjak, D, Straus, SE, Marušić A. Mentoring in academic medicine: a systematic review. *JAMA.* 2006; **296**(9):1103–15.

104. Mann, K, Gordon, J, MacLeod, A. Reflection and reflective practice in health professions education: a systematic review. *Adv Health Sci Educ Theory Pract.* 2009; **14**(4):595–621.

105. Mann, KV. Reflection: understanding its influence on practice. *Med Educ.* 2008; **42**(5):449–51.

106. Cruess, SR, Cruess, RL, Steinert, Y. Role modelling – making the most of a powerful teaching strategy. *BMJ.* 2008; **336**(7646):718–21.

107. Kolb, DA. *Experiential Learning: Experience as the Source of Learning and Development.* Englewood Cliffs, NJ: Prentice-Hall; 1984.

108. Epstein, RM. Reflection, perception and the acquisition of wisdom. *Med Educ.* 2008; **42**(11):1048–50.

109. Wald, HS, Reis, SP, Monroe, AD, Borkan, JM. 'The Loss of My Elderly Patient': interactive reflective writing to support medical students' rites of passage. *Med Teach.* 2010; **32**(4):e178–e184.

110. Wald, HS. Professional identity (trans)formation in medical education: reflection, relationship, resilience. *Acad Med.* 2015; **90**(6):701–06.

111. Polanyi, M. *Personal Knowledge: Towards a Post-Critical Philosophy.* Chicago, IL: University of Chicago Press; 1958.

112. Steinert, Y, Cruess, S, Cruess, R, Snell, L. Faculty development for teaching and evaluating professionalism: from programme design to curriculum change. *Acad Med.* 2005; **39**(2):127–36.

113. Steinert, Y, Cruess, RL, Cruess, SR, Boudreau, JD, Fuks, A. Faculty development as an instrument of change: a case study on teaching professionalism. *Acad Med.* 2007; **82**(11):1057–64.

114. Cruess, RL, Cruess, SR. Professionalism, professional identity, and the hidden curriculum: do as we say and as we do. In Hafferty, FW, O'Donnell, JF, eds. *The Hidden Curriculum in Health Professional Education.* Lebanon, NH: Dartmouth College Press; 2014:171–81.

115. Bebeau, MJ, Faber-Langendoen, K. Remediating lapses in professionalism. In Kalet, A, Chou, CL, eds. *Remediation in Medical Education: A Mid-Course Correction.* New York, NY: Springer; 2014:103–27.

116. Brainard, AH, Brislen, HC. Viewpoint: learning professionalism: a view from the trenches. *Acad Med.* 2007; **82**(11):1010–14.

117. Benbassat, J. Undesirable features of the medical learning environment: a narrative review of the literature. *Adv Health Sci Educ Theory Pract.* 2013; **18**(3):527–36.

118. Lesser, CS, Lucey, CR, Egener, B, Braddock, CH III, Linas, SL, Levinson, W. A behavioral and systems view of professionalism. *JAMA.* 2010; **304**(24):2732–37.

119. Gaufberg, EH, Batalden, M, Sands, R, Bell, SK. The hidden curriculum: what can we learn from third-year medical student narrative reflections? *Acad Med.* 2010; **85**(11):1709–16.

120. Benbassat, J. Changes in wellbeing and professional values among medical undergraduate students: a narrative review of the literature. *Adv Health Sci Educ Theory Pract.* 2014; **19**(4):597–610.

121. Fox, RC. Medical uncertainty revisited. In Albrecht, GL, Fitzpatrick, R, Scrimshaw, SC, eds. *The Handbook of Social Studies in Health & Medicine.* London, UK: SAGE; 2002; 409–25.

122. Janss, R, Rispens, S, Segers, M, Jehn, KA. What is happening under the surface? Power, conflict and the performance of medical teams. *Med Educ.* 2012; **46**(9):838–49.

123. van der Zwet, J, de la Croix, A, de Jonge, LPJWM, Stalmeijer, RE, Scherpbier, AJJA, Teunissen, PW. The power of questions: a discourse analysis about doctor-student interaction. *Med Educ.* 2014; **48**(8):806–19.

124. Bynum, WE IV, Goodie, JL. Shame, guilt, and the medical learner: ignored connections and why we should care. *Med Educ.* 2014; **48**(11):1045–54.

125. LeBlanc, VR. The effects of acute stress on performance: implications for health professions education. *Acad Med.* 2009; **84**(10 Suppl): S25–S33.

126. Yerkes, RM, Dodson, JD. The relation of strength of stimulus to rapidity of habit-formation. *J Comp Neurol.* 1908; **18**(5):459–82.

127. Wear, D, Aultman, JM, Varley, JD, Zarconi, J. Making fun of patients: medical students' perceptions and use of derogatory and cynical humor in clinical settings. *Acad Med.* 2006; **81**(5):454–62.

128. Lingard, L. Language matters: towards an understanding of silence and humour in medical education. *Med Educ.* 2013; **47**(1):40–48.

129. Feudtner, C, Christakis, DA, Christakis, NA. Do clinical clerks suffer ethical erosion? Students' perceptions of their ethical environment and personal development. *Acad Med.* 1994; **69**(8):670–79.

130. Krause, EA. *Death of the Guilds: Professions, States, and the Advance of Capitalism, 1930 to the Present.* New Haven, CT: Yale University Press; 1996.

131. Dunning, AJ. Status of the doctor–present and future. *Lancet.* 1999; **354** Suppl:SIV18.

132. Stevens, RA. Public roles for the medical profession in the United States: beyond theories of decline and fall. *Milbank Q.* 2001; **79**(3):327–53.

133. *Oxford Dictionary of Philosophy.* Oxford, UK: Oxford University Press; 1996.

134. Wynia, MK. The short and tenuous future of medical professionalism: the erosion of medicine's social contract. *Perspect Biol Med.* 2008; **51**(4):565–78.

Chapter

2

Developing a professional identity: a learner's perspective

Robert Sternszus

It was August 2005, and I had just found an empty seat in the auditorium where my first lecture as a McGill medical student would be held. The Dean of the Faculty of Medicine was about to address the class, and his opening words were ones that I still think about to this day: "Today, you begin your transformation from being a lay-person to being a physician." I was very unsettled by this statement, and my mind began to race. What does it mean to be a physician? To be a physician, do I have to stop being who I am? Is being a doctor going to be what I do, or who I am? As unsettling as these questions were, I was intrigued by the notion that I was going to change, and even began to look forward to seeing how this process would unfold. Throughout my training, I learned valuable lessons about the professional values that I needed to adopt, the behaviors that I needed to demonstrate, and the responsibilities that I needed to uphold in order to become a physician. This provided me with an important framework in which to understand medical professionalism; however, my personal transformation from a medical student into a pediatrician, and all of the intermediate steps in between, were rarely formally explored.

Having completed my undergraduate and post-graduate medical training at McGill University in 2009 and 2014 respectively, my professionalism education was based on the work of Cruess and Cruess that influenced much of the teaching of medical professionalism over the last fifteen years.[1,2] At the core of this work were two key principles: (1) medical professionalism needs to be taught explicitly; and (2) the objective of this teaching is to ensure that students understand, demonstrate a commitment to, and internalize the values of the profession. As such, the focus was primarily on the "doing" of professionalism. As has been discussed in Chapter 1, professionalism education hopes to reframe its focus from the

"doing" of professionalism to the "being" of a professional. In other words, ensuring that students understand and demonstrate professionalism is no longer the objective but, rather, an important step in the ultimate goal of supporting learners in the formation of their professional identity.

In this chapter, I will provide a learner's perspective on the benefits and potential pitfalls of curricula focused on the explicit teaching of professional values, roles, and responsibilities, with the hope that readers can learn from my experiences as well as the literature in this area. Furthermore, I will describe how shifting the focus of medical education toward supporting the formation of a professional identity has the potential to respond to many of the potential challenges facing current curricula.

The teaching of medical professionalism: the "doing"

The curriculum

The professionalism curriculum at McGill University, from 2005 to 2014, was designed to both teach the cognitive base of professionalism and reinforce it in authentic learning environments.[1-4] The cognitive base consists of the attributes and values of the medical profession and the relationship between the medical profession and society (i.e., the social contract). In the pre-clinical years (the first two years of medical school), the focus was on teaching the cognitive base through weekly lectures, small group discussions around clinical vignettes, and the creation of a portfolio of reflective essays.[5] Although there was some formal teaching of professionalism in the clinical years (clerkship and residency), the bulk of professionalism training during this period focused on reinforcing the cognitive base through role modeling and

---

Teaching Medical Professionalism, 2nd Edition, ed. Richard L. Cruess, Sylvia R. Cruess and Yvonne Steinert. Published by Cambridge University Press. © Cambridge University Press 2016.

reflection on clinical experiences.[6] Throughout the curriculum, assessment was based on the submission of reflective writing pieces, identifying professionalism issues in clinical situations, and clinical evaluations highlighting outstanding professional behavior as well as lapses in professionalism.[7,8] As such, the curriculum focused on the understanding and demonstration, or the doing, of professionalism.

The learner perspective

The strengths of current approaches

In preparation for writing this chapter, I returned to my medical school portfolio. It begins with a list of terms and attributes with their definitions, such as "healer," "profession," "altruism," and "confidentiality." These principles represent the cognitive base of professionalism, which would be explicitly taught throughout the pre-clinical years of medical school. The remainder of the portfolio comprised a series of reflections on various experiences, such as working with a cadaver and my first patient encounter. In reading through these pieces, it became clear that learning the cognitive base of professionalism provided a framework that guided all of my reflections. By the time I entered the clinical years of training, I was able to use the vocabulary of professionalism in discussing medical issues, identify different

professional attributes that informed ethical dilemmas, understand my own behaviors and worldviews in terms of the tenets of professionalism and the social contract, and articulate a clear vision of what I thought the ideal physician should be.

Prior to entering clerkship, each McGill class composes a pledge that is recited at the "white coat ceremony" (a ceremony honoring the transition from pre-clinical training to clerkship). This pledge represents the commitment that students make to the profession and illustrates the profound understanding of professionalism that can result from its explicit teaching in the pre-clinical years. For example, the McGill 2009 class pledge illustrates an understanding of the responsibility physicians and medical students have to patients, the larger community, and the profession, as well as the importance of ethical practice and lifelong learning (see Figure 2.1).

Although having an understanding of professionalism is important, it does not necessarily mean that it will be incorporated into how one practices medicine. In a reflective piece about my expectations prior to starting clerkship, I wrote:

> It is [in clerkship] that I will become a physician. [...]
> I have always built my life around my core values.
> I brought them with me through my studies,
> have applied them on the sports field and in

Figure 2.1. Class pledge delivered by the McGill Medicine Class of 2009, in 2007, during their White Coat Ceremony

This is our pledge to our patients, community, and profession;
Founded in our desire to care for and learn from others;

To treat every patient as our only patient
To see the wholeness of our patient's spirit beyond the wounded body
To listen to our patients tell their own story in their own time
To remember that there is a time and place for every narrative to be told
To understand our patient's situation within their life story
To guide our patient in the realization of their healing potential

Not to let technology overshadow the importance of humane and individual care
Not to attempt to be infallible, but rather to learn from our mistakes
Not to pretend to be master of our profession, but always an apprentice
Not to permit personal differences to interfere with our duties to our patient
Not to allow expedience, but morality, to guide our decisions
Not to act alone, but as a team, to uphold the dignity of the profession

To our patients, community and profession, we promise to never lose sight of these responsibilities.

relationships. Now, it is of utmost importance that I find a way to integrate them into the way I practice medicine. It is only in doing so, that I can be truly genuine in my practice and with my patients.

I identified clerkship as the time in my training when I would incorporate the cognitive base of professionalism, and my own identity, into my professional practice. Much of what medical students and residents learn about professionalism in the clinical environment results from watching and reflecting on the behaviors, skills, attitudes, and beliefs of their role models.[9,10] What I had learned in the pre-clinical years provided me with a framework for this reflection. Given that much of the role modeling was implicit and most of the reflection was unguided, this framework was essential in shaping my learning. It helped me to differentiate between the positive and negative behaviors I was seeing in the clinical environment and allowed me to understand medical care within the larger social context. As such, the framework that was explicitly taught in the pre-clinical years and the opportunities to apply and internalize it in the clinical years were vital in developing my sense of professionalism.

Areas for improvement in current approaches

The contribution of professionalism education to the formation of medical students and residents over the last fifteen years cannot be overstated. The explicit teaching of the cognitive base of professionalism and its reinforcement through role modeling and clinical experiences are necessary components of professionalism education, and were extremely valuable to my learning and development. However, literature on learners' reactions to professionalism education suggests that although they appreciate its value, they do not always appreciate how it is taught.[9–14] As such, it is important to examine how the delivery of professionalism education can be improved in order to better meet the needs of learners. Based on my experiences, an informal focus group conducted with current McGill pediatric residents, and a review of the literature, there appear to be six issues that can arise in professionalism curricula that merit further discussion: (1) oversimplification of complex content; (2) a focus on negative professionalism; (3) teaching the cognitive base in isolation from the clinical context; (4) insufficient positive role modeling; (5) inadequate focus on periods of transition; and, (6) lack of focus on the individual.

(1) Oversimplification of complex content

One significant challenge in teaching professionalism is navigating the line between highlighting the expectations of the profession and making it seem as though every situation has a clear right and wrong answer. The clinical world is ambiguous and unpredictable, and the explicit teaching of medical professionalism can sometimes feel prescribed. The use of vignettes is one way the core values of the profession are taught. In my experience, scenarios can sometimes be oversimplified by dealing with issues that have clear right and wrong answers, or dealing with more complex issues in which a right or wrong answer is imposed.

Some scenarios that students are asked to reflect upon can deal with obvious violations of professional conduct, such as an attending physician arriving to work drunk or a classmate distributing a stolen copy of the final exam. Students do not need to understand medical professionalism in order to know how to react to these scenarios, and the literature suggests that many students find that these simplistic scenarios make them less likely to engage with professionalism education.[9,13] Conversely, students can also be confronted with challenging vignettes in which the expected response is oversimplified. In these instances, students have learned how to "game the system," and say what they know the "correct" answer is, rather than reflect on the issues in a meaningful way.[11] A common example of this phenomenon is when altruism is addressed, such as when students are given a scenario in which an important personal event conflicts with the needs of a patient. Learners know that the "correct" answer is "altruism," but many, myself included, report struggling with the idea that it is never acceptable to acknowledge and prioritize one's own needs as a person. If students are not challenged to reflect on the complex nature of these issues, valuable educational experiences may be lost.

This concern was further illustrated in a series of focus groups with medical students in the United Kingdom, who reported feeling a tension between themselves as individuals and as professionals, and that rather than reflecting on this tension, the curriculum forced them to conform to the standards of the institution, leading to feelings of resentment.[12] If professionalism education encourages students to reflect on the complexities of professional dilemmas rather than on more simplistic scenarios, it can stimulate learners to reflect on themselves and their work, rather than leaving them feeling patronized and frustrated.[15]

(2) A focus on negative professionalism

As described previously, the main objective of the explicit teaching of professionalism is to produce exemplary physicians who are committed to their patients, their profession, and society. However, efforts to make the teaching of professionalism more explicit have, in some cases, resulted in curricula that are more focused on ensuring that students do not behave unprofessionally than they are on promoting positive professional behavior. The literature suggests that many curricula focus on teaching and enforcing codes of conduct, and employ assessments based exclusively on professionalism lapses. This may result in students associating professionalism education with being judged, scolded, or told how they should behave and, consequently, may lead to frustration.[9,10,13,16]

There are many examples of ways that medical schools can promote positive professionalism rather than only remediate negative professionalism. For example, preceptors at McGill University are given an opportunity to highlight exemplary professional behaviors displayed by students on each rotation evaluation, and outstanding professionalism is recognized at the annual convocation ceremony. These small celebrations of positive professionalism can go a long way in encouraging students to embrace this important part of their education.

(3) Isolating the cognitive base from the clinical context

The cognitive base of professionalism is often taught extensively during the pre-clinical years of medical school.[3] Although doing so provides learners with a framework that they can bring with them into the clinical environment, isolating the explicit teaching of the framework from the clinic can result in the material feeling abstract to the learner. A study of Australian medical students revealed that they believed professionalism should be taught in the practice context and not as an isolated module.[13] These findings were further corroborated by my discussion with current McGill residents who highlighted the importance of continuity between the explicit teaching of professionalism and clinical experiences. These residents also reported that engaging in simulation around issues of professionalism during their training provided them with a safe and authentic environment in which to situate what they were learning.

Therefore, early clinical exposure and the use of simulation in professionalism education, which do not appear to occur uniformly across programs reported in the literature, may help learners better internalize the cognitive base of professionalism by allowing them to situate it within the clinical context.

(4) Insufficient positive role modeling

The gap between what students learn in the classroom and what they see in clinical practice is one of the most significant problems in professionalism education.[9,10,13–15] Role modeling is one of the most important ways students and residents learn about professionalism.[10,17–22] However, role models do not always set the best example. Students at the University of Ottawa reported believing that faculty members needed to enhance the quality of their role modeling.[10] In another study at the University of Ottawa, 36 percent of 255 medical students who responded to an online survey reported having witnessed an example of exemplary professionalism, whereas 64 percent had seen behaviors that they deemed significant lapses in professionalism.[17] I can certainly remember working with negative role models who made me feel like I needed to act "unprofessionally" in order to fit in. These negative role models can also leave students feeling as though there is a double standard between what is expected of them and what is expected of members of the profession.[9,13] All of this contributes to the feelings of resentment and disinterest that many students can express toward professionalism education.

(5) Inadequate focus on periods of transition

In going from a first-year medical student to an attending physician, a medical learner will undergo multiple transitions (e.g., pre-clinical student to clinical clerk, clinical clerk to junior resident, and junior resident to senior resident). Each of these transitions is associated with a change in learning environment, schedule, and, most significantly, role and identity within the clinical team. The transition from medical student to resident was one of the most difficult periods of my training. Overnight, I went from a fully supervised medical student to someone who was trusted to write prescriptions and be left in charge of a care unit. I was also integrating into a new community of pediatric residents, as well as working to earn the trust of the nurses, fellow residents, and clinical supervisors. I had no training on how to navigate this period of transition, and I suffered from insomnia and had difficulty maintaining personal relationships. This period was also critical in developing my identity as a pediatric resident, and in shaping the way I approached my professional life throughout residency training. As such, it represented both a high risk and a tremendously important period in my professional development. However, there was no formal discussion of professionalism or professional identity during this time.

The literature supports the notion that transitions in medical education are both highly stressful and inadequately supported.[23,24] Furthermore, a study of residency program directors identified professionalism as one of the three key areas in which transitioning residents appear to struggle.[25] Although the link between supporting transitions and the promotion of professionalism has not been formally explored (see Chapter 13), I believe that a more explicit focus on navigating periods of transition may increase the degree to which medical students relate to, and benefit from, their professionalism education.

(6) Inadequate focus on the individual

As a college student and young adult, I decided that I wanted to become a physician – a decision that was the product of many influences. Intellectually, I enjoyed learning about biology, physiology, and anatomy. I was also curious, loved solving problems, and enjoyed learning about others. Perhaps even more importantly, this decision was influenced by the values that had been instilled in me throughout my life. I am a second-generation Canadian, whose grandparents came to Canada after having watched the vast majority of their family members perish in World War II. They were denied the right to an education because of their religious background and worked multiple jobs with the hope of being able to provide a better life for their children and grandchildren. Despite the struggles they had in establishing themselves in Canada, they devoted themselves to standing up for the rights of others. This upbringing instilled in me the importance of hard work, social justice, higher education, financial security, family, and generosity. Furthermore, having a grandson become a doctor represented a realization of their dream, and there is no denying the influence that this had on me. Who I was and where I came from had a significant influence on why I wanted to be a doctor.

Who I was and where I came from also had an important influence on how I understood and internalized the professionalism framework that was explicitly taught in medical school. However, the concept of "self" was not often addressed in the curriculum. Going back to when I was asked to reflect on a patient's needs coming into conflict with an important life or family event, my reflection addressed the penultimate importance of altruism. I knew this was the "textbook" answer; however, it was not one that satisfied me. My family history led me to prioritize family over all else, and I felt that there was a tension between this and altruism. I never formally addressed this concern. I simply overlooked my frustration, wrote a reflective piece on altruism, and moved on to the next activity. Had the reflective exercise been focused on how my values interact with the profession, instead of on the interaction between the attribute of altruism and the profession, the learning experience could have been significantly richer.

One of the reasons that professionalism education may sometimes neglect the role of the individual is that it makes assessment less straightforward. It is easier to assess dichotomous answers to questions than complex personal reflections. However, in an essay written by Diane C. Reis, who was a medical student at the University of Wisconsin at the time of publication, she highlights the importance of acknowledging the individual in the process of internalizing the professional values that are taught (p. S112):[11]

> There is little guidance as students attempt to negotiate the balance between altruism and care for self and family. [...] I hope that medical education researchers will consider the role that identity plays in professional decision-making. [...] [If] we limit ourselves to focus on dos and don'ts; I have little confidence that we will, in the process, produce physicians who live the values that we preach.

Multiple publications report that many students feel professionalism curricula do not sufficiently focus on the issues that they face, nor do they adequately help them navigate the tension between their personal and professional selves.[9–13] It appears that this may be the result of curricula that fail to focus on the interaction between the learners' pre-existing identity and the medical profession. The importance of doing so is further reinforced in an essay written together by a first- and final-year medical student who state that "professionalism is cultivated in the individual, not in his [or her] degree."[26]

Summary of the learner perspective

Over the last fifteen years, educators have focused on explicitly teaching professionalism in order to ensure that students understand and internalize the values of the profession. Curricula have provided learners with an excellent cognitive base for understanding professionalism, as well as a framework with which they can interpret their clinical experiences. However, the literature on the learner's perspective suggests that these curricula can sometimes lead to dissatisfaction among learners. As professionalism education moves forward, it will be essential that future curricula respond to the concerns put forth by these learners. The proposed shift toward placing professional identity formation at the center of medical education appears to be an important positive step in that direction.

Supporting professional identity formation: the "being"

If the first day of medical school represents the beginning of one's transformation from lay-person to physician, as was suggested by the Dean of Medicine on my first day, then the notion that the objective of medical education is to support the formation of the learners' professional identity has tremendous face validity. In reflecting on the concept of identity formation, I returned to the questions that circled around in my head on that first day of medical school: Who was I? And how was I going to change?

In order to remember who I was, I read the letter I wrote for my medical school application. In the letter, I discussed many attributes that still describe me today: a hard worker, a leader, a coach, a teacher, and a team player. However, I also described myself in ways that no longer seem relevant: an athlete, a fundraiser, a creative writer, and an optimist. Furthermore, I have also become many things that I was not in 2005: an uncle, a husband, a pediatrician, a master's student, a medical educator, and a researcher. What became evident was that over a ten-year period in my personal and professional life I had gone through a succession of transitions, each of which resulted in shifts in my identity that influenced the person and professional that I have become.

In this section, I will present a learner's perspective on professional identity formation. In particular, I will discuss how focusing professionalism education on the identity shifts that learners experience, and the influence of these shifts on professionalism and professional identity, has the potential to address many of the concerns with current professionalism curricula put forth by students and residents.

Principles of professional identity formation: responding to concerns with professionalism education

In order to discuss professional identity formation, we must first be clear on what it means. Professional identity refers to what a physician is; the editors of this book have defined it as, "a representation of self, achieved in stages over time during which the characteristics, values, and norms of the profession are internalized, resulting in an individual thinking, acting, and feeling like a physician."[27] Identity formation refers to how one becomes a physician and has been defined as "an adaptive developmental process" that occurs both at the level of the individual and as a result of socialization into a clinical role and community of practice.[28] Contained within these definitions are four key principles that should inform any curriculum focused on professional identity: (1) identity formation is a developmental process that occurs in all learners; (2) professional identity is formed in the context of a pre-existing individual identity; (3) professional identity results from socialization into a community of practice; and (4) professional identity results from a series of identity transformations that occur primarily during periods of transition.[27,28]

(1) Professional identity formation is a developmental process

The literature suggests that learners can sometimes feel that professionalism education is overly focused on judgment and negative behaviors.[9,10,13,16] By focusing on professional identity formation, which is a developmental process that necessarily occurs in every learner, professionalism education may be able to change this perception.

Much like every person develops their own individual identity throughout life, every physician will develop their professional identity over the course of their training and career. However, there is no guarantee that all students will develop a professional identity that successfully integrates their values with those of the profession. Therefore, the role of professionalism education should be to guide and support learners in this process of identity formation, rather than ensuring that learners understand medical professionalism and demonstrate professional behaviors.[27,28] This does not mean that the cognitive base of professionalism need not be explicitly taught, but rather, that the focus be shifted from a generic understanding of professionalism[11] to providing learners with a framework with which to understand their own personal identity development.[27] This approach would teach students the basic psychology of identity formation,[27,29-32] as well as the values and attributes of the profession.

Although this may seem similar to current approaches, teaching students the values of the profession in order to help them understand what they can aspire to become is significantly more positive than teaching the values of the profession to make sure that they know how to behave. For example, by recognizing the development of students into clinical clerks through events such as white coat ceremonies, or acknowledging the personal and professional growth of individual learners on longitudinal assessments, curricula focused on professional identity formation can create a culture of support that may be perceived by learners as aspirational rather than punitive. As a result, learners may be more motivated to engage in their professionalism education.

(2) Professional identity is formed in the context of a preexisting individual identity

The literature suggests that some learners become dissatisfied when professionalism curricula oversimplify complex professional issues and fail to adequately guide them in dealing with conflicts between their personal and professional selves.[9,11-13] Professional identity formation acknowledges that one's professional identity is largely influenced by one's individual identity, which in turn is influenced by many factors extrinsic to the profession (e.g., gender, class, ethnicity, religion, family).[27-32] This acknowledgment allows professionalism education to address the real tensions and struggles that learners face in navigating their personal and professional lives. Returning again to the example of a family issue coming into conflict with the needs of a patient, a focus on professional identity formation would have led me to discuss the tension I was feeling between the importance of altruism and responsibility to my family. This would have allowed me to understand the influence of my family history on my personal and

professional life, and encouraged me to think about potential solutions to help overcome this conflict (e.g., turning to another member of the healthcare team to help me meet the needs of my family and of the patient). This deeper and more personal reflection may be more likely to influence the professional behavior of a learner than simply reflecting on the importance of a given professional attribute, such as altruism, to the profession. Although it is clear that the concept of altruism needs to be explicitly taught, if the way in which it was taught operationalized the idea that "professionalism is cultivated in the individual, not in his [or her] degree,"[26] professionalism education could move much closer to addressing the real struggles of today's learners.

(3) Professional identity formation is the result of socialization into a community of practice

Learners have described role modeling and learning in authentic clinical environments as critical to their learning of professionalism.[10] However, there is concern that the cognitive base of professionalism is taught in isolation of the clinical environment and that learners have insufficient access to positive role models.[9,10,13-15]

Professional identity formation highlights the fact that identity is formed as a result of socialization into a clinical and professional role through increasing participation in a community of practice.[33] It is by successfully negotiating individual identity with the expectations of the profession (i.e., the community of practice) that a learner develops a sense of professional belonging.[33] The importance of feeling "a part of the team" when a student is rotating through a clinical service cannot be overlooked. It has a powerful ability to shape behavior, and had a profound impact on my development as a student, a resident, and a pediatrician. As such, if medical education is going to take professional identity formation seriously, programs must adapt to allow students to negotiate the values of the profession with their individual identities in the clinical context by providing them with earlier and more integrated involvement in clinical work environments.

There is also an extensive literature on the importance of role models to the professional socialization of medical students and residents in the clinical setting.[20-22,34-39] It has been suggested that although role modeling is often implicit, effective role models explicitly engage learners in a more active and conscious process.[18,19,38,39] Much in the same way that Cruess and Cruess argued for the explicit teaching of the cognitive base of professionalism,[1,2] faculty development focused on making role modeling more deliberate and explicit may be essential to the success of professionalism curricular reform.

(4) Professional identity results from a series of identity transformations that occur at times of transition

Transitions represent some of the most challenging times for medical trainees.[23] Current curricula may not pay enough attention to the high-risk periods, which can impact learners' academic performance, professional behaviors, and wellness.[40] Developmental psychology suggests that these periods of transition are also critical for identity transformation.[30–32] As such, supporting learners in their formation of a professional identity would require curricula to focus on these periods in order to be successful.

Two potential strategies for supporting transitions could be dedicated transition courses and increased involvement of near-peers in medical training. Some medical schools have short preparatory courses around periods of transition that help learners adapt to their upcoming roles.[40–42] These courses are generally well-received by learners; however, literature suggests that these programs are not present in many schools and may not be as effective as they could be.[43,44] In addition to incorporating these programs more uniformly across medical schools, another way to enhance their efficacy may be to include near-peers. Prior to the beginning of my clerkship, two clinical clerks shared their experiences with the class. I still vividly remember this session because they were talking about the things that concerned me the most. Research has shown that one reason near-peer teaching is highly valuable is that near-peers are better situated to socialize their more

junior colleagues to the institutional culture and to act as "peer-models" since they may be more familiar with the hidden curriculum (i.e., the implicit rules to survive the institution).[45–47] Given the importance of socialization to identity formation, it would follow that using peer-models during transitions would be of benefit. If professionalism education could focus on transitions by helping learners conceptualize them in terms of their own identity development through targeted courses and near-peer teaching, transitions can evolve into a powerful opportunity to support identity formation rather than an ominous threat to professionalism.[23]

Conclusion

The explicit teaching of medical professionalism, with the goal of ensuring that learners understand, internalize, and demonstrate the values of the profession, has contributed greatly to medical education over the last fifteen years. Learners have been provided with a framework to interpret their clinical experiences and a deep understanding of the responsibility physicians have to their patients, the medical profession, and society. However, the literature suggests that professionalism curricula can also sometimes leave learners with negative feelings about professionalism by oversimplifying complex issues, focusing on professionalism lapses, isolating the teaching of professionalism from the clinical context and the individual, not focusing on periods of transition, and not providing learners with enough access to positive role models. Although professional identity formation is still in its early stages of development in the medical education context, it appears to represent a more holistic view of professionalism education that encompasses the current approaches and has the potential to respond to many of the challenges presented in this chapter (see Figure 2.2). If supporting and guiding learners in their formation of a professional identity is to become the

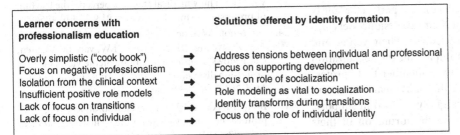

Figure 2.2. Learners' concerns with professionalism education that may be addressed by focusing curricula on identity formation

ultimate goal of medical education, the learners' perspective can provide important lessons for ensuring that future curricula are able to build on what has been accomplished to date.

In a curriculum centered on supporting and guiding learners in the formation of their professional identity, learners need to be explicitly taught a framework for understanding professional identity formation, as well as the cognitive base of professionalism. Doing so will allow them to understand both the transformational process that they will undergo and the nature of the identity that they are expected to develop. Furthermore, this explicit teaching should be done in parallel with exposure to authentic and positive clinical work environments, so that learners can be given opportunities for guided reflection on what they have learned and how it applies to their own personal and clinical experiences. The inconsistent availability of positive learning environments and of positive role models who create positive learning environments poses a significant threat to professionalism education. Investing in faculty development to promote positive role modeling may be an important part of remedying this situation.

It is also vital that professionalism education be framed positively and in such a way that learners can see it as a framework to help them deal with the complex professional challenges that they face. This means actively promoting positive professionalism on clinical evaluation forms and on special occasions such as convocation, as well as recognizing and adequately supporting learners during critical periods of transition.

Finally, in order for curricula focused on professional identity formation to succeed, they need to place the learners at the center. On a macro-level, learners should have a role in curriculum development and be an integral part of the delivery of the curriculum as near-peers, peer-models, and peer-mentors. On a micro-level, the role of the individual learner, their prior experiences, and personal identity in shaping every aspect of their professional development needs to be acknowledged. Their values and choices have a profound impact on the socialization process, and it is only if we remember that "professionalism is cultivated in the individual and not in [the] degree,"[26] that we can fully succeed in supporting and guiding learners in the formation of their professional identity.

References

1. Cruess, RL, Cruess, SR. Teaching medicine as a profession in the service of healing. *Acad Med*. 1997; **72**(11):941–52.

2. Cruess, SR, Cruess, RL. Professionalism must be taught. *BMJ*. 1997; **315**(7123):1674–77.

3. Cruess, RL, Cruess, SR. Teaching professionalism: general principles. *Med Teach*. 2006; **28**(3):205–08.

4. Steinert, Y, Cruess, RL, Cruess, SR, Boudreau, JD, Fuks, A. Faculty development as an instrument of change: a case study on teaching professionalism. *Acad Med*. 2007; **82**(11):1057–64.

5. Boudreau, JD, Cruess, SR, Cruess, RL. Physicianship: educating for professionalism in the post-Flexnerian era. *Perspect Biol Med*. 2011; **54**(1):89–105.

6. Snell, L. Teaching professionalism and fostering professional values during residency: the McGill experience. In Cruess, RL, Cruess, SR, Steinert, Y, eds. *Teaching Medical Professionalism*. New York, NY: Cambridge University Press; 2009:246–62.

7. Wilkinson, TJ, Wade, WB, Knock, LD. A blueprint to assess professionalism: results of a systematic review. *Acad Med*. 2009; **84**(5):551–58.

8. Hodges, BD, Ginsburg, S, Cruess, R, Cruess, S, Delport, R, Hafferty, F, Ho, MJ, Holmboe, E, Holtman, M, Ohbu, S, Rees, C, Ten Cate, O, Tsugawa, Y, Van Mook, W, Wass, V, Wilkinson, T, Wade, W. Assessment of professionalism: recommendations from the Ottawa 2010 Conference. *Med Teach*. 2011; **33**(5):354–63.

9. Leo, T, Eagen, K. Professionalism education: the medical student response. *Perspect Biol Med*. 2008; **51**(4):508–16.

10. Byszewski, A, Hendelman, W, McGuinty, C, Moineau, G. Wanted: role models – medical students' perceptions of professionalism. *BMC Med Educ*. 2012; **12**:115.

11. Reis, DC. Who am I and why am I here? Professionalism research through the eyes of a medical student. *Acad Med*. 2008; **83**(10 Supp.):S111–S112.

12. Finn, G, Garner, J, Sawdon, M. 'You're judged all the time!' Students' views on professionalism: a multicenter study. *Med Educ*. 2010; **44**(8):814–25.

13. Birden, HH, Usherwood, T. "They liked it if you said you cried": how medical students perceive the teaching of professionalism. *Med J Aust*. 2013; **199**(6):406–09.

14. van Mook, WN, de Grave, WS, Gorter, SL, Muijtjens, AM, Zwaveling, JH, Schuwirth, LW, van der Vleuten, CP. Fellows' in intensive care medicine views on professionalism and how they learn it. *Intensive Care Med*. 2010; **36**(2):296–303.

15. Brainard, AH, Brislen, HC. Viewpoint: learning professionalism: a view from the trenches. *Acad Med*. 2007; **82**(11):1010–14.

16. Skinner, C. *Professionalism and Reflective Practice Development across the Curriculum.* Short Communication. Association of Medical Education of Europe annual meeting; 2014.

17. Hendelman, W, Byszewski, A. Formation of medical student professional identity: categorizing lapses of professionalism, and the learning environment. *BMC Med Educ.* 2014; **14**:139.

18. Park, J, Woodrow, SI, Reznick, RK, Beales, J, MacRae, HM. Observation, reflection, and reinforcement: surgery faculty members' and residents' perceptions of how they learned professionalism. *Acad Med.* 2010; **85**(1):134–39.

19. Cruess, SR, Cruess, RL, Steinert, Y. Role modelling–making the most of a powerful teaching strategy. *BMJ.* 2008; **336**(7646):718–21.

20. Wright, SM, Carrese, JA. Excellence in role modelling: insight and perspectives from the pros. *CMAJ.* 2002; **167**(6):638–43.

21. Epstein, RM, Cole, DR, Gawinski, BA, Piotrowski-Lee, S, Ruddy, NB. How students learn from community-based preceptors. *Arch Fam Med.* 1998; **7**(2):149–54.

22. Côté, L, Laughrea, PA. Preceptors' understanding and use of role modeling to develop the CanMEDS competencies in residents. *Acad Med.* 2014; **89**(6):934–39.

23. Teunissen, PW, Westerman, M. Opportunity or threat: the ambiguity of the consequences of transitions in medical education. *Med Educ.* 2011; **45**(1):51–59.

24. Prince, K, Van de Wiel, M, Van der Vleuten, C, Boshuizen, H, Scherpbier, A. Junior doctors' opinions about the transition from medical school to clinical practice: a change of environment. *Educ Health (Abingdon).* 2004; **17**(3):323–31.

25. Lyss-Lerman, P, Teherani, A, Aagaard, E, Loeser, H, Cooke, M, Harper, GM. What training is needed in the fourth year of medical school? Views of residency program directors. *Acad Med.* 2009; **84**(7):823–29.

26. Krych, EH, Vande Voort, JL. Medical students speak: a two-voice comment on learning professionalism in medicine. *Clin Anat.* 2006; **19**(5):415–18.

27. Cruess, RL, Cruess, SR, Boudreau JD, Snell, L, Steinert, Y. Reframing medical education to support professional identity formation. *Acad Med.* 2014; **89**(11):1446–51.

28. Jarvis-Selinger, S, Pratt, DD, Regehr, G. Competency is not enough: integrating identity formation into the medical education discourse. *Acad Med.* 2012; **87**(9):1185–90.

29. Hilton, SR, Slotnick, HB. Proto-professionalism: how professionalisation occurs across the continuum of medical education. *Med Educ.* 2005; **39**(1):58–65.

30. Piaget, J, Inhelder, B. *The Psychology of the Child.* New York, NY: Basic Books; 1969.

31. Kohlberg, L. *The Psychology of Moral Development: Moral Stages and the Life Cycle.* San Francisco, CA: Harper and Row; 1984.

32. Erikson, EH. *The Life Cycle Completed.* New York, NY: WW Norton; 1982.

33. Wenger, E. Communities of practice and social learning systems. *Organization.* 2000; **7**(2):225–46.

34. Kenny, NP, Mann, KV, Macleod, H. Role modeling in physicians' professional formation: reconsidering an essential but untapped educational strategy. *Acad Med.* 2003; **78**(12):1203–10.

35. Sternszus, R, Cruess, S, Cruess, R, Young, M, Steinert, Y. Residents as role models: impact on undergraduate trainees. *Acad Med.* 2012; **87**(9):1282–87.

36. Karani, R, Fromme, HB, Cayea, D, Muller, D, Schwartz, A, Harris, IB. How medical students learn from residents in the workplace: a qualitative study. *Acad Med.* 2014; **89**(3):490–96.

37. Hafferty, FW. Professionalism and the socialization of medical students. In Cruess, RL, Cruess, SR, Steinert, Y, eds. *Teaching Medical Professionalism.* New York, NY: Cambridge University Press; 2009:53–70.

38. Bandura, A. *Social Foundations of Thought and Action: A Social Cognitive Theory.* Englewood Cliffs, NJ: Prentice Hall; 1986.

39. Bandura, A. *Psychological Modeling: Conflicting Theories.* New York, NY: Aldine-Atherton; 1971.

40. Strowd, R, Borgerding, E, Kittner, S, Haddad, D, Fletcher, S, Wofford, M, Lambros, A. *Transitions in Medicine: Four-Year Complementary Process-Oriented Curriculum for Medical Student Guidance.* Washington, DC: MedEdPORTAL; 2014. [Accessed Nov. 1, 2014]. Available from www.mededportal.org/publication/9904.

41. O'Brien, BC, Poncelet, AN. Transition to clerkship courses: preparing students to enter the workplace. *Acad Med.* 2010; **85**(12):1862–69.

42. Poncelet, A, O'Brien, B. Preparing medical students for clerkship: a descriptive analysis of transition courses. *Acad Med.* 2008; **83**(5):444–51.

43. Scicluna, HA, Grimm, MC, Jones, PD, Pilotto, LS, McNeil, HP. Improving the transition from medical school to internship – evaluation of a preparation for internship course. *BMC Med Educ.* 2014; **14**:23.

44. Taylor, JS, Faghri, S, Aggarwal, N, Zeller, K, Dollase, R, Reis, SP. Developing a peer-mentor program for medical students. *Teach Learn Med.* 2013; **25**(1):97–102.

45. Barker, TA, Ngwenya, N, Morley, D, Jones, E, Thomas, CP, Coleman, JJ. Hidden benefits of a peer-mentored 'Hospital Orientation Day': first-year medical students' perspectives. *Med Teach.* 2012; **34**(4):e229–e235.

46. Ten Cate, O, Durning, S. Peer teaching in medical education: twelve reasons to move from theory to practice. *Med Teach.* 2007; **29**(6):591–99.

47. Lockspeiser, TM, O'Sullivan, P, Teherani, A, Muller, J. Understanding the experience of being taught by peers: the value of social and cognitive congruence. *Adv Health Sci Educ Theory Pract.* 2008; **13**(3):361–72.

48. Hafferty, FW. Beyond curriculum reform: confronting medicine's hidden curriculum. *Acad Med.* 1998; **73**(4):403–07.

3

Theoretical insights into the nature and nurture of professional identities

Lynn V. Monrouxe

Introduction

The formation of identities is a process. Our own particular identities enable us to understand our place in the world: in other words, identities enable us to identify others and ourselves in any particular context. Furthermore, identity is not a singular, unchanging entity that we possess. Rather, it is a multifaceted and highly subjective concept that, influenced by many environmental factors, evolves over time and is enacted through language and objects in the social world.[1,2] Likewise, medical professionalism is contextual and evolving and is conceptualized according to a number of different discourses.[3,4] These discourses identify professionalism as an attribute of the individual physician, the interactional exchange, and the wider organizational and social context within which it occurs. Again, professionalism has a temporal aspect, rather than being a static and fixed concept. I will outline a range of theoretical underpinnings for the concept of *professional identities* that seek to explain its nature (i.e., internal cognitive processes) and its nurture (i.e., external social processes). My aim is to simplify, synergize, and contextualize the often complex, conflicting, and abstract notions of identity, identities, and identification in order to inform the ways in which we might consider the nature and nurture of professional identities in our explicit education of professionals. Furthermore, many of the theoretical approaches to identity, and the subsequent research within these approaches, tend to classify individuals into particular *types*. By way of a caveat, I am mindful that, while these are useful classifications for understanding the diverse nature and nurture of professional identities, the stereotyping of people according to such classifications is problematic. Although classifications can be positive or negative, they necessarily overlook the complexity of individuals, and as such are neither true nor false.

Identities and social worlds

Before we begin to think about professional identities, it is useful for us to stand back and consider the broader issue of how we conceptualize the human world within which identities and professionalism emerge, along with the process through which identities are developed. Irrespective of our broader cultural environment, we are all, to some extent, both embodied individuals *and* part of collective worlds, or cultures (e.g., familial, friendship, organizational, national). So, conceptualizing our interrelated position within and across these worlds provides us with the necessary foundation for understanding the formation of professional identities. In this way, Jenkins[5] has argued that it is useful for us to think about the social world according to three distinct, yet interrelated world *orders*:[5] (1) the *individual* order, comprising embodied individuals and their psychological–cognitive worlds; (2) the *interactional* order, comprising relationships among those individuals and what happens between them; and (3) the *institutional* order, comprising patterns and organization of established ways of doing things. To these orders, I add the *national* order, comprising the set of norms, behaviors, beliefs, and customs that are learned by virtue of being a member of the population of a nation.

These orders enable us to consider different perspectives of the same phenomenon, as they necessarily occupy the same physical and intersubjective (collective conscious) space.[5] They also enable us to understand the various ways in which identities have been conceptualized and researched: typically, individual theories pay attention to one aspect of the social

Teaching Medical Professionalism, 2nd Edition, ed. Richard L. Cruess, Sylvia R. Cruess and Yvonne Steinert.
Published by Cambridge University Press. © Cambridge University Press 2016.

order, downplaying the others in the process.[6] Thus, the challenge for educators of medical professionalism is to consider the relationship *between* the orders, and the internal–external processes through which identities and professionalism are constituted. A consideration of these processes of self-identification – how we come to know, represent, and express who we are – will enable us to have a better understanding of how professional identities might be developed and supported across students' undergraduate years and into practice. However, before we go into more detail regarding the theoretical perspectives across the various social worlds, let us consider the very early, core identities that we develop. These early identities form the basis of our understanding of who we are, from which we develop our later professional identities.

Self-identification: primary identities

Identification is a *process of socialization* through which we come to understand others and ourselves: in other words, it is the process through which our identities are thought to evolve and through which our identities become embodied (part of ourselves). As infants, during the initial stages of our self-recognition, we begin to have an awareness of others as being separate from ourselves. This *mirror stage* occurs from around six months of age, when we realize that the reflected image in front of us is that of our body, separate from that of our caretaker.[7] From this point forward, the process of self-identification begins – *who am I?* – and this continues throughout our lives. Among the earliest of identities developed (so-called primary identities) are selfhood (understanding ourselves as separate to others), gender–sex, ethnicity–race, and disability–impairment.[5]

Furthermore, the process of identification is ongoing. Our identities are continually *rewritten* throughout our lives as we draw on the environment, from people and from objects for their content. For example, we present ourselves to others (through clothes, mannerisms, language) in a certain way.[8] The reaction of others to this presentation informs both *their* identity of *us,* and our *own* self-identity: through our internal debate of how we see ourselves, of how we think others see us, and of how we identify with those others.[5] Indeed, we might feel validated by others in terms of how we present ourselves, or feel partially accepted or rejected. From this, our identities are further refined and developed. It is important to

know that how we receive feedback, and how that is incorporated into the process of our self-identification, is unlikely to be under our full control. And while all identities are reasonably malleable, our primary identities are relatively stable and resistant to change.[5] This resistance to change is important when we come to later consider the nature and nurture of professional identities within the national order.

Identity as a moral process

The development of a professional identity is not only an intellectual and social process; it is also a moral process.[9] Indeed, the origins of professional codes are ethical in nature (e.g., Code of Hammurabi in 2,000 B.C., Hippocratic Oath in the fifth century B.C.). Thus, as the nature of our professional identity incorporates a strong element of our moral identity as a prerequisite, it is important to understand how this develops over time and its relative primacy within our repertoire of identities. Around the age of eighteen months, children display an awareness of a *moral world* in which actions have consequences.[10,11] Due to these early beginnings in the development of our moral identity, many researchers believe that moral identity comprises one of our primary identities. However, because it develops over a protracted timeframe, with some believing it to be linked with more general cognitive development,[12] it is generally conceived of as a gradual form of self-realization that moves from an understanding of *right* from *wrong,* to the development of practical wisdom: *phronesis.*[13] This practical wisdom can take years to establish. So, unlike other primary identities, our moral identities remain relatively fluid as we seek to define who we are and how we view our social world.[14] Such an exploration can continue throughout our early adult lives and beyond.

The consequence of this protracted development is that we are subject to many different moral influences as we develop our identities. During this period of identity formation we can therefore take many paths. For example, we might conform to the prevailing moral norms within a world order (interactional, organizational, national); we might deviate positively from them; or we might deviate negatively from them. This means that it is entirely possible that we might conform to prevailing interactional or organizational norms that excuse – or even espouse – morally questionable behavior.[15–19] Furthermore, when complying with requests to participate in professionalism lapses,[15,18] through the process of self-identification, we might infer from our behavior a moral identity that deviates from the ideal. So, the influence of the informal and hidden curricula[20,21] – those unwritten, unofficial, and unintended messages that students implicitly and sometimes explicitly pick up during unplanned educational interactions – are of utmost importance in understanding the development of professional identities. Thus we can see that both the process of identification (and in particular, self-identification) and the development of our moral selves are important concepts for the understanding of our professional identities.

Having established a framework through which we can conceptualize the nature and nurture of professional identities, I now take each layer in turn. My aim is to consider the range of theoretical perspectives across the individual, interactional, institutional, and national orders that seek to inform us how physicians come to possess the concepts and structures that contribute to their professional identities. In doing so, I will highlight the relevance for medical educators of considering a particular lens through which to view identity. However, it is important to note that my classification is relatively pragmatic; in reality, things are not so clear cut. My aim in presenting them in this way is to clarify, within each perspective, the *location* of identity that each theory asserts.

Identities and the individual order

For many, the starting point for considering identity – and professionalism – is the self (I use the term *identity* as researchers here tend to use the singular, rather than plural form). By this I mean that identity and professionalism are conceived as being *situated in our minds* and are thought of as something we "have," to a greater or lesser degree. In terms of professionalism, this comprises a set of individual attributes – of attitudes, values, and behaviors – that exist in individuals and which are context-independent. Either we possess them or we do not. Such attributes include having integrity and good communication and decision-making skills and being trustworthy, empathic, honest, and patient-centered. From this perspective, the aim of educators is to select incoming students who possess the right attitudes and values and to instill, develop, and maintain those desired attributes in medical students as they become doctors. With this in mind, we now consider three (of the many) related theories of

individual identity formation, along with a range of empirical evidence that contributes to our understanding of professional identities and the consequence of this for medical educators.

Erikson's identity crisis

Erik Erikson is arguably the forefather of identity theorists in this camp. His psychoanalytic approach to understanding identity proposes eight stages of psychosocial development through which we pass from infancy to late adulthood.[22] Each stage is described as being a *psychosocial crisis* between our conflicting biological and sociocultural forces (here, crisis is the period of conscious questioning and of active struggling as we form our coherent identity). Although identity formation is a life-long process, the stage in which identity is key occurs during adolescence (originally thirteen – nineteen years but nowadays thought to end somewhere in our twenties). This stage has been termed *Identity Cohesion vs. Role Confusion*. The existential question associated with this stage is, "Who am I and who and what can I be?" Indeed, Erikson suggests that two main issues faced by people during this phase are career choice and ideology formation. So the obvious significance for medical educators is that the *identity crisis* stage spans at least the early years of most medical students' undergraduate education, and for some, its entirety.

To understand Erikson's theory, it is useful to draw on Freud's notion of the *id*: the primal, instinctive, and unconscious component of the self. The id comprises the biological aspect of the self (including the life instinct *Eros,* and the death instinct *Thanatos*). Because the id is chaotic and instinct driven, and because we are primarily social animals, we need a mechanism through which we can realistically satisfy our drives: this is called the *ego*. The ego has a particular meaning within psychodynamic theories. The ego is the decision-making and reasoning component of the self. Developed from the id, it acts as a mediator between the id's unrealistic demands and the social world. Thus Erikson's[22] theory emphasizes the equal weight of the interplay between our biology, psychology, social recognition, and response to these within a historical context. In doing so, he recognizes the importance of acknowledging the range of social orders (our personal historical context being important, and related to all of them) and the importance of key relationships, while focusing on the interior, psychosocial, nature of identity.

Erikson used the term *ego-identity* to refer to our conscious sense of uniqueness, alongside our unconscious need for consistency through change (thereby being the *same* person). Within each of his proposed stages, we are thought to confront, and, it is hoped, to master, new life challenges before moving on to the next stage. Successful reconciliation between biological and sociocultural forces results in positive outcomes for our ego-identity and the acquisition of a new virtue (e.g., hope, purpose, wisdom). The result is a reformulation of all that we have been into a core of what we are to become. As such, our "healthy" ego-identity provides us with a strong sense of well-being: "… a feeling of being at home in one's body, a sense of knowing where one is going, and an inner assuredness of anticipated recognition from those who count."[22] (p. 165) Social relationships are highly important to us during this stage, and *those who count* are our peers and role models. However, unsuccessful management of a stage can result in an "unhealthy" ego-identity (potentially leading to struggles around our identity and a sense of unease, which sometimes can continue throughout our lives).

Marcia's identity status model

Erikson's understanding of identity development across our lives, articulated approximately fifty years ago, has laid the foundation for others to build upon. Marcia's identity status model,[23,24] Berzonsky's[25,26] social cognitive model, and McAdams's[27] concept of narrative identity are well-known examples, drawing on different aspects of Erikson's theory and operationalizing it empirically. For example, based on Erikson's ideas, Marcia identifies two criteria used to examine the processes through which we develop our identities: *exploration* (originally *crisis*) and *commitment*.[23] The exploratory period comprises an active investigation of different meaningful identity actions (e.g., going to medical school) or beliefs (e.g., personal ideology), with commitment being the amount of personal investment we have in our chosen identity action or belief. Using the Identity Status Interview,[23] Marcia classified individuals into one of four identity statuses: *identity achievement* (commitment through high exploration), *foreclosure* (commitment following little or no exploration), *moratorium* (lengthy exploration but struggling to commit), and *identity diffusion* (little or no exploration or commitment).

But why does this matter for the education of medical professionalism? To answer this I draw on a plethora of research (including numerous meta analyses) identifying personal and interpersonal patterns and behavioral outcomes relevant to medical education that have been associated with people classified according to Marcia's identity statuses. For example, people classified as identity-achievers have been shown to be low in neuroticism and high in conscientiousness (which has been linked with professionalism)[28] and extroversion;[29] have a high internal locus of control;[30] use high levels of moral reasoning in terms of justice and care;[31] have the ability to perform well under stress;[23] and engage in planned and logical, rational, and systematic decision-making strategies more than people classified to other identity statuses.[32]

For people classified as identity-foreclosed, the values and roles they accept are typically grounded in parental values, with which a strong identification has already been formed. Marcia suggested that identity-foreclosed individuals often have their career choice limited due to family expectations to carry on their family tradition (legacy), typically around entering into the professions or family businesses, and a desire to be accepted. Such people have been shown to score high in authoritarianism,[33] tending to prefer to follow strong leaders unquestioningly; they are inclined to be closed to new experiences;[29] and, along with those classified to identity-diffusion and moratorium statuses, tend to use intuitive and indecisive decision-making styles.[32]

In terms of research specifically within medical education, there have been surprisingly few studies. From the little work that has been done, albeit using methods of data collection that somewhat differ from validated scales, research suggests that preclinical students could still be classified within the identity-diffusion group, or at least that they display very tentative professional identities,[34] but later are more likely to be classified in either the identity-achievement or -foreclosure groups.[35] This developmental movement from one classification to another echoes the body of research that has examined developmental patterns, suggesting that these classifications should not be considered as fixed trait, but rather states of individuals that might shift over time.[33]

Berzonsky's social cognitive model

Although echoing Erikson's original work, such as the need for continuity and dealing with identity conflicts, the social–cognitive approach to identity formation differs from psychosocial accounts in many ways.[25,36] This approach considers our identity as a cognitive structure or self-theory "which provides a personal frame of reference for interpreting self-relevant information, solving problems, and making decisions."[36] (p. 55) Our self-theory is also said to provide us with a conceptual framework within which we encode, organize, and comprehend our experiences in relation to our identity. Thus, the regularities that our brains detect as we experience events become organized into personal constructs (concepts) that are then synthesized into higher-order cognitive structures (personal theories).[25,36,37] This approach is based on constructivist epistemological assumptions: we actively construct new understandings of our world through the interaction of our prior beliefs and the new events and activities that we encounter. This construction is not always a conscious process. Thus our self-theory comprises everything we require for us to manage and adapt to aspects of our daily lives, including our core values, ways of knowing the world, aspirations, and ideals. Thus, negative feedback sometimes might signal the need for us to readjust aspects of our self-theory, and so our identity continuously evolves. In sum, the social–cognitive approach focuses on the nature of the cognitive *processes* through which we engage – and sometimes avoid – identity conflicts and issues.

Following Marcia's theory of identity statuses,[23,24] three different types of identity theorists have been posited, each having a specific method through which we might resolve our conflicts.[25] First, there is the *informational* orientation. Such individuals approach resolution in an open and informed manner, employing formal reasoning strategies. These skeptical self-explorers are open to new ideas, to learning new things about themselves (akin to Marcia's identity-achieved or moratorium statuses), and to engaging in problem-focused coping strategies.[38–40] Their reasoning focuses on personal values, goals, and standards; they are highly self-efficacious, self-regulating, and emotionally intelligent; and they value emotional and academic autonomy.[41–44]

Second, there are individuals who use a *diffuse-avoidant* approach, typically avoiding or delaying resolution. This approach is associated with a reluctance to deal with identity conflicts, leading to temporary behavioral or verbal compliance when required (i.e., strategic avoidance and impression management), rather than more stable, structural revisions of their self-theory. They can be impulsive, having little personal control over events: their reasoning tends to emphasize social attributes of themselves such as their reputation, popularity, and how others view them.[41,45] Additionally, conscientiousness has been negatively linked with this approach.[39,40,46]

Finally, individuals can be classified as having a *normative* orientation, typified by an inflexible and closed approach to conflict resolution. Reasoning tends to focus on collective aspects of their world such as their family, religion, and nationality. Individuals using this approach can be highly influenced by significant others and referent groups. Thus, in a relatively automatic and uncritical manner, they adopt their values or goals in an attempt to reduce ambiguity, to maintain a structure in their lives, and to achieve cognitive closure (akin to Marcia's foreclosed-identity status). Informational and normative styles are associated with characteristics and resources such as self-discipline, frustration tolerance, and conscientiousness.[36,39,40,46]

Identities, the individual order, and implications for medical education

So what practical implications for medical education can we draw from our understanding of how identities are shaped, developed, and represented when they are viewed within the individual order? What we can say is that certain identities are more malleable than others. The good news in terms of professional identities is that our moral identity continues to form over much of our adulthood. During this period, our moral selves are very much shaped through core relationships with our peers, in-groups, role models, and organizational cultures. Alongside this knowledge, and considering the existential questions of the developing medical student within their identity crisis stage[22] – "*Who am I and who and what do I want to be?*" – experiences during undergraduate medical school seem to be of great importance. Although this takes some of the pressure away from medical school selection processes, it does mean that we might focus our attention on faculty development programs, educational activities within clinical teams, interprofessional teaching and learning, and leadership. In this respect, role models are of utmost importance. It is therefore crucially important that educational leaders, who role model values and behaviors in the workplace, understand this key role that they play. This is because "responsiveness to modelling influences is largely determined by three factors ... these include the characteristics of the models ... those who have high status, prestige and power are much more effective in evoking matching behavior in observers than models of low standing."[102] (p. 18) Indeed, as we have seen, individuals who have been classified as *identity-foreclosed* within Marcia's model[23,24] or as having a *normative* orientation within Berzonsky's model,[36] tend to follow strong leaders unquestioningly.[33]

Furthermore, research on identities from within the individual order suggests that while individuals might be classified according to one approach to conflict resolution, exploration, and commitment at one point in time, this is not necessarily a fixed trait,[35] although some caution is required, because research tends to be cross-sectional rather than longitudinal. However, if this is the case, then perhaps there are things we can do within medical education to encourage our students to actively explore who they are and who they want to be (so helping to move them from the state of moratorium, foreclosure, or diffusion). Such encouragement could begin early on, ideally in facilitated small-group settings, and include students' exploration of who they are in terms of what they believe is right and wrong, how they approach situations that involve ethical and professional conflicts, and how they develop and maintain a commitment to their values. Furthermore, medical schools might consider how they support students during this exploration and students' commitment to becoming ethical doctors, especially during times of conflict.

Identities and the interactional order

Having considered the nature of a professional identity from psychodynamic, psychosocial, and social-cognitivist perspectives, I now move on to discuss a very different way of understanding the nature of professionalism and *identities* within the interactional order. Here, assumptions about the nature of mind, and of correlational relationships with other psychological constructs (e.g., self-efficacy, personality traits, thinking and reasoning styles, and so on) are considered inadequate for the understanding of our complex and diverse identities. Instead, grouped under the interactional order, are theoretical perspectives that draw largely on social constructionism. From this perspective, the nature of professional identities is

constructed and co-constructed through language, artifacts, and action, rather than cognitively constructed within an individual's mind. This is not to say that identity is not embodied and has no place in our "mind" – indeed, Harré uses the metaphor of *cognition as conversation*.[47] Rather than our professional identity being stored mentally (e.g., as a cognitive structure or *self-theory*), this approach suggests that professional identities are "often part of a complex pattern of interpersonal actions and relationships"[47] (p. 613), and, as such, they are socially constructed, emerging in the moment. From this perspective, professional attributes such as trust and patient-centeredness are culturally defined, distributed, and enacted. During this process of collective enactment, a form of collective socialization occurs through which our consciousness is shaped.

There are obvious implications for facilitating the development of professional identities: from this perspective, the moral style of any culture and the expectations for the profession are understood through discourses. Such discourses can include dominant, "capital-D," discourses (e.g., messages about what a doctor *should be*, which are culturally available, historically derived, and socially negotiated),[48–50] and "little-d" discourses, comprising the minutiae of interactive systems (e.g., the pronoun system – *I, we, you, them*)[51] through which important aspects of professional identities are expressed.[52,53] Furthermore, there is often a tension between competing discourses in society and how these discourses "fit" within our current sense of self. Therefore, discourses are drawn upon and used very differently by different people as we negotiate and construct our unique identities. From this perspective, researchers have examined language and interaction across a wide variety of activity types such as teaching practices, joint problem-solving and decision making, and storytelling.[48,51,53–57] Once again, a range of different theories has been utilized for the understanding of how professional identities are negotiated and the impact that this has upon medical students as they go through their training. Here, I will touch on the broad perspective – narrative discourse analyses – to illustrate this.

Narrative identities

In terms of storytelling, researchers have been drawn to the analyses of narratives to understand the nature of, and the process through which, professional identities are accomplished. Narrative theory comprises a range of approaches to examine how we construct our professional identities through the stories we tell and our interactions with others. Some theories belong to the individual, psychological perspective, suggesting that through narratives we can classify people into types: often relating them in some way to Erikson's or Marcia's classifications.[27] However, narrative theory within a social constructionist perspective examines how identities are influenced and asserted through language as we draw on character tropes (conceptual figures of speech, e.g., lazy nurses, scary surgeons, heroic doctors) and dominant discourses (or master narratives) from society. It is through these tropes and discourses that we identify and classify one another. In other words, through narrative, we position others and ourselves as particular persons in relation to one another, and in doing so we construct aspects of our (developing) identities: including the values we hold and our moral character.[15–17,50,58–60] Across this broad perspective, the general finding is that individuals experience identity *struggles* or *tensions* as we draw upon and utilize competing societal messages in order to make sense of ourselves through various life transitions (e.g., becoming a doctor).[15,50,59,61]

In a review of the literature, Frost and Regehr[50] considered the competing discourses around diversity and standardization in the training of doctors and their effect on medical student identities. The discourse of *diversity* highlights the need to respect and value individuals' uniqueness in terms of a range of demographic factors (e.g., socioeconomic status, education, gender, religiosity, ethnicity). This contrasts starkly with the discourse of *standardization*, which emphasizes uniformity and consistency within the profession in terms of what it means to be a doctor (e.g., values, knowledge, and skills).[62] They found that, influenced by the force of discourses toward creating a homogeneity of what it means to be professional, along with fears of appearing different, some medical students appear to resolve their conflicts.[63,64] Sometimes they do so by negotiating "trade-offs" and downplaying or suppressing certain aspects of their personal identities (e.g., sexuality) that seem incompatible with their developing professional identity. However, some students consider their individuality to be of critical importance to them, and resist the pressure to conform. This might entail emphasizing their personal and cultural identities (e.g., as gay or as an American Indian), by constructing an "alternative" professional identity based around these aspects.[65] Others construct hybrid identities: selecting different aspects across the discourses that enable them to construct a professional identity that retains enough of their present identities to maintain their individuality.[66]

The role of dominant discourses in identity construction

Other research has considered the range of discourses medical students draw upon when constructing their identities, the process through which this construction occurs, and the impact that these discourses have on students when dealing with illness and death.[48,59,61,67] For example, in a longitudinal audiodiary study of medical students' experiences of becoming a doctor, I examined how they positioned themselves with respect to social and institutional discourses of what it means to be a doctor.[48] I identified eight complementary and competing discourses that participants drew upon when constructing their developing identities, including the "Good Doctor," the "Healing Doctor," and the "Detached Doctor" narratives. As they negotiated their journeys through medical school, participants encountered events that challenged these discourses: the very discourses that sometimes initially inspired them to study medicine.

In terms of the "Good Doctor," participants narrated admiration when encountering a physician who fit this mold, but shock and dismay when doctors acted counter to these expectations. They also narrated how idealized notions of being a "Good Doctor" were negotiated within their own developing identities, occasionally causing anxiety, especially in the face of their own feelings of inadequacies.[59] Likewise, tensions were also found as students compared the "Healing Doctor" discourse – highlighting the curing role of the doctor – to what they found in reality: very often the role of the doctor is to manage illness and death.[48,59,61,67] Furthermore, the "Detached Doctor" discourse – to be professional one must not become emotionally involved – caused problems when students were placed in traumatic situations, such as the unexpected death of a patient.[59,61] One participant drew upon the metaphor of climbing a mountain with an unreachable, *unachievable* summit as she struggled to understand the death of a young man in a motorbike accident.[61] Indeed, the process of narrating these tensions between idealized discourses, reality, and identities within an audio-diary was complex, with students' narratives "oscillating between the literal and the more elaborate metaphorical, between the diagnostic and the reflective, between the physical and the metaphysical."[61] (p. 98) This process sheds light onto the very nature of participants' identity negotiation through narrative and the indivisibility of students as *clinicians-to-be* and students as *themselves*: although developing separately, they interact reciprocally.[59] However, some of these discourses were so culturally embedded that it seemed exceptionally difficult for students to re-story them. So from the perspective of narrative research within a social constructionist framework, the formation of professional identities is a complex and highly personal journey: one that is paradoxically informed, facilitated, and constrained by larger discourses around who a doctor is and the personal and professional roles they are expected to assume.

The role of little-d discourses in identity construction

Other work from a social constructionist perspective examines in detail the implicit socialization of students through aspects such as role modeling practices. Rather than examining the capital-D discourses of stories, this analytical method focuses on language-in-use during social interaction to examine the co-creation of identities *in situ*. Indeed, it has been argued that at all times educators need to adopt a role modeling consciousness,[68] recognizing the importance of this for the teaching and learning of professionalism and the impact, both positive and negative, that this has on students' professional identities. Furthermore, recent research examining students' narratives of professionalism dilemmas – situations in which they witness or participate in something they believe to be unethical or "wrong" – highlights the impact that being exposed to negative role models has on students' professional identities.[15,17,19,69] But these were narratives of events, not the events themselves. What about the actual interaction between doctors and students? One place in which medical students learn to become doctors is within bedside teaching encounters. Within these activities, physicians teach medical students a range of skills and values required for them to become doctors,[51,55–57] including aspects of professionalism such as patient-centeredness,

ethical practice (e.g., consent), and values (e.g., honesty and trust). It is to these activities that we now turn.

Developing identities through interaction

Patient-centeredness has often been constructed as an individual value and a competence within professionalism; something we possess and which can be measured.[70] A review of the conceptual and empirical literature has led to the identification of five key dimensions of patient-centeredness: adopting a biopsychosocial perspective, understanding the patient-as-person, sharing power and responsibility, the therapeutic doctor-patient alliance, and the doctor-as-person.[71] Likewise, trust is typically viewed within an individual perspective: either someone is trustworthy or not, and trust is something that one person bestows on another (e.g., a patient places his or her trust in a doctor). However, within a social constructionist approach, the concepts of patient-centeredness and trust are achieved, in and through interaction.[55,56,72]

In terms of patient-centeredness, the sharing of power and responsibility advocates an egalitarian doctor-patient relationship.[71] Related to this are notions of *user involvement* and *patient empowerment* in medical education. Thus, the teaching and learning of the specific dimension of sharing power and responsibility through language and social practice within hospital and general practice (family medicine) bedside teaching encounters has been examined across a number of related studies in the United Kingdom and Australia.[51,55,73] For example, drawing on Goffman's dramaturgy theory,[8] which uses a theatre metaphor to examine the different roles in which people are empowered and disempowered through language and artifacts (including the roles of actor, director, audience, nonperson, and prop), Monrouxe and Rees[55] examined the extent to which patients were included as members of the teaching team within hospital-based bedside teaching encounters.[55] They found that patients were commonly positioned in less active roles (audience, nonperson, prop), even when they actively rejected these passive roles. Thus, linguistically bounded *front-stage* and *back-stage* environments were constructed through paralanguage (e.g., doctors spoke to students in fast-paced, hushed tones, thereby constructing a back-stage impression and excluding the patient). Exclusion also occurred through pronominal talk (e.g., the use of *I* and *me*), anatomizing the patient (e.g., the liver), using medical jargon, and the continual use of yes/no questions and directives (instructions or orders). However, empowerment of patients was also found. This was constructed through doctors' talking *to* (rather than about) the patient, using the pronouns *we* and *us* to include all present in the teaching team, referring to the patient's body and body parts as belonging to them (e.g., *your* liver), and explaining medical jargon and prioritizing patients' narratives of their own illness (e.g., "in his own words").

In terms of trust, using conversation analysis, Elsey et al.[56] examined trust as a *reciprocal* shared process between doctor (or medical student) and patient within the context of bedside teaching encounters. From this perspective, the successful achievement of a medical encounter requires the "trust" of all parties to act in an appropriate, relevant, coherent, and understandable manner: doctors expect patients to provide information about their health and access to their bodies, while patients expect doctors to provide an interactional environment (e.g., asking guiding questions) in which such disclosures are made or relevant concerns shared. Furthermore, due to the medical student presence disrupting the normal doctor–patient consultation, trust is in need of careful management by doctors (or the students) to restore or recreate patients' understanding of the reconfigured consultation process.

Demonstrating how trust is established through verbal and bodily interaction, Elsey et al.[56] show how sensitive management of the interactional environment (e.g., through physical positioning of all parties involved and occasionally averting eye contact) provided patients with additional space and opportunities to reveal previously unmentioned, potentially embarrassing, concerns. Furthermore, the students' presence in the consultation meant that trust between doctor and patient had to be worked on, and made visible, rather than taken for granted and left to chance. In order to do this, the notion of clinicians adopting a role modeling consciousness is paramount.[68]

Identities, the interactional order, and implications for medical education

In this section, we have seen a number of different ways in which language is used to construct and co-construct identities *in situ*. We began by considering societies' dominant discourses around what it means to be a doctor: doctors are constructed through professionalism codes of practice in a reasonably standardized manner, doctors are "good" and are detached, and they heal the sick. These dominant ways in which doctors are constructed have implications on students who, for example, do not fit the mold.

Reflecting on this interactional order, educators need to find ways to facilitate students' understandings of what it means to become a professional and how this developmental process is not about *replacing* their current identities: it is about understanding who they are and what they bring as individuals. It is about helping students find their way on their journey to become a doctor. And as Frost and Regehr[50] say (p. 1574), "We cannot continue to leave students to their own devices as they attempt to reconcile competing discourses.... Educators might become explicitly and intentionally involved in this process." This includes reminding students that doctors are just people who are no more special than other professional groups or patients. Furthermore, building on the place of role models within the interactional space, as educators we could reflect on the influence of the dominant discourses we draw on in our *own* understandings of the world, including the various character tropes we convey in our everyday interactions with students, and the implicit conceptualizations we have in terms of what it means to be a doctor.

Finally, as identities are co-constructed through the use of language, artifacts, and physical positioning of ourselves and others, educators might reflect on the ways in which they role model aspects of professionalism, such as patient-centeredness and trust, during teaching encounters with patients. This might start by considering the various ways in which the patient can be included in both teaching and student feedback. By role modeling patient-centeredness in this way, not only do students and trainees learn *how* to empower patients within an educational setting, they also begin to develop their own identities as patient-centered professionals internally and relationally.

Identities and the institutional order

Following on from examining the nature of professional identities as residing in and through interaction, I now outline a number of ways in which identities are located or formed in and through institutions and the consequences of this for professional identities. As can be seen, the theoretical perspectives outlined here overlap with those discussed elsewhere and can cut across different social orders. What makes these theories part of the institutional order is the *location* of identities and the forces through which identities are constructed (e.g., within the workplace). However, some theorists consider institutional identities to be located in the individual, others in the interaction, and others still in the location or institutional setting.[74,75] For the sake of simplicity, I address all theoretical perspectives that specifically consider the role of the institution (or workplace) in this section.

Institutions are typically associated with organizational settings or physical buildings and are inherently imbibed with notions of power. Such power is not necessarily embodied by individuals, nor always oppressive. When viewed as an interactional accomplishment, power can be *productive*, enabling individuals to resist as well as comply with institutional norms. Nevertheless, institutional and organizational identities are intrinsically shaped by these norms. Moreover, there is a symbiotic relationship between our organizational identities and the organization; our collective sense of who we are within an organization (along with who we are not, or who we *might* be) forms the psychological foundation of the organization itself. From this perspective we can see that the professional values inherent within any organization do not only *live through* the individuals within the system, but are (in part) constituted *by* them.[75] Against this backdrop of interdependence, I now outline the nature of professional identity formation within the institutional order, drawing heavily on the theoretical perspectives of social identity and self-categorization theories.[76,77]

Social identity and self-categorization theories

From the perspective of social identity and self-categorization theories, our social identities refer to the way in which we understand ourselves to be a member of a group, along with an emotional attachment to our group membership(s). As such, group membership is a very central aspect within all of our identities.[76] In the context of work-based relationships, the organization in which we work and learn contributes to our social identity in a number of ways: through our developing sense of self as a member of

the organization (e.g., hospital X, university Y) or profession (e.g., physician, nurse, researcher) as a whole, and as a member of the specific team or department in which we work (e.g., surgery, pediatrics, emergency medicine). Furthermore, the specific activities in which we engage within the organization, and the level to which we are included, also contribute to our concept of our professional identities: it is all about our perception of *fit*.

In terms of *fit* and the structure of our identities, self-categorization theory asserts that we hold a mental representation of specific organizations and groups. We then categorize ourselves as being more or less similar to those in that category, depending on how meaningful our role is in terms of category-related expectations (so-called *normative fit*).[77] We are also motivated to reduce uncertainty, so we seek to identify with social groups that afford us the highest source of self-concept clarity. So, a first-year medical student is likely to categorize herself as being a student rather than a doctor. However, if she is in her final year, she might categorize herself as a doctor, more than a student. This is particularly so if she is afforded that status within the medical team in which she is learning through, for instance, being given greater levels of responsibility for patient care over time.[78] But sometimes a group stereotype is unavailable to us. This can be the case with transient groups (including situations in which a range of professionals come together to form an ad-hoc team). In such cases we use a method of *comparative fit*: considering the extent to which differences among members of a group are perceived as smaller than those between members of other groups. However, it is important to remember that this categorization process is highly context dependent and so our identities are continuously being renegotiated.

Importantly, social identity theory considers the processes through which we categorize ourselves into groups. Once we have identified with a particular group, we then make social comparisons between our group (the in-group) and other groups (the out-groups). Social identity theory suggests that the value we gain from belonging to a group depends on the extent to which we positively evaluate our own group against out-groups. This provides us with the motivation to develop, and maintain, our sense of positive group uniqueness.[79] This has direct implications within medical education, particularly when we consider the difficulties faced when introducing interprofessional learning programs. For example, a study of year 1 UK medical students found that they identified different characteristics for doctors and nurses, believing nurses to be more caring, but with lower academic ability, competence, and status than doctors.[80]

In addition to individuals, organizations themselves can be seen as being *collective social actors*,[81] capable of holding an identity through which individuals may carry out social roles. In this light, organizations can be seen as a frame of reference for self-categorization. As organizations tend to assert (explicitly or implicitly) a particular organizational culture, they can be said to have an *organizational moral identity*. From this we can see how organizational contexts serve to strengthen (or undermine) the formation of a moral identity for those who work, or are learning, within that organization. Furthermore, due to the emotional attachment that we have to our group membership, along with our own moral identities, the process of this identification can be complex. For example, when our organization's moral identity appears to be in harmony with our own professional values, we are more likely to identify with it, thereby strengthening our moral actions in concordance with the organization's values, ideologies, and culture;[82] thus, individual values are coordinated and become shared, distributed values. However, when one's own (developing) professional identity appears to be at odds with that of the prevailing organizational moral identity, distress occurs,[83] sometimes resulting in a *morally numb* response to ethically challenging situations, disengagement, burnout, and even leaving the profession.[84–89] In essence, the nature of our professional identity is intimately entwined with the institutional order in which we learn and work. To my knowledge, there has been little work undertaken specifically drawing on the theories of social identity and self-categorization within medical education.

Identities, the institutional order, and implications for medical education

Perhaps one of the most difficult areas to address in terms of implications for medical education is the institutional order, because becoming a professional within institutions is much more of a collective endeavor. We all know how hard it is to influence the culture of the workplace through merely developing

rules and regulations, including curricula design. For this aspect of identity development, I draw on self-categorization theory and the notions of normative and comparative fit (matching ourselves to our mental representations of specific organizations and groups), as well as being mindful of ourselves as collective social actors. Within this institutional frame, the notions of ethical teamwork and understanding the status of students within teams are key. By finding ways to appropriately engage students as legitimate members of medical teams at all stages in their learning, we can facilitate the development of their identities as ethical and moral medical students. Furthermore, through being given greater levels of responsibility for patient care progressively over time, these students can gradually develop their embodied professional identities.

Identities and the national order

Having examined a range of theoretical perspectives on the nature and nurture of professional identities classified across individual, interactional, and institutional social orders, I now conclude by considering professional identities and the national order. In terms of medical professionalism, the Physician Charter sets out the "fundamental and universal principles and values" required to be a doctor.[90] The Charter has been translated into 12 languages and endorsed by more than 130 organizations worldwide. At its heart, it holds the fundamental principles of the primacy of patient welfare, patient autonomy, and social justice (among others). However, the Charter itself has been developed within an individualist Western culture of norms, values, and habits; a culture that is different from that found predominately in the East. From this perspective we might ask a number of questions around the nature and nurture of professional identities, including the extent to which Western traditions of professionalism can be embodied by individuals originating from, or learning within, non-Western cultures.[91]

Individualism versus collectivism

There has been a great deal of research that has examined the differences between typically Eastern and Western cultures. Synthesizing approximately thirty years of this work, Maleki and de Jong[92] identify nine cross-cutting clusters of cultural dimensions, the most powerful of these being individualism versus collectivism. This cultural dimension highlights the extent to which people within a society are inculcated from birth into a set of values that emphasize the relative interrelatedness between people: key concepts include autonomy, whereby everyone is expected to look after themselves first and foremost (individualism). This contrasts with embeddedness, in which members of a society are integrated into cohesive in-groups, often comprising extended families (collectivism). Additionally, specific cultures differ according to hierarchy (so-called vertical cultures) and equality (so-called horizontal cultures). Thus, we see differences across vertical and horizontal collectivist cultures, and similarly between vertical and horizontal individualist cultures.[93] Maleki and de Jong[92] highlight further complexities across this East–West divide. For example, team working can be considered to be a relatively high priority in collective cultures (the group being their main concern). However, some individualistic cultures can be extremely high in team working (e.g., Nordic countries) with some collectivistic cultures (e.g., Iran, Colombia) being low.[92]

From a psychological perspective, the terms *allocentrism* and *idiocentrism* have been used to refer to personality types that are believed to be the result of growing up and living within collectivist and individualist cultures respectively. From this perspective it has been demonstrated that allocentric people internalize in-group norms to a high degree; their self-esteem is based more on harmony and getting along (helping others is viewed as a duty), and a high value is placed on equality. On the other hand, idiocentric people base their self-esteem on getting ahead; helping others is seen as a choice (and influenced by how much a person is liked), and they place a high value on equity.[93] However, these so-called trait approaches to identities, focusing on habitual patterns of behavior and cognition, ignore the fact that individuals can act and even think differently in different social contexts.[94] This is particularly so for individuals within collectivist cultures whose practices, institutions, and traditions tend to foster a high level of responsivity to others, and where social context is an important aspect of daily life (e.g., communication relies heavily on contextual cues for interpretation).[92,95] Furthermore, these contingent identities can be viewed within the Eastern philosophical concept of *dialecticism*: a state of attunement to variations within one's sense of self, along with an acceptance

that such inconsistency is normal and natural.[96] Indeed, research has demonstrated that, rather than holding a fixed-trait approach to personality (a particularly Western propensity), East Asians tend to conceptualize it as being open to change.[97] Furthermore, in terms of group identities, it has been argued that people within a collectivist culture hold a perspective of the self as being interconnected and relational. This is distinct from Western in-group categorization (as specified in social identity theory). People are connected to each other though stable and visible relationships, in-group harmony is valued, and all groups (even out-groups) are conceptualized as an entity unto itself (group *entitativity*).[98]

The caring practitioner across Eastern and Western cultures

In addition to cultural differences around fundamental values within societies, conceptions of the self, and groups, there are also differences within the practice of medicine in terms of both how medicine is practiced and what it means to be a caring practitioner. Thus, on a basic level, Western medicine is derived from observation and analyses: bringing the scientific method into healthcare practice and decision-making process. However, by contrast, sometimes Eastern approaches to medicine – for example, traditional Chinese medicine – are not based on the scientific method and often are idiosyncratic in practice. Echoing the philosophy dialecticism, traditional Chinese medicine includes many contradictory yet complementary elements (such as wood, fire, earth, metal, water) and the dualities of Yin and Yang. To add further complexity, within the indigenous contexts in which Eastern medicine is practiced, it is ever more likely that Western medicine now coexists (if not dominates). Likewise, professionalism differs from Western frameworks. For example, whereas Western notions emphasize the primacy of patients and of separating doctors' personal and professional lives, Confucian cultural traditions appear to support the harmonization of these roles.[99] Furthermore, in a survey of medical practitioners from across the United Kingdom, Europe, North America, and Asia, Chandratilake et al.[100] found stark differences around the appropriateness of some professional attributes. For example, only Asian participants demonstrated high agreement with the attributes of punctuality and being adaptable to change. These cultural differences can be explained by considering the wider culture within which these doctors inhabit, such as Asians valuing strict discipline and being more open to change.[96,101]

Given such cultural differences in approaches to medicine, professionalism, and identities, alongside the ever-increasing Western influence within Eastern cultures, a number of questions come to mind regarding the nature and nurture of professional identities: How do students in Eastern societies negotiate and assimilate their professional identities if they learn within a predominately Westernized framework of professionalism? In such situations, to what extent do they reconstruct or negotiate their own cultural propensity in order to fully embody their new professional identities, or can these identities only be enacted? For example, how do the individualistic principles of patient autonomy and confidentiality translate within a collectivist culture? What are the consequences of these students' developing identities, based on Western values, in terms of their own emotional well-being and patient care? Furthermore, in our increasingly multicultural world, what are the processes and consequences of developing professional identities for Eastern students learning within Western cultures? To my knowledge, these questions are under-theorized and under-researched areas within medical education.

Identities, the national order, and implications for medical education

Finally, I turn to how we might address the development of professional identity within the national order. Medical education across the world has a number of challenges relating to issues such as the learning and practicing of medical professionalism within and across different cultural (philosophical) spaces. Although I have tried to cover a range of key identity theories, there are necessarily omissions. One particular absence, with relevance to cultural differences, are intersectionality theories.[103] This group of theories asserts that identities are uniquely multidimensional, comprising numerous interconnecting identities (race, gender, cultural, professional, relational) with a *transformational* (rather than *additional*) effect. Think of colors: blue and red make purple. Medical education research has yet to embrace this theoretical perspective. Given that much of the research undertaken by identity theorists comes

from within a predominately Western individualist culture, this perspective could prove a fruitful way forward for researchers attempting to understand the processes through which professional identities are shaped, experienced, replicated, or resisted within our burgeoning, diverse, multicultural systems of medical education.

Lessons learned and future directions

In this chapter, I have provided an overview of some of the main theoretical perspectives shedding light onto the nature and nurture of professional identities in which identities are complex and considered to be situated within individuals, and through interaction, organizations, and national cultures. In short, I have shown how professional identities emerge from and through social action and interaction. I have also highlighted how this process is not about replacing one identity with another; rather it is a transformational process: who we are and who we are becoming interact reciprocally. The challenge for educators is to consider the relationships between these social orders and the implication this has for the development of appropriate medical professional identities. However, this challenge is not the only one; an even greater challenge lies ahead.

It is true that research so far has shed light onto how professional identities comprise elements of continuity and change: how aspects of our personal identities are brought into our professional identity, which is also shaped though interpersonal, societal and contextual factors. On this basis, I have highlighted the findings from some of this research that might shed light onto this process and have suggested ways in which students' professional identities might be nurtured within and across the different social orders. But there is so much we do not yet know. First, much of the programmatic and theoretical research in the domain of identity, identities, and identification has been conducted on university students, mainly employing cross-sectional study designs. What research has been conducted with medical students and doctors often comprises small-scale individual studies in which researchers attempt to develop their own "theories" of how students develop their professional identity, within which there is often little or no engagement, critical examination, or development of existing knowledge. This is our greatest challenge. Without a better understanding of the processes through which our students develop their professional identities, any suggestions for nurturing this process can only be very tentative. Indeed, even among identity and career theorists, there is a paucity of research examining the efficacy of targeted interventions in terms of strengthening professional identities and how such interventions affect later career and life trajectories.[104] We know not what works, for whom, and how.

In short, what is now needed is to develop a strong programmatic body of applied research around identities developed within our field of medical education; a body of work that both draws upon, and builds on, the theoretical approaches developed within the social sciences. So, rather than reinventing the wheel, I urge us all to work within the particular theoretical framework that resonates with our own ontological and epistemological perspective; to fully engage with those theories and to understand the evidence base from which they originate; and, finally, to critically evaluate and develop them to build our evidence base together. Only in this manner will we better understand how best to facilitate the process of professional identity formation within and across the different social worlds in which today's medical students and trainees learn to become tomorrow's doctors.

References

1. Monrouxe, LV. Identity, identification and medical education: why should we care? *Med Educ.* 2010; 44(1):40–49.

2. Monrouxe, LV. Identity, self and medical education. In Walsh, K, ed. *Oxford Textbook of Medical Education.* Oxford, UK: Oxford University Press; 2013:113–23.

3. Hafferty, FW, Castellani, B. A sociological framing of medicine's modern-day professionalism movement. *Med Educ.* 2009; 43(9): 826–28.

4. Monrouxe, LV, Rees, CE, Hu, W. Differences in medical students' explicit discourses of professionalism: acting, representing, becoming. *Med Educ.* 2011; 45(6):585–602.

5. Jenkins, R. *Social Identity.* Third edition. New York, NY: Routledge; 2008.

6. Schwartz, SJ, Luyckx, K, Vignoles VL, eds. *Handbook of Identity Theory and Research.* New York, NY: Springer; 2011.

7. Lacan, J. The mirror stage. In du Gay, P, Evans, J, Redman, P, eds. *Identity: A Reader.* London, UK: SAGE Publications; 2000; 44–50.

8. Goffman, E. *The Presentation of Self in Everyday Life.* New York, NY: Anchor; 1959.

9. Egan, EA, Parsi, K, Ramirez, C. Comparing ethics education in medicine and law: combining the best of both worlds. *Ann Health Law.* 2004; 13(1):303–25.

10. Narvaez, D, Lapsley, DK. The psychological foundations of everyday morality and moral expertise. In Lapsley, DK, Power, FC, eds. *Character Psychology and Character Education.* Notre Dame, IN: University of Notre Dame Press; 2005; 140–65.

11. Kagan, J. Human morality and temperament. In Carlo, G, Pope-Edwards, C, eds. *Moral Motivation through the Life Span (Volume 51 of the Nebraska Symposium on Motivation).* Lincoln, NE: University of Nebraska Press; 2005; 1–32.

12. Kohlberg, L. *Essays on Moral Development, Volume One: The Philosophy of Moral Development.* San Francisco, CA: Harper and Row; 1981.

13. Frank, AW. Ethics as process and practice. *Intern Med J.* 2004; 34(6): 355–57.

14. Blasi, A. Moral cognition and moral action: a theoretical perspective. *Dev Rev.* 1983; 3(2):178–210.

15. Monrouxe, LV, Rees, CE. "It's just a clash of cultures": emotional talk within medical students' narratives of professionalism dilemmas. *Adv Health Sci Educ Theory Pract.* 2012; 17(5):671–701.

16. Monrouxe, LV, & Rees CE. Hero, Voyeur, Judge: Understanding medical students' moral identities through professionalism dilemma narratives. In Kenneth Mavor, Michael Platow and Boris Bizumic (Eds.) *Self and Social Identity in Learning and Educational Contexts.* Psychology Press; in press.

17. Monrouxe, LV, Rees, CE, Endacott, R, Ternan, E. 'Even now it makes me angry': health care students' professionalism dilemma narratives. *Med Educ.* 2014; 48(5):502–17.

18. Rees, CE, Monrouxe, LV, Ajjawi, R. Professionalism in workplace learning: understanding interprofessional dilemmas through healthcare student narratives. In Jindal-Snape, D, Hannah, ESF, eds. *Exploring the Dynamics of Personal, Professional and Interprofessional Ethics.* Bristol, UK: Policy Press; 2014: 295–310.

19. Rees, CE, Monrouxe, LV, McDonald, LA. 'My mentor kicked a dying woman's bed…' Analysing UK nursing students' 'most memorable' professionalism dilemmas. *J Adv Nurs.* 2015; 71(1):169–80.

20. Hafferty, FW, Franks, R. The hidden curriculum, ethics teaching, and the structure of medical education. *Acad Med.* 1994; 69(11):861–71.

21. Witman, Y. What do we transfer in case discussions? The hidden curriculum in medicine... *Perspect Med Educ.* 2014; 3(2):113–23.

22. Erikson, EH. *Identity: Youth and Crisis*. New York, NY: WW Norton; 1968.

23. Marcia, JE. Development and validation of ego-identity status. *J Pers Soc Psychol*. 1966; **3**(5):551–58.

24. Marcia, JE, Waterman, AS, Matteson, DR, Archer, SL, Orlofsky, JL. *Ego Identity: A Handbook for Psychosocial Research*. New York, NY: Springer; 1993.

25. Berzonsky, MD. The self as theorist: individual differences in identity formation. *International Journal of Personal Construct Psychology*. 1989; **2**(4):363–76.

26. Berzonsky, MD. Self construction across the life-span: a process view of identity development. In Neimeyer, GH, Neimeyer, RA, eds. *Advances in Personal Construct Psychology*. Greenwich, CT: JAI Press; 1990:155–86.

27. McAdams, DP. *The Stories We Live By: Personal Myths and the Making of the Self*. New York, NY: Guildford Press; 1993.

28. Chaytor, AT, Spence, J, Armstrong, A, McLachlan, JC. Do students learn to be more conscientious at medical school? *BMC Med Educ*. 2012; **12**:54.

29. Clancy, SM, Dollinger, SJ. Identity, self, and personality: I. Identity status and the five-factor model of personality. *J Res Adolesc*. 1993; **3**(3):227–45.

30. Lillevoll, KR, Kroger, J, Martinussen, M. Identity status and locus of control: a meta-analysis. *Identity: An International Journal of Theory and Research*. 2013; **13**(3):253–65.

31. Jespersen, K, Kroger, J, Martinussen, M. Identity status and moral reasoning: a meta-analysis. *Identity: An International Journal of Theory and Research*. 2013; **13**(3):266–80.

32. Bacanli, F. An examination of the relationship amongst decision-making strategies and ego identity statuses. *Education and Science*. 2012; **37**(163):17–18.

33. Ryeng, MS, Kroger, J, Martinussen, M. Identity status and authoritarianism: a meta-analysis. *Identity: An International Journal of Theory and Research*. 2013; **13**(3):242–52.

34. Niemi, PM, Vainiomäki, PT, Murto-Kangas, M. "My future as a physician" – professional representations and their background among first-day medical students. *Teach Learn Med*. 2003; **15**(1):31–39.

35. Beran, T Hecker, K, Coderre, S, Wright, B, Woloschuk, W, McLaughlin, K. Ego identity status of medical students in clerkship. *Can Med Educ J*. 2011; **2**(1): e4–e10.

36. In Schwartz, SJ, Luyckx, K, Vignoles, VL, eds. Berzonsky, *M. D. A social-cognitive perspective on identity construction. Handbook of Identity Theory and Research*. New York, NY: Springer; 2011:55–76.

37. Kelly, GA. *The Psychology of Personal Constructs*. New York, NY: WW Norton; 1955.

38. Berzonsky, MD, Sullivan, C. Social-cognitive aspects of identity style: need for cognition, experiential openness, and introspection. *J Adolesc Res*. 1992; **7**(2):140–55.

39. Dollinger, SMC. Identity styles and the five-factor model of personality. *J Res Pers*. 1995; **29**(4):475–79.

40. Dollinger, SJ, Dollinger, SMC. Individuality and identity exploration: an autophotographic study. *J Res Pers*. 1997; **31**(3):337–54.

41. Berzonsky, MD, Kuk, LS. Identity style, psychosocial maturity, and academic performance. *Pers Individ Dif*. 2005; **39**(1):235–47.

42. Hejazi, E, Shahraray, M, Farsinejad, M, Asgary, A. Identity styles and academic achievement: mediating role of academic self-efficacy. *Soc Psychol Educ*. 2009; **12**(1):123–35.

43. Seaton, CL, Beaumont, SL. Individual differences in identity styles predict proactive forms of positive adjustment. *Identity: An International Journal of Theory and Research*. 2008; **8**(3):249–68.

44. Jakubowski, TG, Dembo, MH. The relationship of self-efficacy, identity style, and stage of change with academic self-regulation. *Journal of College Reading and Learning*. 2004; **35**(1):7–24.

45. Soenens, B, Berzonsky, MD, Vansteenkiste, M, Beyers, W, Goossens, L. Identity styles and causality orientations: in search of the motivational underpinnings of the identity exploration process. *Eur J Pers*. 2005; **19**(5):427–42.

46. Duriez, B, Soenens, B. Personality, identity styles and authoritarianism: an integrative study among late adolescents. *Eur J Pers*. 2006; **20**(5):397–417.

47. Harré, R. Public sources of the personal mind: social constructionism in context. *Theory Psychol*. 2002; **12**(5):611–23.

48. Monrouxe, LV. Negotiating professional identities: dominant and contesting narratives in medical students' longitudinal audio diaries. *Current Narratives*. 2009; **1**(1):41–59.

49. Whitehead, CR. *The Good Doctor in Medical Education 1910–2010: A Critical Discourse Analysis*. Toronto, ON: Leslie Dan Faculty of Pharmacy, University of Toronto, 2011.

50. Frost, HD, Regehr, G. "I am a doctor": negotiating the discourses of standardization and diversity in professional identity construction. *Acad Med*. 2013; **88**(10):1570–77.

51. Rees, CE, Monrouxe, LV. 'Is it alright if I-um-we unbutton your pyjama top now?' Pronominal use in bedside teaching encounters. *Commun Med*. 2008; **5**(2):171–82.

52. Bamberg, M. Stories: big or small. Why do we care? *Narrat Inq*. 2006; **16**(1):139–47.

53. Bamberg, MGW, De Fina, A, Schiffrin, D, eds. *Selves and Identities in Narrative and Discourse*. Amsterdam, the Netherlands: John Benjamins; 2007.

54. Davies, R, Harré, R. Positioning: the discursive production of selves. *J Theory Soc Behav*. 1990; **20**(1):43–63.

55. Monrouxe, LV, Rees, CE, Bradley, P. The construction of patients' involvement in hospital bedside teaching encounters. *Qual Health Res*. 2009; **19**(7):918–30.

56. Elsey, C, Monrouxe, LV, Grant, A. The reciprocal nature of trust in bedside teaching encounters. In Pelsmaekers, K, Jacobs, G, Rollo, C, eds. *Trust and Discourse: Organizational Perspectives*. Amsterdam, the Netherlands: John Benjamins; 2014:45–70.

57. Rizan, C, Elsey, C, Lemon, T, Grant, A, Monrouxe, LV. Feedback in action within bedside teaching encounters: a video ethnographic study. *Med Educ*. 2014; **48**(9):902–20.

58. Watson, C. Small stories, positioning analysis, and the doing of professional identities in learning to teach. *Narrat Inq*. 2007; **17**(2):371–89.

59. Monrouxe, LV, Sweeney, K. Between two worlds: medical students narrating identity tensions. In Figley, C, Huggard, P, Rees, CE, eds. *First Do No Self-Harm: Understanding and Promoting Physician Stress Resilience*. Oxford, UK: Oxford University Press; 2013:44–66.

60. Monrouxe, LV, Rees, CE. Theoretical perspectives on identity: researching identities in healthcare education. In Cleland, A, Durning, SJ, eds. *Researching Medical Education*. Oxford, UK: Wiley Blackwell; 2015:129–40.

61. Monrouxe, LV. Solicited audio diaries in longitudinal narrative research: a view from inside. *Qual Res*. 2009; **9**(1):81–103.

62. Swick, HM. Toward a normative definition of medical professionalism. *Acad Med*. 2000; **75**(6):612–16.

63. Finlay, SE, Fawzy, M. Becoming a doctor. *Med Humanit*. 2001; **27**(2):90–92.

64. Beagan, BL. Neutralizing differences: producing neutral doctors for (almost) neutral patients. *Soc Sci Med*. 2000; **51**(18):1253–65.

65. Buckley, A. Does becoming a professional mean I have to become white? *J Am Indian Educ*. 2004; **43**(2):19–32.

66. Geraci, AP. Earring etiquette in medical school. *JAMA*. 1994; **271**.(9):716.

67. Monrouxe, LV, Sweeney, K. Contesting narratives: medical professional identity formation amidst changing values. In Pattison, S, Hannigan, B, Thomas, H, Pill, R, eds. *Emerging Values in Health Care: The Challenge for Professionals*. London, UK: Jessica Kingsley; 2010:61–77.

68. Cruess, SR, Cruess, RL, Steinert, Y. Role modelling—making the most of a powerful teaching strategy. *BMJ*. 2008; **336**(7646):718–21.

69. Rees, CE, Monrouxe, LV, McDonald, LA. Narrative, emotion and action: analysing 'most memorable' professionalism dilemmas. *Med Educ*. 2013; **47**(1):80–96.

70. Hudon, C, Fortin, M, Haggerty, JL, Lambert, M, Poitras, ME. Measuring patients' perceptions of patient-centered care: a systematic review of tools for family medicine. *Ann Fam Med*. 2011; **9**(2):155–64.

71. Mead, N, Bower, P. Patient-centredness: a conceptual framework and review of the empirical literature. *Soc Sci Med*. 2000; **51**(7):1087–1110.

72. Elsey, C, Monrouxe, LV, Grant, A. *Role-Modelling Patient-Centredness within Bedside Teaching Encounters: A Video Ethnographic Study*. Association for the Study of Medical Education annual scientific meeting: Brighton, UK; 2012.

73. Rees, CE, Ajjawi, R, Monrouxe, LV. The construction of power in family medicine bedside teaching: a video observation study. *Med Educ*. 2013; **47**(2):154–65.

74. Benwell, B, Stokoe, E. *Discourse and Identity*. Edinburgh, UK: Edinburgh University Press; 2006.

75. Haslam, SA, Ellemers, N. Identity processes in organizations. In Schwartz, SJ, Luyckx, K, Vignoles VL, eds. *Handbook of Identity Theory and Research*. New York, NY: Springer; 2011:715–44.

76. Tajfel, H, Turner, JC. The social identity theory of intergroup behavior. In Jost, JT, Sidanius, J, eds. *Political Psychology: Key Readings*. New York, NY: Psychology Press; 2004:367–90.

77. Turner, JC, Hogg, MA, Oakes, PJ, Reicher, SD, Wetherell, MS, eds. *Rediscovering the Social Group: A Self-Categorization Theory*. Oxford, UK: Blackwell; 1987.

78. Zabarenko, RN, Zabarenko, L. *Doctor Tree: Developmental Stages in the Growth of Physicians*. Pittsburgh, PA: University of Pittsburgh Press; 1978.

79. Tajfel, H, ed. *Differentiation between Social Groups: Studies in the Social Psychology of Intergroup Relations*. London, UK: Academic Press; 1978.

80. Rudland, JR, Mires, GJ. Characteristics of doctors and nurses as perceived by students entering medical school: implications for shared teaching. *Med Educ*. 2005; **39**(5):448–55.

81. Whetten, DA. Albert and Whetten revisited: strengthening the concept of organizational identity. *Journal of Management Inquiry*. 2006; **15**(3):219–34.

82. Kramer, RM, Brewer, MB, Hanna, BA. Collective trust and collective action: the decision to trust as a social decision. In Kramer, RM, Tyler, TR, eds. *Trust in Organizations: Frontiers of Theory and Research*. Thousand Oaks, CA: SAGE; 1996:357–89.

83. Monrouxe, LV, Rees CE, Dennis I & Wells SE (2015) Professionalism dilemmas, moral distress and the healthcare student: Insights from two online UK-wide questionnaire studies. *BMJ Open.* 5(5).

84. Chiu, PP, Hilliard, RI, Azzie, G, Fecteau, A. Experience of moral distress among pediatric surgery trainees. *J Pediatr Surg.* 2008; **43**(6):986–93.

85. Førde, R, Aasland, OG. Moral distress among Norwegian doctors. *J Med Ethics.* 2008; **34**(7):521–25.

86. Kälvemark, S, Höglund, AT, Hansson, MG, Westerholm, P, Arnetz, B. Living with conflicts-ethical dilemmas and moral distress in the health care system. *Soc Sci Med.* 2004; **58**(6):1075–84.

87. Lomis, KD, Carpenter, RO, Miller, BM. Moral distress in the third year of medical school; a descriptive review of student case reflections. *Am J Surg.* 2009; **197**(1):107–12.

88. Mobley, MJ, Rady, MY, Verheijde, JL, Patel, B, Larson, JS. The relationship between moral distress and perception of futile care in the critical care unit. *Intensive Crit Care Nurs.* 2007; **23**(5):256–63.

89. Sundin-Huard, D, Fahy, K. Moral distress, advocacy and burnout: theorizing the relationships. *Int J Nurs Pract.* 1999; **5**(1):8–13.

90. ABIM Foundation, American Board of Internal Medicine; ACP-ASIM Foundation, American College of Physicians-American Society of Internal Medicine; European Federation of Internal Medicine. Medical professionalism in the new millennium: a physician charter. *Ann Intern Med.* 2002; **136**(3):243–46.

91. Ho, MJ. Culturally sensitive medical professionalism. *Acad Med.* 2013; **88**(7):1014.

92. Maleki, A, de Jong, M. A proposal for clustering the dimensions of national culture. *Cross Cult Res.* 2014; **48**(2):107–43.

93. Triandis, HC. *Individualism and Collectivism.* Boulder, CO: Westview Press; 1995.

94. Tafarodi, RW, Lo, C, Yamaguchi, S, Lee, WWS, Katsura, H. The inner self in three countries. *J Cross Cult Psychol.* 2004; **35**(1):97–117.

95. English, T, Chen, S. Culture and self-concept stability: consistency across and within contexts among Asian Americans and European Americans. *J Pers Soc Psychol.* 2007; **93**(3):478–90.

96. Peng, K, Nisbett, RE. Culture, dialectics, and reasoning about contradiction. *Am Psychol.* 1999; **54**(9):741–54.

97. Chiu, CY, Hong, YY, Dweck, CS. Lay dispositionism and implicit theories of personality. *J Pers Soc Psychol.* 1997; **73**(1):19–30.

98. Yuki, M. Intergroup comparison versus intragroup relationships: a cross-cultural examination of social identity theory in North American and East Asian cultural contexts. *Soc Psychol Q.* 2003; **66**(2):166–83.

99. Ho, MJ, Yu, KH, Hirsh, D, Huang, TS, Yang, PC. Does one size fit all? Building a framework for medical professionalism. *Acad Med.* 2011; **86**(11):1407–14.

100. Chandratilake, M, McAleer, S, Gibson, J. Cultural similarities and differences in medical professionalism: a multi-region study. *Med Educ.* 2012; **46**(3):257–66.

101. Schwartz, SH. A theory of cultural values and some implications for work. *J Appl Psychol.* 1999; **48**(1):23–47.

102. Bandura, A. *Social Learning Theory.* New York, NY: General Learning Press; 1973.

103. Monrouxe, LV. When I say... intersectionality in medical education research. *Med Educ.* 2015; **49**(1):21–22.

104. Skorikov, VB, Vondracek, FW. Occupational identity. In Schwartz, SJ, Luyckx, K, Vignoles VL, eds. *Handbook of Identity Theory and Research.* New York, NY: Springer; 2011:693–714.

Chapter 4

Socialization, professionalism, and professional identity formation

Frederic William Hafferty

History is opaque. You see what comes out, not the script that produces events, the generator of history.[1]

Introduction

In this chapter, we will examine issues of professionalism and professional identity formation through the particular lens of socialization theory. The fundamental assumption driving this chapter is my belief that current discussions about professionalism, and to a lesser extent professional identity formation, contain a bevy of unexamined assumptions about what happens to learners as they move from the social and social–psychological status of lay outsiders to full members in a particular occupational group – in this case, medicine. The largely tacit nature of these suppositions, in turn, may block or otherwise distort meaningful efforts by medical educators to optimally link medical education with the principles and practices of professionalism and identity formation. Until these disconnects and contradictions are made more explicit, efforts to develop and deploy effective educational interventions will be less than optimal.

To facilitate this examination, I treat medicine's current professionalism movement as *discourse* and analyze "how the specialized language of academic medicine disciplines has defined, organized, contained, and made seemingly immutable a group of attitudes, values, and behaviors subsumed under the label of 'professionalism.'"[2] My principal focus will be on the discourse of professionalism that has emerged since the mid 1980s, a period I consider to be the general launching point for organized medicine's modern-day professionalism movement. This discourse is marked by calls for physicians to recommit themselves to an ethic of professionalism – an ethic grounded in selfless service (e.g., altruism) and an ethic calling for the transformation of practitioners at the level of core values and self-identity.

This discourse identifies medical schools as the primary change agent with medical students being the principal foci. While this discourse has evolved to include calls for changing educational institutions at the level of organizational culture, there are few details about how to link the structure, process, and content of education with the called-for changes in outcomes. Perhaps most consequentially, this discourse is awash with often inconsistent and conflicting references to professionalism across a broad variety of social–cognitive entities such as behaviors, attitudes, values, motives, and tendencies. In bringing these inconsistencies to the surface, I argue that approaching and defining professionalism at the level of values and self-identity (for example) calls for a fundamentally different educational enterprise, and thus a fundamentally different process of professional identity formation, than approaching professionalism at the level of attitudes and behavior. In short, *how* we conceptualize professionalism, and in turn, professional identity formation, must be an explicit part of how we structure our pedagogical practices to such ends.

In preparing this chapter, I sought to understand exactly how professionalism is being handled within medicine's modern-day professionalism literature.[2,3] Thus, if a given article referred to "professional attitudes," I asked, "In what way is professionalism treated as an attitude?" Conversely, if a given article specified "professional values," I wanted to understand how the author actually framed professionalism as a value. As the reader might anticipate, it is not unusual, in fact it is unsettlingly common, for authors to refer to professionalism as a value *and* as an attitude (among other things), and to do so in largely tacit ways that imply that the entities listed (attitudes, values) are interchangeable. While values, attitudes, and other dimensions of social life certainly coexist in a complex web of mutualities, they are not synonyms. Although there is nothing inherently wrong with approaching professionalism as

Teaching Medical Professionalism, 2nd Edition, ed. Richard L. Cruess, Sylvia R. Cruess and Yvonne Steinert.
Published by Cambridge University Press. © Cambridge University Press 2016.

behavior – the question of whether it really matters what one *believes* as long as one *acts* professionally being a not uncommon one in medicine – I do argue in this chapter that the fundamental uncertainties that underscore clinical decision making, and the ambiguities that permeate medical practice, require a professional presence that is best grounded in who one *is* rather than what one *does*.[4]

I organize this chapter in four parts. First, I present a brief overview of medicine's modern-day professionalism movement and its emergent discourse of professionalism. I then subject this discourse to a critical review by highlighting its tacit assumptions and conceptual weaknesses. Second, and taking an "if-then" form of argument, I conclude that if professionalism is to be conceptualized as values, then this calls for a particular framing of medical education – in this case, education-as-socialization as opposed to education-as-training, with the latter's focus on the transmission of knowledge and skills and their affirming behaviors. To this end, I briefly review some principles of socialization and apply them to the particular case of medical education as professional preparation. Third, I take a more explicit look at professionalization as a form of social control and the implications of such a framing for a socialization approach to medical education. I close with some thoughts on how better to conceptualize medical education as socialization, including what it means to prepare physicians *as professionals*, along with how socialization theory fits within the emerging discourse of professional identity formation.

Medical professionalism: a truncated history

Professionalism can be defined for all time as the means by which individual doctors fulfill the medical profession's contract with society. The specific attributes that have long been understood to animate professionalism include altruism, respect, honesty, integrity, dutifulness, honour, excellence, and accountability.[5]

This version of professionalism is now moribund.[6]

As will become evident in this chapter, the nature (and characterization) of professionalism has become, even within organized medicine itself, a highly contested construct.

Background

For the purposes of this chapter, the rise of a modern professionalism literature within medicine can be traced to the 1980s and 1990s, with the emergence of what has been termed a "nostalgic" form of professionalism.[7] This particular discourse emerged from a consensus among medical leaders that medicine had "strayed" from its "traditional commitments" to patient welfare and had violated its social contract with society. Consequently, leaders called for a "rediscovery of" and subsequent "recommitment to" "traditional values" and "core professional principles."[8-11] In turn, and across a broad number of initiatives, medicine began to develop definitions, assessment tools, standards and competencies, and curricula.[5,12-32] As a general rule, this movement identified "market forces" and "market incentives" as *the* primary threat to professionalism.[33]

In addition to being framed as something essential to the identity of both medicine and its practitioners, professionalism was cast as something central to sustaining the public's trust in the medical profession by emphasizing the "primacy of patient welfare and the subordination of self-interest."[5,17,19] Writers referred to "avowed standards" and listed "core characteristics" such as altruism, respect, and honesty. Physicians, meanwhile, were expected to "pledge... fidelity to their professional ethic" and to "pursue their professional prerogatives in the public interest."[5]

Warnings about commercialism were a key element in this discourse. Medical leaders saw a rise in unprofessional behavior, with professionalism being marginalized by the "irreconcilable ethics of the marketplace."[5] The fear was that medicine would evolve into "just another business," as physicians became increasingly disillusioned, frustrated, and cynical.

In addition to creating definitions, codes, statements of standards, and tools for assessment, the emerging discourse of professionalism identified medical education as *the* principle agent of remediation. Organized medical education responded. The Association of American Medical Colleges (AAMC) launched its Medical School Objectives Project (MSOP). Graduate medical education (GME) and continuing professional development (CPD) responded as well. The Accreditation Council for Graduate Medical Education (ACGME), in conjunction with the American Board of Medical Specialties (ABMS), identified professionalism as one of six "core competencies" and tied residency accreditation and maintenance of certification (MOC) to meeting these competencies. Formal coursework in professionalism became ubiquitous throughout medical schools in the United States, Canada, and the United Kingdom.

Targets for change included admissions practices and an emphasis on small group and experiential learning, along with calls to "purge" educational environments of "unprofessional practices" and related tacit messages.[5,34–36] Even personality factors came under the gun. Former AAMC president Jordan Cohen, for example, insisted that physicians, not unlike humans in general, were "hard-wired for self-interest," leading to "self-serving decisions under the guise of respectability."[5] For these and related reasons, Cohen called for "substantial change in the culture and environment of medical education" and for medical educators to "assume greater responsibility and accountability for strengthening the resolve of future doctors to sustain their commitment to the ethics of professionalism."[5] Educators were encouraged to develop learning experiences that would enable trainees to "inculcate" and "internalize" those principles.

This movement, while impressive in its collective breadth, energy, and commitment, was not without opposition. Some medical school faculties, for example, expressed reservations that "something like professionalism" could actually be taught to medical students and residents.[37–40] Students, in turn, complained that the sudden infusion of professionalism materials within the formal curriculum was "unnecessary," "too rule driven," or "just another way to keep us in line."[41–43] Data from the AAMC's Graduation Questionnaire (GQ) identified professionalism as one of the few subjects students felt to be "excessively taught."[44] Moreover, new generations of students appeared to embrace alternative definitions of professionalism by emphasizing issues of lifestyle and balance over traditional medical concerns with altruism and "selfless service to others."[7,43,45] Older faculty, in turn, found themselves bewildered by what they saw as a younger generation of trainees who "no longer want to work hard."[46] Meanwhile, and operating somewhat in the background relative to these more pressing student–faculty conundrums, was the trickle of ongoing calls for a "new professionalism," with this term coming to embrace a variety of related themes such as "civic engagement" and "patient-centered care."[47–50]

More recently, issues of professionalism have been tied to a number of other movements and their related discourses, including (1) physician and trainee "burnout";[51,52] (2) medical student, resident, and faculty "wellness" and "well-being";[53,54] (3) remediating professionalism (largely dominated by the term "lapses");[55,56] (4) using the humanities and ethics to promote professionalism;[57] (5) the aforementioned rise of a literature on professional identity formation;[58–63] (6) how professional societies, as organizational entities, might promote professionalism;[64] and (7) how organizations and organizational settings can foster or hinder the professionalism of their members, including being considered professional entities in their own right.[65,66]

Where, then, do things stand with respect to professionalism and organized medical education? On the one hand, we have today a genuinely broad-based movement with considerable progress in defining and assessing professionalism and in establishing curricula and standards.[35,67] On the other hand, there also appears to be some measure of student and faculty resistance to the ways in which professionalism is represented within the movement.[68] Finally, there appear to be disconnects between the discourse of professionalism and what we expect from our underlying medical educational system if, in fact, we are going to formally prepare physicians based upon what is called for within that discourse. For example, if commercialism is antithetical to professionalism, and the traditional professionalism literature is quite specific on this point, then the pedagogical task is not how to be a professional *in principle*, but rather how to be a professional within a den of industry iniquity. After all, pedagogy shorn of context is little more than rhetoric.

In summary, the problem we are addressing here is not so much a lack of definition(s) within the medical professionalism literature as it is an ongoing vagueness about the underlying *nature* to which we aspire. In turn, confusions about this nature have direct implications for, and impact on, the integrity of the educational mission as we seek to translate our professionalism ideals into educational outcomes.

Deconstructing the discourse

What, then, are we to make of these calls to professionalism – particularly the calls for necessary and substantial changes in the culture of the educational enterprise and the internalization of core values by trainees?

First, we need to agree upon what it is we are dealing with – and thus what we seek to address. Are we talking about "professional values," "professional attitudes," "professional attributes," "character traits," or, perhaps more restrictively, "professional behaviors?" For example, Cohen,[5] and he is hardly alone, references all five, often interchangeably, along with using professionalism as an adjective attached to a wide variety of entities. The implication is that all of the above terms are equivalent entities – which, of course they are not.

Second, regardless of our target (e.g., professionalism), what are we asking medical educators to do? Teach? Instruct? Transmit? Inform? Guide? Support? Model? Inculcate? Transform? Or perhaps we anticipate structuring student learning across multiple fronts and expect medical schools to stress one modality of learning at one time and others at different phases or stages of the educational process? Cohen's use of the noun "inculcation," for example, posits change at the level of self-identity. Inculcation, however, is a fundamentally different social act than calling upon students to *learn the principles* of professionalism" (italics mine) or to *master* behavioral skills or competencies, or to have students *model* themselves upon exemplary faculty. The same types of disconnects exist for faculty. Calling upon faculty to *guide* student learning is a fundamentally different task than mandating them to *shape* the learning process.

Third, and related, what do we expect from students? Do we expect them to *learn* about professionalism, *appreciate* key professionalism principles, *behave* in professionally appropriate ways? Or, do we expect them to *identify* with the precepts of professionalism, *be* or *become* professionals, and make these precepts part of their core identity? Knowing, behaving, and identification are very different ends.

Fourth, what about professionalism's "core expectation" to subordinate self-interest in deference to the interest of others? This call to altruism is a key element in virtually all statements of nostalgic professionalism, yet there appear to be substantive shifts in how the newest cohorts of students and practitioners view what it means to practice medicine. Can one actually be professional without being altruistic? Is it possible – or perhaps preferable – to approach altruism as a behavior rather than as a core attribute of one's personality or character? Teaching students to *act* or behave in an altruistic fashion calls for a different set of pedagogical practices than developing learning environments to promote altruism as a matter of being or identity.

Fifth, what about marketplace ethics and their threat as a "corrupting influence"? What exactly is being corrupted – and how? And at what level does "corruption" operate? Does it function more as a surface phenomenon, which may change what you do but not who you are, or does it operate more at the level of character and identity, with a corresponding invisibleness to the social actor? I understand that the framing of commercialism as antithetical to professionalism is often more a rallying cry than nuanced analytical distinction within the medical literature, but efforts by faculty and students to tease out the social–psychological nature of this altercation has important implications for how best to assist students to counter its influences.

Finally, while this example clearly is U.S.-centric in its specific references to market forces, there are a host of parallel concerns and issues within other healthcare systems, particularly national healthcare systems, around issues of professionalism and its "antitheticals" or "corrupting influences." From a professional identity formation perspective, it is not enough to understand the "good stuff" (e.g., professionalism) and its respective trajectory of loss and then redemption. Any adequate theory of professional identity formation also requires that equal attention be paid to the system-specific "threats to professionalism," the nature of those threats, and how they might be operating within the context of identity formation.

To summarize, the call within medicine's modern-day professionalism literature for trainees to *embrace* the principles and practices of professionalism, and for educators to "strengthen the resolve" of their trainees "to the ethics of professionalism,"[5] have fundamental implications for how we structure our educational opportunities. To further raise the pedagogical stakes, this literature also calls for such a re-affirmation in the face of social forces (including commercialism, corporatization, and bureaucratization and managerialism) deemed anti-professional in nature, and to do so in the presence of trainees who are viewed by some as "hard-wired" for selfishness. Finally, all this remediation and redemption is to take place within an educational milieu populated with role models and mentors whom themselves, according to organized medicine, have wandered somewhat afield from medicine's core values and mission.

The medical school as a site of occupational socialization

Professional schools are an institutional context in which the organized profession can exert significant control. They are perhaps the sole sites where the professions' standards of good work set the agenda for learning. Professional schools are not only where expert knowledge and judgment are communicated from advanced practitioner to beginner; they are also the place where the profession puts its defining values and exemplars on display, where future practitioners can begin both to assume and critically examine their future identities. This is a complex educational process, however, and its value depends, in large part, on how well the several aspects of professional education are understood and woven into a whole.[69]

The notion of the medical school as a special place permeates the medical education and professions literatures. One hallmark of medicine's status as a profession is that it controls both the selection and education of future physicians. As such, and as noted in the above quotation, medical schools and residency training programs are formidable – and formative – settings that structure and shape how future physicians will think, act, and identify themselves with core occupational values.

Although neither uses the concept directly, both Sullivan (as quoted directly above) and Cohen (as quoted earlier) consider medical education as a locus of occupational socialization and the medical school as a setting of deep learning.[70] Sullivan (who co-directed the Carnegie Foundation's Preparation for the Professions Program) and Cohen, along with others, also frame the learning process as multifaceted, and thus, at least implicitly, recognize that *becoming* a doctor requires educators to take explicit steps to coordinate the multiplicity of learning environments that make up medical education, and in doing so produce a professionally infused tapestry of physicianhood.

If we heed Sullivan's call, and if we frame the educational undertaking at the level of identity, and do so utilizing "defining values and exemplars," then we are talking about socialization. If we accept Cohen's framing, and conceptualize the medical school as a site of occupational culture, then we are talking about having to make changes in the structure and process of occupational socialization. While there will always be room (see below) for educators to decide whether we wish to emphasize a professionalism of attitudes or behaviors versus a professionalism of values and identity, the fact remains that if we wish to frame the formation of future physicians at the level of identity and at the level of organizational culture, then we are dealing, at a fundamental level, more with norms and values than with attitudes and behaviors.

To date, and at least within this chapter, we have seen professionalism cast as a little bit of everything (e.g., attitude, identity, value, norm, behavior, attributes, and perception), sometimes in the same document and oftentimes interchangeably. While it certainly is reasonable for educators to identify "professional attitudes" *and* "professional values" as dually important objects of pedagogy, attitudes and values are different social–psychological creatures with different implications for how we transform neophyte outsiders into well-established insiders.

One approach to this conceptual conundrum is to examine medical education from within the framework of socialization theory.

Socialization theory

There is no singular or universal theory of socialization. Core meanings and foci have evolved over time and across academic disciplines.[71,72] Within the medical education literature, references to "socialization" have a moderate presence, but most often what readers encounter is the isolated term without explanation or explication. In some instances, "socialization" appears to be used as a throwaway term, often as a synonym for "medical education" – which it most certainly is not, or as a vague reference to an unspecified social process. (See Fineberg et al.[73] as an exception.) Similarly, one also encounters references to the term "professional socialization" in the medical education literature, but without understanding whether the author is referring to the training of a particular occupational group (e.g., professionals), or to a particular or special type of socialization. Recognizing the distinction between a particular occupational group and a particular type of socialization is critical because it directs our attention either to the *product* of a social process (e.g., the socialization of professionals), or to the process itself (e.g., socialization). As Wentworth notes in his detailed analysis of socialization theory, contemporary writings on socialization tend to stress product over process, thus narrowing our understanding – and appreciation – of the social dynamics that underscore this particular form of social learning.[71]

Differences in time and discipline notwithstanding, there are some basic principles of socialization theory we can draw upon in exploring issues of medical education and professionalism. First, while the socialization literature does address issues of behavior and attitudes, socialization fundamentally involves training for self-image and identity. One can behave in certain respects because of underlying beliefs and one can have attitudes about the objects involved in the process, but the underlying dimension of socialization is personal transformation. Furthermore, while any occupational training involves learning new knowledge and skills, it is the melding of knowledge and skills with an altered sense of self that differentiates "training" from "socialization."

Second, much of what takes place during socialization, whether that be as child or adult, takes place at a tacit or unconscious level.[74–76] While agency and intentionality are a fundamental part of any process of socialization, particularly in the case of adult socialization in general and occupational socialization in particular,[77] the purpose of socialization is to take that which is unusual, nonroutine, or discordant (to an outsider) and render it commonplace and taken for granted by those within the group one seeks to join. In short, socialization works best when it unfolds in a subtle and incremental fashion rather than under the scrutiny of reflection at the group or personal level. How this "nature of" socialization dovetails with the recent emphasis within the professionalism literature on promoting reflection[78] and mindfulness[79] within the educational context, however, will not be explored in this chapter.

Third, the identification of medical education as a site of occupational culture links us directly to the concept of socialization.[80] Furthermore, while there is great value in attending to organizational ceremonies and rituals in the transmission of group values and norms, the role of the less dramatic, routine and taken-for-granted nature of everyday social life in the transmission and reinforcement of group values and normative standards has been underappreciated within the occupational training literature.[81] Finally, distinctions between the recognized and taken for granted, the formal and tacit, or the espoused and underlying, echo properties of the formal, informal, and hidden curriculum.[82] The informal curriculum, for example, is awash with usualness. In turn, the hidden curriculum is closely aligned with Schein's model of occupational culture, including, as Schein's three basic levels of organizational culture, the identity-shaping presence of artifacts, espoused values, and basic underlying assumptions.[80]

Fourth, while references to medical education as transformational are common within the medical education literature, explicit references to the nature of medicine as a moral community and the medical school as sites of moral acculturation are relatively rare.[83,84] In contrast to other arenas of professional and occupational training, such as the military[85–88] and the ministry,[89,90] medicine appears relatively reluctant to formally identity itself as a locus of personal and moral transformation. The consequence, for medical students at least, is not so much an absence of normative messages within the educational process but rather a deluge of them – often at the individual (e.g., "this is how *I* do things around here...") rather than group (e.g., "this is what *we* do...") level. This focus on the individual rather than the group results in a learning experience that is more disjointed and chaotic than unifying and directive. None of this is to imply that physicians should think like soldiers or profess like ministers, but it is to challenge the notion that medicine is best exemplified at the level of individually based knowledge and skills.

Finally, and attention to issues of student "wellness" and "balance" notwithstanding, the experience of medical education is hardly a benign process. Some consider it "challenging," others "stressful," and still others rife with "bullying,"[91,92] mistreatment,[93,94] and "abuse."[33] Moreover, and independent of such environmental pressures, medical students are a tense, anxious, and highly goal-directed lot. They are high achievers, placed within settings of considerable tension and ambiguity, and where all – quite intensely – want to become in-group members (e.g., physicians). As such, and to invoke the imagery of a perfect storm with its massive turbulence and kinetic energy, medical students are the "perfect objects" for socialization. They are social and financial captives in a strange land, and a land in which "fitting in" and "not rocking the boat" are deemed essential strategies by these doctors-in-the-making[95,96] who conjointly seek to both "survive" and "join the club." This "readiness for socialization" is heightened by a medical culture that devalues (at least until recently) introspection and reflection.

Finally, and returning to the quote that opens this chapter, if we are to accept the characterization of professional schools as "the sole sites where the professions' standards of good work set the agenda for learning" and "where the profession puts its defining values and exemplars on display," then we should be able to go to medical schools, residency programs, and teaching hospitals and see these standards, defining values, and exemplars not only in action, but in high relief – even to outsiders.

In sum, if the object of our pedagogical attention is socialization (as opposed to other types of learning), then we are committing ourselves to working with a pedagogical sandbox of values and personal and group identity rather than some other focus of learning. This framing, in turn, has appreciable implications for how we structure the medical learning process.

Professionalism as a form of social and self-control

There are other reasons to place the concept of socialization at the forefront of any discussion of professionalism and medical education. Whether our referent literature is sociology or medicine, the concept of professionalism is linked indelibly to the notion of social control. While the specifics of medicine's rise as a profession have been detailed elsewhere,[97–99] medicine's ascendancy as a profession, its acquisition of occupational autonomy, and its promise to act as a fiduciary rest on two promises about, and related forms of, social control. The first is medicine's own widely cited promise to police itself in the public's interest. This is the concept – and promise – of peer review. This is social control at a collective level. An ineffective, dysfunctional, or otherwise corrupt process of peer review significantly weakens medicine's claim to professional status.

The second form of social control, taking place at the level of the individual (e.g., self-review) is more foundational, yet only recently has it become the object of analytic attention within the medical professions literature.[100–104] This form of social control involves both the ability (based on identified skill sets) and willingness (with the nature of this "willingness" being a core issue in this chapter) of individuals to regulate their own selves and do so in the public's interest. Examples include calls for medical education to promote critical and humanistic reflection.[105]

Self-regulation, in the form of self-review and reflection, is a precursor for, and condition of, peer review. Peer review sans self-review is ritualized social action. It is the promise without the product. At a fundamental and definitional level, professionals are professionals because they *self*-regulate. Moreover, they do so not because of external rules or the threat of sanctions, but rather because this is who they are. In short, self-review functions (or should function) as a core value within the overall normative framework of what it means to be a professional. In this respect, the notion of the physician-as-professional revolves around the internalization of core occupational values that include a work ethic linked to a committed, concerned, and continuous self-monitoring on the public's behalf. Professionals, by definition, and at least as represented within the medicine's modern-day professionalism literature, do not require the same types of external controls afforded, for example, by bureaucratic structures. Once again, we have core theoretical reasons within both sociology and the medical professionalism literatures for treating professionalism as the product of deep learning and internalization, something that functions at the level of personality and self-identity. Professionals regulate themselves because this is who they are and because of the special nature of their work – in that they work on behalf of "others" (the patient). Finally, our focus on self-review also returns us to issues of self-reflection, which itself is a core topic within the emergent professional identity formation literature.[106]

Considerable work still needs to be done to better link self to peer review, and then self and peer review to the social contract, the social contract to broader issues of professionalism, and broader issues of professionalism to the nature of social control – particularly the control of work.[96] Nonetheless, the necessity of such work does not detract from the core argument that links self-regulation to socialization.

Medical education as resocialization

As noted above, socialization is hardly a monolithic entity. There are many different types of socialization, along with a multiplicity of dimensions to this process. Some types are widely referenced in the literature (primary/secondary; child/adult; political; gender; religious) while others are less visible (e.g., anticipatory,[107] emotional,[108,109] and resocialization).[110,111]

On a most general level, professional socialization is a type of adult socialization. Nonetheless, because of its structure (hierarchical, extended), its setting (something often linked to Erving Goffman's concept of the "total institution"[112]), and its cognitive and emotional demands (intensive, stressful), it is reasonable to frame medical education as special or a particular type of adult socialization.[113] The image of medical education as stressful and self-altering is a ubiquitous part of the medical education literature, as well as a prominent message within autobiographical accounts of physician training[114,115] – even if the framing of training as "self-altering" never appears on the printed page.

Framing medical education as resocialization moves us away from the seduction of imagining medical training as a simple augmentative or additive process in which a new set of occupationally specific knowledge, behaviors, and dispositions "simply" are layered onto previously existing ones. Moreover, it moves us away from a characterization of socialization that is a "natural" addendum to the the educational process and thus something that already exists in some nonproblematic fashion. Instead, postulating medical education as resocialization forces us to view it as a more intentional, purposeful, and prescriptive social process whereby certain aspects of one's prior self are *replaced* by new ways of thinking, acting, and valuing. The concept of resocialization allows us to view certain types of occupational preparation as involving a process not simply of moving into a new occupational role or status, but also as moving away from old ways of thinking and being. This symbiotic interface of entering–embracing and exiting–rejecting has been observed in studies of medical education, including educational experiences as early as the first few months of medical school.[116,117]

Relevant to this linking of resocialization and occupational preparation is the long-standing association of resocialization with brainwashing, including intentional efforts to reshape the identities (and ideologies) of "deviants" such as political prisoners or the "reprogramming" of "rescued" religious cult members. Although rarely used within the medical education literature, the concept has been considered germane to the study of certain types of occupational preparation including professions (law and medicine), along with certain occupations (soldiers, firefighters, police officers) in which the educational process itself is considered arduous (mentally or physically), the work is considered dangerous or even life threatening, and that danger to self is accompanied by some kind of service ethic (e.g., to the public). As such, resocialization involves a degree of intentionality as well as a reorientation or restructuring of self-identity. It is not something that "just happens" or is the "natural byproduct" of an educational system focused on the occupational reproduction of knowledge and skills. This dimension of intentionality or

deliberateness has implications for medical education and is a theme we will revisit at the end of this chapter.

The concept of resocialization also raises, once again, the role of environmental stresses (often purposefully manipulated in the case of resocialization) and the corresponding (and often causally linked) anxieties experienced by the learner–socializee. Resocialization is most effective when the subject is repeatedly and purposefully stressed. Even extreme forms of psychological "readjustment" such as the Stockholm Syndrome can be explained within the framework of resocialization theory. Resocialization thus becomes a concept within which we can link the various descriptors of medical education (from "difficult," "challenging," and "exacting" to "intimidating," "traumatizing," and "abusive" – all underscored by sleep deprivation and fatigue) to the process of socialization. Resocialization is a process – for better or for worse – to change hearts *and* minds.

Finally, viewing medical education as resocialization more directly raises issues of agency and determination, and the degree to which we may (tacitly) hold an over-socialized versus an under-socialized version of the educational enterprise. While no one today really believes that medical schools form their learners via some cookie-cutter, homogeneous assembly line, the degree that trainees exhibit agency, choice, self-determination, and individuality versus conformity to group norms is very much an issue. There is a certain almost romantic and perhaps nostalgic notion that socialization is all about helping students become "all that they want to be." At an extreme, this kind of rendition transforms socialization into little more than a process of self-actualization in which trainees become "all that they can be" or aspire to be upon first contemplating life as a physician. Lest we forget, and according to medicine itself, becoming a physician is supposed to be a *transformative* process, and if we adhere to socialization theory, a transformation that largely takes place, for better and for worse, in tacit and unconscious ways.

Conclusion

The preceding discussion about social/self-control and professionalism returns us to the concept of socialization and our core arguments linking professionalism, professional identity formation, and socialization. Without attempting to minimize what is, after all, an exhaustively broad topic about the nature of social and occupational preparation, it is vitally important that we periodically pause and ask, "What exactly are we talking about when we use the term 'medical education'"? Are we in the business of imparting basic knowledge, skills, and requisite behaviors, or are we, foundationally speaking, imparting beliefs, behaviors that are normative in scope and, most important, values? What is our verb? Are we an enterprise driven by "learning about," "appreciating," "behaving," and "acting," or are we in the "being," "internalizing," and "embracing" business? Moreover, do we actually believe – really and truly – calls from educational leaders for "substantial change in the culture and environment of medical education" and for medical educators to "assume greater responsibility and accountability for strengthening the resolve of future doctors to sustain their commitment to the ethics of professionalism"?[5] If yes, then such an affirmation moves us down one pedagogical path. If no, then another. To date, the choice remains medicine's, given its continued control over the selection and education of future physicians. The Carnegie Foundation's comparative study of professional education in medicine, nursing, law, engineering, and clergy is quite specific in noting that the "common aim of all professional education (is) specialized knowledge and professional identity."[69] Do we agree? One's fundamental position on this issue carries different implications for how we structure and deliver medical education.

Socialization, at root, is learning to be an insider, and in this chapter we have focused on one set of social process involved in what it means to become (and be) an insider-as-professional. While I do not wish to disparage an educational model that emphasizes knowledge and skills, it should be fairly clear from our brief review of the socialization literature that socialization is, at root, more about deep than surface learning, and more about identity transformation than practices of situational adjustment. When we talk about socialization, the behaviors of record are normative, not idiosyncratic, and the attitudes of import have to do with core beliefs and values rather than the more ephemeral aspects of social life, such as one's all-time favorite *American Idol* winners, or even something directly germane to the world of medicine, such as how one feels about physician pay-for-performance. Moreover, while the process of socialization is not an unequivocal top-down or prescriptive process, and thus individual agency is always in play,

socialization always involves, as a core element, adopting a collective and shared sense what it means to be an in-group versus an out-of-group member. In this respect, becoming a group member does restrict the autonomous free agent and thus limits individual choice. Finally, the material in this chapter on resocialization is included, in part, to provoke further thinking about issues of intentionality and purpose. As reviewed in this chapter, optimizing the linkages among professionalism, socialization, and professional identity formation should not rest on good intentions or from having desired outcomes be the incidental or serendipitous byproducts of other-focused educational practices. Professional identity formation should be intentionally conceptualized and cultivated, and we, as medical educators, should be able to point to our learning environments and explain how all this is taking place. Good outcomes may be accidental; occupational socialization, particularly in the context of culture change, is not.

With these framings in mind, a particular challenge for medical educators, given the presence of medicine's professionalism project, is to wrestle with and reconcile the ambiguous and discordant conceptions of the physician-as-professional that still exist within the broader medical culture of medicine and to then infuse these newer understandings into a series of learning environments that are intentionally designed to reinforce and promote the types of physicians (as professionals) we wish to produce. Until recently, becoming a professional was thought to be little more than a byproduct of an educational process. One *was* a professional by virtue of *becoming* a physician. While medical educators no longer accept this rather benign, passive, and essentially insipid view of professionalism, they have yet to articulate a collective vision of how the process should change to better reflect the emerging literature on professional identity formation.

What then am I calling for in terms of educational design – or more specifically, redesign? I will limit myself to two sets of initiatives – and thus hopefully avoid the distractions that can arise from within a longer list of specifics. The necessary first step is to answer the three primal questions that underscore this chapter. Are we in the business of educating professionals or technicians? Are we engaged in transformation or augmentation? Do we seek to educate individuals qua individuals, or a collectivity? I ask these questions neither rhetorically nor presumptively.

Their answers, whatever they are, set a direction for subsequent educational design and practices. As a first step, these questions need to be answered by leadership.[118] In turn, and based on their answers (now, hopefully, functioning as Leadership), what must follow is a process of faculty development in which the goal is to bring faculty onboard as a collectivity, thus creating a Faculty that sees itself engaged in a cooperative endeavor infused with a new sense of collegiality. Professionalism, socialization, and professional identity formation, at least as represented in this chapter, are group processes. All three involve conjoint activities by one community (Faculty), toward another (trainees), on behalf of a third (the public). The identity I speak of is a collective identity. Furthermore, it is an identity reflected in work on behalf of others. Finally, it is worth noting that to sidestep this first step and avoid answering the three questions is to locate one's sentiments more in the individual–augmentative–technician camp than in the collective–transformational–professional camp.

What follows? The second step is to take our answers, along with our newly energized Leadership–Faculty partnership, and move beyond the traditional focus of curricular reform and integration[82] and situate our remedial efforts more squarely within the framework of learning environments.[34,119] Here, the goal is to dissect the overall milieu of learning (which is different than the overall milieu of teaching) using the lens of professional identity formation. Technically speaking, we still have not left our opening three questions, and thus the possibility that Leadership–Faculty have decided that they are committed to an augmentation, technical preparation, and individual formation model. Both camps, in turn, now will, it is hoped, be involved in some deliberative and intentional fashion, with identity formation. However, if Leadership–Faculty tilt more to the professionalism side of the aisle, then we are talking about *professional* identity formation, and thus the issue of how what we do (including formal and other-than-formal learning experiences) contributes to the formation of a collective group identity as professionals. No one claims that identity, particularly the identity that accompanies professional formation, can take place sans the acquisition of occupationally specific knowledge and skills. At the same time, few of us can point to specifics in our current learning systems in which the acquisition of such knowledge and skills explicitly is being framed from an identity formation perspective (e.g., "and here is how this all fits into what it means to be a

physician") – all of which means collective work in the service of others.

Finally, and as a capstone to this second step, we need to examine how such a newly framed learning environment might indeed be formative in nature and thus how the learning environments we provide for our learners reflect the emergent nature of socialization processes and identity formation. Milestones[118] represents one possible model, and although probably not perfect for our purposes, we might want to address how we structure the *formative* elements of identity *formation*, recalling, once again, that our operational goal remains the collective and not the individual.

Issues of medical education, socialization, and professionalism are, of course, a great deal more complicated and nuanced than the characterizations represented in this chapter. In some very real respects, I have been restrictive in both my questions and answers. Nonetheless, I believe the issue as framed ("What does it mean to be a physician-as-professional?") is more foundational than asking how to best define or measure professionalism. At root, we want our definitions and measures to reflect core meanings rather than to dictate them ex post facto.

Finally, there is the issue of authenticity. When we label something "professional," are we referring to something that is the product of deep or of surface learning? The issue is not one of semantics or aesthetics. Medicine trains for the usual and commonplace as well as the unusual and idiosyncratic. It is *relatively* easy to *be* professional, and even easier to *appear* so, within the usualness of everyday medical life. All medical settings, including those infused with crisis (e.g., the EDs and ICUs), have routines that fill the vast majority of "what goes on." At the same time, every work setting has its "black swans,"[1] the unanticipated and often unanticipatable events that truly stretch the boundaries of an occupation's knowledge, skills, and values. This is why training in professionalism functions – and should function – at the level of socialization and thus at the level of values and identity. Case studies are important pedagogical tools. They help students to grasp particulars. So too is the situated learning that takes place on the job as individuals "learn the ropes" and "the way things are done around here." However, medical practice is riddled with the unexpected. This is the nature of our beast. This is why, when the unusual surfaces, the hope is that practitioners will return to their knowledge bases, their skills, and their collective identity as professionals to tease out *new* answers, come up with *innovative* responses, all grounded in their sense of *being* physician–professionals.

Efforts to lay bare the variety and types of learning that go on during this transformation of lay outsiders to medical insiders is an iterative process. We may seek to move some aspects of the informal and hidden curriculum more under the spotlight of formal educational activities. Nonetheless, there will always be those aspects of any occupational learning, particularly workplace learning, that remain counter to and even antithetical to what is being formally proffered. Counterfactuals are part of the richness and messiness of social life and thus there is an omnipresent and ongoing need to reflectively ask ourselves, "What does it mean to be a physician-as-professional" – and then to fold our answers back into the structure and process of medical education. After all, the iterative process of linking reflection with subsequent action speaks to a type of integrity that is the hallmark of what it means to be a profession.

References

1. Taleb, NN. *The Black Swan: The Impact of the Highly Improbable*. New York, NY: Random House; 2007.

2. Wear, D, Kuczewski, MG. The professionalism movement: can we pause?. *Am J Bioeth*. 2004; **4**(2): 1–10.

3. Hafferty, FW, Castellani, B. A sociological framing of medicine's modern-day professionalism movement. *Med Educ*. 2009; **43**(9):826–28.

4. Hafferty, FW. Professionalism: the next wave. *N Engl J Med*. 2006; **355**(20): 2151–52.

5. Cohen, JJ. Professionalism in medical education, an American perspective: from evidence to accountability. *Med Educ*. 2006; **40**(7):607–17.

6. Horton, R. What's wrong with doctors? *New York Rev Books*. 2007; **54**(9): 16–20.

7. Castellani, B, Hafferty, FW. The complexities of professionalism: a preliminary investigation. In Wear, D, Aultman, JM, eds. *Professionalism in Medicine: Critical Perspectives*. New York, NY: Springer; 2006:3–23.

8. Lundberg, GD. Promoting professionalism through self-appraisal in this critical decade. *JAMA*. 1991; **265**(21):2859.

9. Relman, AS. Shattuck lecture–the health care industry: where is it taking us? *N Engl J Med*. 1991; **325**(12):854–59.

10. Ring, JJ. The right road for medicine: professionalism and the new American Medical Association. *JAMA*. 1991; **266**(12): 1694.

11. Todd, JS. Professionalism at its worst. *JAMA*. 1991; **266**(23): 3338.

12. Reynolds, PP. Reaffirming professionalism through the educational community. *Ann Intern Med*. 1994; **120**(7):609–14.

13. Frank, JR, Jabbour, M, Tugwell P. Skills for the new millennium: report of the Societal Needs Working Group. CanMEDS 2000 Project. *Ann R Coll Physicians Surg Can*. 1996; **29**(4):206–16.

14. Wynia, MK, Latham, SR, Kao, AC, Berg, JW, Emanuel, LL. Medical professionalism in society. *N Engl J Med*. 1999; **341**(21):1612–16.

15. Swick, HM, Szenas, P, Danoff D, Whitcomb, ME. Teaching professionalism in undergraduate medical education. *JAMA*. 1999; **282**(9):830–32.

16. Rothman, DJ. Medical professionalism–focusing on the real issues. *N Engl J Med*. 2000; **342**(17):1284–86.

17. Swick, HM. Toward a normative definition of medical professionalism. *Acad Med*. 2000; **75**(6):612–16.

18. General Medical Council. *Good Medical Practice*. London, UK: GMC; 2001.

19. ABIM Foundation, American Board of Internal Medicine; ACP-ASIM Foundation, American College of Physicians-American Society of Internal Medicine; European Federation of Internal Medicine. Medical professionalism in the new millennium: a physician charter. *Ann Intern Med*. 2002; **136**(3):243–46.

20. Arnold, L. Assessing professional behavior: yesterday, today, and tomorrow. *Acad Med*. 2002; **77**(6):502–15.

21. Barondess, JA. Medicine and professionalism. *Arch Intern Med*. 2003; **163**(2):145–49.

22. Blank, L, Kimball, H, McDonald, W, Merino, J; ABIM Foundation; ACP Foundation; European Federation of Internal Medicine. Medical professionalism in the new millennium: a physician charter 15 months later. *Ann Intern Med*. 2003; **138**(10):839–41.

23. Inui, TS. *A Flag in the Wind: Educating for Professionalism in Medicine*. Washington, DC: Association of American Medical Colleges; 2003.

24. Ginsburg, S, Regehr, G, Lingard, L. Basing the evaluation of professionalism on observable behaviors: a cautionary tale. *Acad Med*. 2004; **79**(10 Suppl):S1–S4.

25. Coulehan, J. Viewpoint: today's professionalism: engaging the mind but not the heart. *Acad Med*. 2005; **80**(10):892–98.

26. Papadakis, MA, Teherani, A, Banach, MA, Knettler, TR, Rattner, SL, Stern, DT, Veloski, JJ, Hodgson, CS. Disciplinary action by medical boards and prior behavior in medical school. *N Engl J Med*. 2005; **353**(25):2673–82.

27. Stern, DT. *Measuring Medical Professionalism*. New York, NY: Oxford University Press; 2006.

28. Cruess, RL. Teaching professionalism: theory, principles, and practices. *Clin Orthop Relat Res.* 2006; **449**:177–85.

29. Cruess, RL, Cruess, SR. Teaching professionalism: general principles. *Med Teach.* 2006; **28**(3):205–08.

30. Wear, D, Aultman, JM, eds. *Professionalism in Medicine: Critical Perspectives.* New York, NY: Springer; 2006.

31. Goldie, J, Dowie, A, Cotton, P, Morrison, J. Teaching professionalism in the early years of a medical curriculum: a qualitative study. *Med Educ.* 2007; **41**(6):610–17.

32. ABIM Foundation, American College of Physicians, Institute on Medicine as a Profession. *Advancing 21st Century Medical Professionalism: A Multi-Stakeholder Approach.* Roundtable discussion. Philadelphia, PA: ABIM Foundation; 2009. Summary available from www .abimfoundation.org/~/media/Foundation/Initiatives/ Multi-Stakeholders%20Meeting%20Recap.ashx?la=en.

33. Hafferty, FW. Professionalism and commercialism as antitheticals: a search for "unprofessional commercialism" within the writings and work of American medicine. In Parsi, K, Sheehan, MN, eds. *Healing as Vocation: A Medical Professionalism Primer.* Lanham, MD: Rowman & Littlefield; 2006:35–59.

34. Benbassat, J. Undesirable features of the medical learning environment: a narrative review of the literature. *Adv Health Sci Educ Theory Pract.* 2013; **18**(3):527–36.

35. Birden, H, Glass, N, Wilson, I, Harrison, M, Usherwood, T, Nass, D. Teaching professionalism in medical education: a Best Evidence Medical Education (BEME) systematic review. BEME Guide No. 25. *Med Teach.* 2013; **35**(7):e1252–e1266.

36. Bleakley, A. Gender matters in medical education. *Med Educ.* 2013; **47**(1): 59–70.

37. Cruess, RL, Cruess, SR. Professionalism must be taught. *BMJ.* 1997; **315**(7123):1674–77.

38. Rowley, BD, Baldwin, DC Jr, Bay, RC, Cannula, M. Can professional values be taught? A look at residency training. *Clin Orthop Relat Res.* 2000; **378**:110–14.

39. Collier, R. Professionalism: can it be taught? *CMAJ.* 2012; **184**(11):1234–36.

40. Symonds, IM, Talley, NJ. Can professionalism be taught? *Med J Aust.* 2013; **199**(6):380–81.

41. American Medical Student Association. *AMSA'S 2007 PharmFree Scorecard.* Washington, DC: AMSA; 2007.

42. Goldstein, EA, Maestas, RR, Fryer-Edwards, K, Wenrich, MD, Oelschlager, AM, Baernstein, A, Kimball, HR. Professionalism in medical education: an institutional challenge. *Acad Med.* 2006; **81**(10):871–76.

43. Ross, S, Lai, K, Walton, JM, Kirwan, P, White, JS. "I have the right to a private life": medical students'

44. Association of American Medical Colleges. *Medical School Graduation Questionnaire: 2013 All Schools Summary Report.* Washington, DC: AAMC; 2013. [Accessed May 19, 2014.] Available from www .aamc.org/download/350998/data/2013gqallschools summaryreport.pdf.

45. Hafferty, FW. What medical students know about professionalism. *Mt Sinai J Med.* 2002; **69**(6):385–97.

46. Smith, LG. Medical professionalism and the generation gap. *Am J Med.* 2005; **118**(4):439–42.

47. Irvine, D. The performance of doctors: the new professionalism. *Lancet.* 1999; **353**(9159):1174–77.

48. Smith, R. Medical professionalism: out with the old and in with the new. *J R Soc Med.* 2006; **99**(2): 48–50.

49. Christmas, S, Millward, L. *New Medical Professionalism: A Scoping Report for the Health Foundation.* London, UK: The Health Foundation; 2011. [Accessed May 14, 2014.] Available from www.health.org.uk/publication/ new-medical-professionalism.

50. Evetts, J. A new professionalism? Challenges and opportunities. *Curr Sociol.* 2011; **59**(4):406–22.

51. Dyrbye, LN, Massie, FS Jr, Eacker, A, Harper, W, Power, D, Durning, SJ, Thomas, MR, Moutier, C, Satele, D, Sloan, J, Shanafelt, TD. Relationship between burnout and professional conduct and attitudes among U.S. medical students. *JAMA.* 2010; **304**(11):1173–80.

52. Shanafelt, TD, Boone, S, Tan, L, Dyrbye, LN, Sotile, W, Satele, D, West, CP, Sloan, J, Oreskovich, MR. Burnout and satisfaction with work-life balance among U.S. physicians relative to the general U.S. population. *Arch Intern Med.* 2012; **172**(18):1377–85.

53. Kligler, B, Linde, B, Katz, NT. Becoming a doctor: a qualitative evaluation of challenges and opportunities in medical student wellness during the third year. *Acad Med.* 2013; **88**(4):535–40.

54. West, CP, Dyrbye, LN, Rabatin, JT, Call, TG, Davidson, JH, Multari, A, Romanski, SA, Hellyer, JM, Sloan, JA, Shanafelt, TD. Intervention to promote physician well-being, job satisfaction, and professionalism: a randomized clinical trial. *JAMA Intern Med.* 2014; **174**(4):527–33.

55. Hickson, GB, Pichert, JW, Webb, LE, Gabbe, SG. A complementary approach to promoting professionalism: identifying, measuring, and addressing unprofessional behaviors. *Acad Med.* 2007; **82**(11):1040–48.

56. Papadakis, MA, Paauw, DS, Hafferty, FW, Shapiro, J, Byyny, RL; Alpha Omega Alpha Honor Medical Society Think Tank. Perspective: The education community must develop best practices informed by

evidence-based research to remediate lapses of professionalism. *Acad Med.* 2012; **87**(12):1694–98.

57. Doukas, DJ, McCullough, LB, Wear, S, Lehmann, LS, Nixon, LL, Carrese, JA, Shapiro, JF, Green, MJ, Kirch, DG; Project to Rebalance and Integrate Medical Education (PRIME) Investigators. The challenge of promoting professionalism through medical ethics and humanities education. *Acad Med.* 2013; **88**(11):1624–29.

58. Holden, M, Buck, E, Clark, M, Szauter, K, Trumble, J. Professional identity formation in medical education: the convergence of multiple domains. *HEC Forum.* 2012; **24**(4):245–55.

59. Brody, H, Doukas, D. Professionalism: a framework to guide medical education. *Med Educ.* 2014; **48**(10):980–87.

60. Crigger, N, Godfrey, N. From the inside out: a new approach to teaching professional identity formation and professional ethics. *J Prof Nurs.* 2014; **30**(5):376–82.

61. Cruess, RL, Cruess, SR, Boudreau, JD, Snell, L, Steinert, Y. Reframing medical education to support professional identity formation. *Acad Med.* 2014; **89**(11):1446–51.

62. Cruess, RL, Cruess, SR, Boudreau, JD, Snell, L, Steinert, Y. A schematic representation of the professional identity formation and socialization of medical students and residents: a guide for medical educators. *Acad Med.* 2015; **90**(6):718–25.

63. Nothnagle, M, Reis, S, Goldman, RE, Anandarajah, G. Fostering professional formation in residency: development and evaluation of the "forum" seminar series. *Teach Learn Med.* 2014; **26**(3):230–38.

64. Wynia, MK, Papadakis, MA, Sullivan, WM, Hafferty, FW. More than a list of values and desired behaviors: a foundational understanding of medical professionalism. *Acad Med.* 2014; **89**(5):712–14.

65. Lesser, CS, Lucey, CR, Egener, B, Braddock, CH 3rd, Linas, SL, Levinson, W. A behavioral and systems view of professionalism. *JAMA.* 2010; **304**(24):2732–37.

66. Egener, B, McDonald, W, Rosof, B, Gullen, D. Perspective: Organizational professionalism: relevant competencies and behaviors. *Acad Med.* 2012; **87**(5):668–74.

67. Hodges, BD, Ginsburg, S, Cruess R, Cruess, S, Delport, R, Hafferty, F, Ho, MJ, Holmboe, E, Holtman, M, Ohbu, S, Rees, C, Ten Cate, O, Tsugawa, Y, Van Mook, W, Wass, V, Wilkinson, T, Wade, W. Assessment of professionalism: recommendations from the Ottawa 2010 Conference. *Med Teach.* 2011; **33**(5):354–63.

68. Birden, HH, Usherwood, T. "They liked it if you said you cried": how medical students perceive the teaching of professionalism. *Med J Aust.* 2013; **199**(6):406–09.

69. Sullivan, WM, Colby, A, Wegner, JW, Bond, L, Shulman, LS. *Educating Lawyers: Preparation for the Profession of Law.* San Francisco, CA: John Wiley & Sons; 2007.

70. Atherton, JS. *Learning and Teaching: Deep and Surface Learning.* [Accessed Feb. 21, 2015.] Available from www.learningandteaching.info/learning/deepsurf.htm.

71. Wentworth, WM. *Context and Understanding: An Inquiry into Socialization Theory.* New York, NY: Elsevier; 1980.

72. Tierney, WG. Organizational socialization in higher education. *J Higher Educ.* 1997; **68**(1): 1–16.

73. Fineberg, IC, Wenger, NS, Forrow, L. Interdisciplinary education: evaluation of a palliative care training intervention for pre-professionals. *Acad Med.* 2004; **79**(8):769–76.

74. Polanyi, M. *Personal Knowledge: Towards a Post-Critical Philosophy.* London, UK: Routledge & Kegan Paul; 1958.

75. Helmich, E, Bolhuis, S, Dornan, T, Laan, R, Koopmans, R. Entering medical practice for the very first time: emotional talk, meaning and identity development. *Med Educ.* 2012; **46**(11):1074–86.

76. Monrouxe, LV. Identities, self and medical education. In Walsh, K, ed. *Oxford Textbook of Medical Education.* New York, NY: Oxford University Press; 2013:113–23.

77. Goldie, J. The formation of professional identity in medical students: considerations for educators. *Med Teach.* 2012; **34**(9):e641–e648.

78. Wong, A, Trollope-Kumar, K. Reflections: an inquiry into medical students' professional identity formation. *Med Educ.* 2014; **48**(5): 489–501.

79. de Vibe, M, Solhaug, I, Tyssen, R, Friborg, O, Rosenvinge, JH, Sørlie, T, Bjørndal, A. Mindfulness training for stress management: a randomised controlled study of medical and psychology students. *BMC Med Educ.* 2013; **13**:107.

80. Schein, EH. *Organizational Culture and Leadership.* Second edition. San Francisco, CA: Jossey-Bass; 1992.

81. Van Maanen, J, Barley, SR. Occupational communities: culture and control in organizations. In Staw, BM, Cummings, LL, eds. *Research in Organizational Behavior. Volume 6.* Greenwich, CT: JAI Press; 1984:265–87.

82. Hafferty, FW. Beyond curriculum reform: confronting medicine's hidden curriculum. *Acad Med.* 1998; **73**(4):403–07.

83. Pellegrino, ED. The medical community as a moral community. *Bull N Y Acad Med.* 1990; **66**(3):221–32.

84. Hafferty, FW, Franks, R. The hidden curriculum, ethics teaching, and the structure of medical education. *Acad Med.* 1994; **69**(11):861–71.

85. Hays, K. *Practicing Virtues: Moral Traditions at Quaker and Military Boarding Schools*. Berkeley, CA: University of California Press; 1994.

86. Janowitz, M. *The Professional Soldier: A Social and Political Portrait*. New York, NY: Free Press; 1960.

87. Leahy, JF. *Honor, Courage, Commitment: Navy Boot Camp*. Annapolis, MD: Naval Institute Press; 2002.

88. Lipsky, D. *Absolutely American: Four Years at West Point*. New York, NY: Houghton Mifflin; 2003.

89. Kleinman, S. Women in seminary: dilemmas of professional socialization. *Sociol Educ*. 1984; 57(4):210–19.

90. Foster, CR, Dahill, L, Golemon, L, Tolentino, BW. *Educating Clergy: Teaching Practices and Pastoral Imagination*. San Francisco, CA: Jossey-Bass; 2005.

91. Quine, L. Workplace bullying in junior doctors: questionnaire survey. *BMJ*. 2002; 324(7342):878–79.

92. Mukhtar, F, Daud, S, Manzoor, I, Amjad, I, Saeed, K, Naeem, M, Javed, M. Bullying of medical students. *J Coll Physicians Surg Pak*. 2010; 20(12):814–18.

93. Mavis, B, Sousa, A, Lipscomb, W, Rappley, MD. Learning about medical student mistreatment from responses to the medical school graduation questionnaire. *Acad Med*. 2014; 89(5):705–11.

94. Sklar, DP. Mistreatment of students and residents: why can't we just be nice? *Acad Med*. 2014; 89(5):693–95.

95. Freidson, E. *Professionalism: The Third Logic*. Cambridge, UK: Polity; 2001.

96. Knight, JA. *Medical Student: Doctor in the Making*. New York, NY: Appleton-Century-Crofts; 1973.

97. Poirier, S. *Doctors in the Making: Memoirs and Medical Education*. Iowa City, IA: University of Iowa Press; 2009.

98. Starr, P. *The Social Transformation of American Medicine: The Rise of a Sovereign Profession and the Making of a Vast Industry*. New York, NY: Basic Books; 1982.

99. Starr, P. Social transformation twenty years on. *J Health Polit Policy Law*. 2004; 29(4):1005–19.

100. Niemi, PM. Medical students' professional identity: self-reflection during the preclinical years. *Med Educ*. 1997; 31(6):408–15.

101. Epstein, RM. Mindful practice. *JAMA*. 1999; 282(9):833–39.

102. Sobral, DT. An appraisal of medical students' reflection-in-learning. *Med Educ*. 2000; 34(3):182–87.

103. Carr, SE, Johnson, PH. Does self reflection and insight correlate with academic performance in medical students? *BMC Med Educ*. 2013; 13:113.

104. Duke, P, Grosseman, S, Novack, DH, Rosenzweig, S. Preserving third year medical students' empathy and enhancing self-reflection using small group "virtual hangout" technology. *Med Teach*. 2015; 37(6):566–71.

105. Branch, WT. Teaching professional and humanistic values: suggestion for a practical and theoretical model. *Patient Educ Couns*. 2015; 98(2):162–67.

106. Nothnagle, M, Reis, S, Goldman, RE, Anandarajah, G. Fostering professional formation in residency: development and evaluation of the "forum" seminar series. *Teach Learn Med*. 2014; 26(3):230–38.

107. Harvill, LM. Anticipatory socialization of medical students. *J Med Educ*. 1981; 56(5):431–33.

108. Hochschild, AR. *The Managed Heart: Commercialization of Human Feeling*. Berkeley, CA: University of California Press; 1983.

109. Pollak, LH, Thoits, PA. Processes in emotional socialization. *Soc Psychol Q*. 1989; 52(1): 22–34.

110. Feldman, DC. Socialization, resocialization, and training: reframing the research agenda. In Goldstein, IL, ed. *Training and Development in Organizations*. San Francisco, CA: Jossey-Bass; 1989:376–416.

111. Egan, JM. Graduate school and the self: a theoretical view of some negative effects of professional socialization. *Teach Sociol*. 1989; 17(2):200–07.

112. Goffman, E. *Asylums: Essays on the Social Situations of Mental Patients and Other Inmates*. New York, NY: Doubleday; 1961.

113. Morrison, L. Resocialization. In Ritzer, G, ed. *Blackwell Encyclopedia of Sociology*. Oxford, UK: Blackwell; 2007. Blackwell Reference Online. [Accessed May 19, 2014.] Available from www.blackwellreference.com/subscriber/uid=1714/tocnode?id=g9781405124331_chunk_g978140512433124_ss1–59.

114. Gawande, A. *Complications: A Surgeon's Notes on an Imperfect Science*. New York, NY: Metropolitan Books; 2002.

115. Collins, MJ. *Hot Lights, Cold Steel: Life, Death and Sleepless Nights in a Surgeon's First Years*. New York, NY: St. Martin's Press; 2005.

116. Hafferty, FW. *Into the Valley: Death and the Socialization of Medical Students*. New Haven, CT: Yale University Press; 1991.

117. Sinclair, S. *Making Doctors: An Institutional Apprenticeship (Explorations in Anthropology)*. New York, NY: Berg; 1997.

118. Louis KS, Leithwood, K, Wahlstrom, KL, Anderson, SE, Michlin, M, Mascall, B, Gordon, M, Strauss, T, Thomas, E, Moore, S. *Investigating the Links to Improved Student Learning*. New York, NY: Wallace Foundation; 2010. [Accessed May 19, 2014.] Available from www.wallacefoundation.org/knowledge-center/school-leadership/key-research/Documents/Investigating-the-Links-to-Improved-Student-Learning.pdf.

119. Nasca, TJ, Philibert, I, Brigham, T, Flynn, TC. The next GME accreditation system–rationale and benefits. *N Engl J Med*. 2012; 366(11):1051–56.

Chapter 5

Educational theory and strategies to support professionalism and professional identity formation

Yvonne Steinert

There is nothing so practical as a good theory.[1]

As the chapters in this book demonstrate, professionalism and professional identity formation are promoted in diverse and complex ways. Indeed, the past decade has witnessed a significant increase in the teaching and learning of professionalism in undergraduate and postgraduate medical education,[2–4] and the support of professional identity formation has gained importance.[5–8] However, despite this renewed interest, few authors have described the educational frameworks that underpin their work in this area,[9] even though teachers and educators all hold different assumptions about *what* we should teach and *how* we should try to achieve our goals.

With regard to the teaching and learning of professionalism, one contemporary school of thought has emphasized that professionalism needs to be taught explicitly, either by defining core content or outlining professionalism as a list of traits or characteristics.[10–12] From this perspective, the goal is to ensure that every physician understands the nature of professionalism, its basis in morality, the reasons for its existence, its characteristics, and the obligations necessary to sustain it. Other educators have stated that the teaching of professionalism should be approached primarily as a moral endeavor, emphasizing altruism and service, the importance of role modeling, self-awareness, community service, and other methods of experiential knowledge.[13–15] In this school of thought, explicit teaching receives less attention and learning is embedded in an authentic activity. Although both approaches are needed to promote the teaching and learning of professionalism,[16] as teachers and educators we must clarify the assumptions that we hold and try to answer the following question: What is our guiding theory or educational framework as we work to promote professionalism and support identity formation?

With regard to professional identity formation, a number of authors have described developmental theories (e.g., Erikson;[17] Kegan;[18] Marcia[19]) that could inform our thinking. Others have described the process of socialization and how it unfolds in a medical context.[20,21] Jarvis-Selinger et al.[7] (p. 1186) have described identity formation as an adaptive, developmental process that "happens simultaneously at two levels: (1) at the level of the individual, which involves the psychological development of the person and (2) at the collective level, which involves a socialization of the person into appropriate roles and forms of participation in the community's work." Interestingly, however, although different theoretical frameworks regarding the development of professional identity formation have been put forward,[22,23] little attention has been given to the *educational* frameworks that can guide the design and implementation of educational programs.

The goal of this chapter is to situate the teaching and learning of professionalism, and the support of professional identity formation, in an educationally relevant theoretical context, to review the key features of instructional design, and to describe a number of educational strategies that can guide our work in this area. Both the teaching of professionalism and the support of professional identity formation often occur in a spontaneous, unplanned fashion. By describing several relevant theoretical frameworks, this chapter is designed to help facilitate a more systematic approach.

Why theory?

Theory has been defined as "a conception or mental scheme of something to be done; a systematic statement of rules or principles to be followed."[24] In diverse ways, theories represent various aspects of reality in an understandable way.[25] That is, they simplify reality by ignoring a large number of variables

Teaching Medical Professionalism, 2nd Edition, ed. Richard L. Cruess, Sylvia R. Cruess and Yvonne Steinert.
Published by Cambridge University Press. © Cambridge University Press 2016.

(like a map) and they often stress the importance of certain variables by giving them special names or stressing their importance in words, figures, or formulas. However, theory is not simply a summary of the data; rather, it is a specification of loosely construed mechanisms that give rise to observed effects.[26]

The particular theory we subscribe to, whether consciously or not, is likely to dictate how we work.[27] Thus, an awareness of different theoretical frameworks will allow us to make informed choices about how we approach teaching and learning; it will also enable us to share what we do in a scholarly manner. Without theoretical frameworks to guide our practice, there is a danger that there will be too much reliance on intuition or "common sense." Theory can help to ensure that interactions are intentional.

In summary, theory can influence practice, provide a structure for interactions that move toward identifiable outcomes, and create the shared understanding and terminology that is a necessary prerequisite for discussion and debate. "New" theories can also pave the way for progress and innovation when "old" theories are found wanting.[28]

A theoretical framework to guide the support of professionalism and professional identity formation

Although a number of educational theories can be applied to this important content area (e.g., social learning theory;[29] self-efficacy;[30] figured worlds[31]), we have chosen to carefully examine situated learning[32,33] and communities of practice[34,35] as two overarching and interrelated sociocultural frameworks, both of which fall under a constructivist paradigm.[36,37] The choice of these frameworks seems to be particularly appropriate, as identities are constructed and co-constructed through language, artifacts, and action over time (as highlighted in Chapter 3), and both frameworks relate to learning in the workplace,[38–41] the context in which professional behaviors and identities are acquired. Principles of adult learning, experiential learning, and instructional design, which are also pertinent to the design and delivery of educational programs, will be described in a separate section.

Situated learning

Situated learning is based upon the notion that knowledge is *contextually situated* and fundamentally influenced by the *activity, context,* and *culture* in which it is used.[32] This view of knowledge as situated in authentic contexts has important implications for our understanding of teaching and learning professionalism as well as the support of professional identity formation in both work-based and classroom settings.

We have chosen to describe situated learning theory for a number of reasons. Although we are aware of only two articles in the literature that have specifically addressed educational theories and the teaching and learning of professionalism, both have referred to principles of situated learning.[16,42] As Maudsley and Strivens[42] have observed, situated learning theory offers a powerful model that can help to explain the transformation of students from members of the lay public to expert members of a profession who possess specific skills and a commitment to a common set of values. It has also been said that situated learning is particularly appropriate to educating the professions that are communities or cultures joined by "intricate, socially constructed webs of belief"[32] (p. 33); this description is particularly relevant to the formation of professional identities.

Situated learning theory brings together the cognitive base and experiential learning that are needed to facilitate the acquisition of professional behaviors and identities. That is, it bridges the gap between the "know what" and the "know how" of teaching and learning by embedding learning in authentic activities. It also helps to transform knowledge from the abstract and theoretical to the useable and useful.[16] Proponents of situated learning suggest that there should be a balance between the explicit teaching of a subject and the activities in which the knowledge learned is used in an authentic context – essential principles in the teaching and learning of professionalism and the support of professional identity formation.

Key components of situated learning include cognitive apprenticeship, collaborative learning, reflection, practice, and articulation of learning skills.[33]

Cognitive apprenticeship, a fundamental element of situated learning, has particular relevance to clinical teaching and learning, and therefore to professionalism and professional identity formation. Apprenticeship is a familiar and pervasive method of learning in medicine.[43] Cognitive apprenticeship builds on this traditional form of learning and consists of four distinct phases: modeling, scaffolding, fading, and coaching (all of which will be detailed below).

In traditional apprenticeship, the expert shows the apprentice how to do a task, watches as the apprentice practices the task, and then turns over more and more responsibility until the apprentice is proficient enough to accomplish the task independently.[44] Cognitive apprenticeship differs from a more traditional approach in that the process of carrying out the task that is to be learned is not always observable; learning is not always situated in the workplace (and thus the value of the final product is not always evident); and transfer of skills to new situations is required. In order to translate the model of traditional apprenticeship to cognitive apprenticeship, teachers need to *identify the processes* of the task and make them visible, or explicit, to the learner; *situate* abstract tasks in authentic contexts, so that learners understand the relevance of the work; *vary* the diversity of learning situations; and *articulate* common aspects so that students and residents can transfer their new knowledge and learning to new situations.[33]

In *modeling*, learners observe and then mimic the teacher in the performance of a task. Modeling is most effective when teachers make the target processes visible, often by explicitly showing the learner, or apprentice, what to do. Through modeling, learners observe normally invisible processes and begin to integrate *what* occurs with *why* it happens.[45] As outlined in Chapter 6, modeling is one of the strongest influences on professional identity formation.

Scaffolding refers to the support teachers give learners in carrying out specific tasks. This can range from almost completing the entire task to giving occasional hints as to what to do next. Scaffolding supports and simplifies a task as much as necessary to enable learners to manage their learning, allowing them to accomplish otherwise difficult tasks with optimal challenge. Too little challenge will prove boring; too much challenge will foster frustration.[46] By supporting the integration of established understanding and know-how, scaffolding facilitates the transfer of what learners already know to the task at hand.[47] This is relevant to both the acquisition of professional behaviors and professional identities.

Fading is the notion of slowly removing support, giving the learner more and more responsibility. It is a critical step in the trajectory of becoming an independent practitioner.

Coaching is the thread that runs through the entire apprenticeship experience and involves helping individuals while they attempt to learn or perform a task.

It includes directing learner attention, providing ongoing suggestions and feedback, structuring tasks and activities, and providing additional challenges or problems. Coaches explain activities in terms of the learners' understanding and background knowledge, and they provide additional directions about how, when, and why to proceed; they also identify errors, misconceptions, or faulty reasoning in learners' thinking and help to correct them. In situated learning environments, advice and guidance help students and residents to maximize use of their own cognitive resources and knowledge,[45] an important component in becoming a professional.

Collaborative learning is another important feature of situated learning and cognitive apprenticeship. Brown et al.[32] identified the following strategies to promote collaborative learning: collective problem-solving, displaying and identifying multiple roles, confronting ineffective strategies and misconceptions, and developing collaborative work skills. Small group work, peer teaching, and group projects can also facilitate the acquisition of collaborative skills. As interprofessional teamwork is an essential component of healthcare (as outlined in Chapter 10), collaborative learning should be incorporated whenever possible into the teaching and learning of professionalism as well as the support of professional identity formation.

Reflection, an essential ingredient of situated learning, has received significant attention in the medical literature;[48–50] it is also viewed as a core skill in professional competence.[51] In practice, there are three kinds of reflective activity. Schön[50] describes a spontaneous reaction (i.e., "thinking on your feet") as "reflection *in* action." This type of reflection, which is frequently described as a subliminal process of which the participant is only partially aware, most likely involves pattern recognition; as well, it is usually triggered by recognition that "something doesn't seem right."[50,52] Thinking of a situation after it has happened, and initiating the ability to reevaluate the situation, is referred to as "reflection *on* action." This type of reflection, in which the participant is fully aware of what has occurred, allows the individual to mentally reconstruct the experience, paying particular attention to context. Reflection on action also forms a bridge between the relived situation and knowledge retrieved from internal memory or other external sources.[53] While the development of the capacity to reflect "in" and "on" action has become an important feature of medical practice, "reflection *for* action"[54] forms an additional avenue for professional training and improvement of practice. As Lachman and Pawlina[54] (p. 460) observed, "The benefits of reflective practice, whilst meeting the objectives of new and revised curricula, extend beyond the construct of a medical curriculum. The process of reflection and its basis of critical thinking allows for the integration of theoretical concepts into practice; increased learning through experience; enhanced critical thinking and judgment in complex situations; and the encouragement of student-centred learning." Clearly, these benefits are vitally important in the promotion of professionalism and the acquisition of a professional identity.

Boud et al.[55] describe three elements critical to the reflective process. All of these can help to promote the teaching and learning of professionalism as well as the formation of a professional identity:

- *Returning to experience* – This refers to the recollection of salient events, the replaying of the initial experience in the mind of the learner, or the recounting to others of the key features of the experience.
- *Attending to feelings* – This includes utilizing positive feelings and removing negative feelings, both of which are needed for learning to occur
- *Reevaluating experience* – This is clearly the most important phase and relies on the completion of the other two phases. Reevaluation involves a reexamination of the original experience in light of the learner's goals, associating new knowledge with that which is already processed, and integrating new knowledge into the learner's conceptual framework.

According to Roth,[56] a truly reflective process implies an educational process that provides the opportunity to keep an open mind about "what," "how," and "why" things are being done. From this perspective, the learning of professionalism can be achieved through questioning, investigating, evaluating, analyzing, theorizing, seeking feedback, and incorporating the ideas and viewpoints of team members. Professional identity formation is also nurtured and enhanced by this process,[57] which is integral to all of the theoretical perspectives described in this chapter.[49,58]

Practice is another central component of situated learning. Repeated practice serves to test, refine, and extend skills into a web of increasing expertise in a social context of collaboration and reflection.[33] Practice also enables skills to become deeply rooted

and mobilized as needed. In the clinical setting, practice consists of working with patients[59] and interacting with colleagues,[57] both of which are fundamental to the acquisition of a professional identity. The notion of experiential learning (outlined below) is also closely tied to the concept of practice.

Articulation includes two aspects.[33] First, it refers to the concept of articulating or separating out different component skills in order to learn them more effectively. An example of this can be seen as students learn to communicate effectively with patients. Second, articulation refers to clearly enunciating knowledge, reasoning, or problem-solving processes in a specific domain. By articulating problem-solving processes, students and residents can come to a better understanding of their thinking processes and can improve their ability to explain things to themselves and others. This is relevant to the attainment of both professional behaviors and professional identities. Articulation can also help to make learning – and reflection – visible.

In summary, situated learning is based upon the idea that knowledge is contextually situated and fundamentally influenced by the activity, context, and culture in which it is used. Adherence to a situated learning model can also lead to different perceptions of the teacher's role. From this perspective, teachers can assume the role of *coach* in addition to that of pedagogue while acting as a *model* for learners.[60] At the same time, students and residents can become *experts* and engage in reciprocal teaching,[61] while the roles of *apprentice* and *master* are shared. In many ways, situated learning (and its key components of apprenticeship, collaboration, reflection, practice and articulation of skills) provides a useful framework by which to understand how professionalism can be taught and learned and how identity formation can be promoted. An understanding of this sociocultural model can also help to guide the design and delivery of diverse educational programs and activities. As Mann[62] (p. 60) has reflected, "viewing medical education through the lens of situated learning suggests teaching and learning approaches that maximize participation and build on community processes to enhance both collective and individual learning."

Communities of practice

Closely tied to the notion of situated learning is that of communities of practice.[35] Barab et al.[63] (p. 495) defined a community of practice as a "persistent, sustaining, social network of individuals who share and develop an overlapping knowledge base, set of beliefs, values, history, and experiences focused on a common practice and/or mutual enterprise." As outlined in Chapter 1, becoming a member of a community of practice is one of the major ways in which students begin to acquire their professional identities, often through a process of "legitimate peripheral participation."[34] This social practice, which combines "learning by doing" (also known as experiential learning) and apprenticeship into a single theoretical perspective, is the process by which a novice becomes an expert. That is, from a situated learning perspective, learners build new knowledge and understanding through gradual participation in the community of which they are becoming a part. As learners, they begin at the edge – or periphery – of the community, where because of their status as learners, they have what is called "legitimate peripheral participation."[53] Mann[43] provides a useful example. As students in a clinical rotation, or residents at the beginning of their training, gain experiences, they slowly become involved in a community of physicians; at the same time, they gradually participate in more of the community's work and move from the periphery toward the center. They also take on increasing responsibility for the work of the community, namely the care of patients. In the process, they learn to "talk the talk" and "walk the walk." A key element of participation in the community is the opportunity to see and join in the framing of problems and understanding of how knowledge is structured.

According to Wenger,[35] social participation within the community is the key to informal learning. It is embedded in the practices and relationships of the workplace and helps to create identity and meaning. It also complements, and can substitute for, formal learning mechanisms. Informal learning is often not acknowledged as learning within organizations; rather, it is typically regarded as being "part of the job" or a mechanism for "doing the job properly." However, "learning at work" – most often in a community of practice – is a key component of medical education, and there is value in rendering this learning as visible as possible so that it can be valued as an important curricular component.

As a number of authors have suggested, "professional formation occurs most powerfully through participation in a community of practice – by observing how others behave and how they embody the values and behaviors of the profession."[64] (p. S5) Lave and Wenger[34] suggest that the success of a community of practice depends on five factors: the existence and

sharing by the community of a common goal; the existence and use of knowledge to achieve that goal; the nature and importance of relationships formed among community members; the relationships between the community and those outside it; and the relationship between the work of the community and the value of the activity. A community also requires a shared repertoire of common resources, including language, stories, and practices.[35] Awareness of these factors and their influence on professional identity formation is important in the design of all educational programs interested in promoting professional behaviors and identity among students and faculty members. Cognizance of how to cultivate such communities,[65] which can include designing for evolution, opening a dialogue between inside and outside perspectives, inviting different levels of participation, developing public and private community spaces, combining familiarity and excitement, and creating a rhythm for the community, can also be of benefit.

Work-based learning

As stated above, professional behaviors and identities are primarily acquired in the workplace, as students and residents engage in clinical work and learn from their role models and peers. In fact, it is in the everyday workplace where learning most often takes place. Work-based learning, perhaps the signature pedagogy of health professions education, has been defined as learning *for* work, learning *at* work, and learning *from* work,[66] with an emphasis on observation, participation, and expert guidance in an authentic environment.[38] Fundamental to the notion of work-based learning is a view of learning as a socially mediated constructive process,[67] the value of "participation in work" as a catalyst for learning,[68] and the complexity of this process in an ever-changing environment. Billett[67] proposed a curriculum for work-based learning that accounts for the "constructive nature of learning through problem-solving" and consists of two key components: activities and guidance. From this perspective, we need to *sequence* workplace activities that are of increasing complexity and, in so doing, permit the learner to experience more responsible goals and tasks, and *create a pathway* that affords learners the opportunity to access the outcomes of their work activities so that they will understand what they have achieved. Clearly, the sequencing of activities and the delineation of learning pathways to achieve specific goals are critical factors in the development of students and residents, as is the process of engagement, without which learning may be superficial or, at worst, non-existent. Engagement is also dependent upon the congruence between the individual's interests and values and those of the workplace.[39]

Research by Boud and Middleton[40] identified a range of informal learning that occurs in the workplace and illustrates the complexities of learning. For example, there is a diverse range of people that we learn from at work, very few of whom are recognized by the organization as individuals with a role in promoting learning. In a large organization, the range and diversity of communities of practice in which we legitimately participate increases with seniority; as a result, the range of opportunities for informal learning also increases. Some learning networks manifest features of communities of practice; others do not build identity and meaning. Awareness of these networks, often labeled part of the informal or hidden curriculum, is fundamental to our understanding of where the teaching and learning of professionalism, and the acquisition of a professional identity, takes place.

In summary, it is important to understand the nature of work-based learning (where learning takes place), which promotes situated learning (comprised of modeling, scaffolding, coaching, and fading), and the setting in which this process unfolds, often a community of practice. These frameworks also parallel the processes identified by Jarvis-Selinger et al.[7] – at the individual and the collective level – which underpin professional identity formation.

The cycle of instructional design

Figure 5.1 summarizes the key steps in designing an educational activity, course, or curriculum. The main components include defining educational goals and objectives, identifying core content, selecting educational strategies and methods, and evaluating outcome. Each of these steps will be explained below. However, two additional conceptual frameworks will influence the design of activities in this area and they will be addressed first: principles of adult learning and experiential learning.

Some have argued that the principles of instructional design are not compatible with situated learning because instructional design refers to a systematic process that follows a step-wise progression – and this is not always the case in work-based learning. As well,

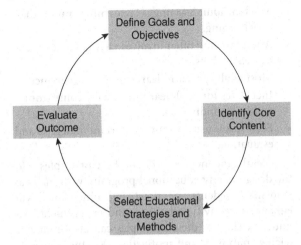

Figure 5.1. The instructional design cycle

the theoretical framework of instructional design assumes that what people learn is relatively stable across situations and that people apply what is learned in a logical, planned way.[60] However, the two perspectives are not incompatible; teachers and educators need to plan for student "apprenticeships" and create learning experiences that are situated in the real world. At the same time, the basic premises of instructional design *can* be maintained in a situated learning model.[60] For example, teaching strategies must still be based on what is known about the students and what they have to master; they must also be chosen rationally and modified as needed. Most importantly, thinking about instructional design forces us to think about how we can facilitate learning in authentic contexts.

Principles of adult learning

Although some have argued that adult learning is not a theory but rather a mere description of the adult learner,[70] others believe that principles of adult learning (also referred to as andragogy) form an important theoretical construct.[71] In either case, andragogy captures essential characteristics of adult learners and offers important guidelines for planning instruction.

Knowles[72,73] first introduced the concept of andragogy, defining it as "the art and science of helping adults learn." Key principles include the following:

- Adults are independent.
- Adults come to learning situations with a variety of motivations and clear expectations about particular learning goals and teaching methods.
- Adults demonstrate different learning styles.

- Much of adult learning is "relearning" rather than new learning.
- Adult learning often involves changes in attitudes as well as skills.
- Most adults prefer to learn through experience.
- Incentives for adult learning usually come from within the individual.
- Feedback is usually more important than tests and evaluations.

Clearly, the incorporation of these principles into the design of any educational program, with medical students, residents, or practicing physicians, will enhance receptivity, relevance, and engagement. An understanding of these principles can also influence pacing, meaning, and motivation. Kaufman et al.[74] outlined a number of recommendations for program planning based on principles of adult learning that are equally relevant in the context of acquiring professional behaviors as well as a professional identity. To paraphrase these authors, teachers and educators should try to:

- Establish an effective learning climate, so that learners will feel "safe" and be able to express themselves without judgment or ridicule.
- Involve learners in the planning of curricular content and methods, to enhance "buy in," collaboration, and relevance.
- Enable learners to diagnose their own needs and formulate their own learning objectives, to ensure motivation and meaningful learning.
- Encourage learners to identify available resources and devise strategies to achieve their objectives.
- Help learners to carry out their learning plans and try to ensure successful completion of necessary tasks.
- Involve learners in the evaluation of learning, an essential step in self-directed learning.

In many ways, adult learning theory offers us a means of thinking about student learners "in a way that is consistent with what is known about learning and development."[74] (p. 6) Interestingly, the criteria of self-directedness, learning from experience, and self-assessment, which are key to effective learning, are also essential aspects of the practice of medicine.

The experiential learning cycle

Kolb and Fry[75] provided a description of the learning cycle that highlights the role of experience in the

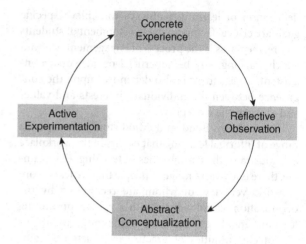

Figure 5.2. The experiential learning cycle[75]

learning process. More specifically, they describe how experience is translated into concepts, which in turn guide the choice of new experiences.[55] In this model, which should be considered in the design of all instructional events, learning is viewed as a four-stage cycle (outlined in Figure 5.2). Immediate concrete experience is the basis for observation and reflection; observations are then assimilated into a personal theory, from which new implications for action can be deduced; and all of these steps eventually lead to new experiences. According to Kolb and Fry,[75] learners need opportunities to experience each step of the learning cycle. That is, they need the ability to experience diverse situations (in both the classroom and the clinical setting); observe and reflect on what they have learned (often in a large group session); develop their own theory and understanding of the world; and experiment new ways of being in order for learning to occur. Attention to the experiential learning cycle will facilitate both the teaching *and* the learning of professionalism and ensure that different learning styles are respected and nurtured as learners develop their professional identities.

Steps to instructional design

In the last section of this volume, we offer examples of educational programs that have been created to support professionalism and professional identity formation. In carefully examining these case studies, we see that a number of principles (or steps) of instructional design have been incorporated, some of which are detailed below.

Defining goals and objectives

The goals (and objectives) for teaching and learning in this area must be carefully determined, in collaboration with learners (at all levels of the educational continuum), their teachers, and other members of the healthcare team. Often, a formal (or informal) analysis of needs will guide the articulation of goals and objectives; at other times, the requirements of licensing or accrediting bodies will determine the learning outcomes. Irrespective of the process, a thorough needs assessment is critical in determining goals and objectives, which serve as the roadmap for educational planning.

Identifying core content

The needs of the learners, their teachers, and other members of the healthcare team will also help to define the core content to be addressed. Core content includes the competencies underlying professionalism as well as the process of socialization that leads to professional identity formation. Chapter 1 provides an overview of the cognitive base of professionalism as well as the core content that guides professional identity formation; other chapters in this book address specific components of identity formation and the attitudes and skills that underpin professional behavior. In each situation, core content must be chosen in line with learner needs, the institutional context, available time, and accessible resources. Moreover, the determination of content is a critical step in the design process, as it will determine educational strategies and methods.

Selecting educational strategies

Once the core content has been identified, teachers and educators must select the strategies they wish to use in light of their goals and objectives as well as learners' capabilities, prior knowledge, and skills. For example, interactive lectures and large group sessions can be used to convey the cognitive base of professionalism. Case vignettes and small group discussions allow for an exploration of personal beliefs, values, and assumptions, fundamental to professional identity formation. Clinical and simulated teaching environments enable skill acquisition, practice, and feedback.

It has been said that professional identity arises "from a long term combination of experience and reflection on experience."[76] (p. 63) The choice of educational strategies should therefore ensure stage-appropriate opportunities for gaining experiences and reflecting upon them; these methods should also provide students, residents, and practitioners with structured occasions to discuss, reflect on, and internalize professional issues in a safe environment.[42,77,78] In addition, the choice of educational strategies should be influenced by the notion that multiple instructional modes are considered to be more effective than a single method,[79] and that active learning methods are more effective than passive ones.[80,81] With this in mind, educators should consider a variety of strategies to meet diverse objectives.

Evaluating outcome

Evaluating outcome includes the assessment of learning (and thereby the evaluation of students) as well as program evaluation (and whether the goals and objectives have been met). Student learning can be measured in a number of ways, including written assessments (e.g., essays; multiple choice questions); clinical assessments (e.g., global rating scales; oral examinations); clinical simulations (e.g., Objective Structured Clinical Examinations; standardized patients); and multi-source assessments (e.g., peer assessments; self-assessments; portfolios). It is beyond the scope of this chapter to describe diverse methods of student assessment. However, a review by Epstein[82] can be a very useful resource. Chapter 11 also provides a rich description of how to assess professionalism and professional identity formation among students and residents. These methods should be incorporated into the design of any instructional program focusing on this core aspect of professional development.

To evaluate the educational activity, be it a one-time event or a curricular unit, teachers should consider available data sources (e.g., students; peers; patients); common methods of evaluation (e.g., questionnaires; focus groups; observations); resources to support assessment; and models of program evaluation (e.g., goal attainment; decision facilitation).[83,84] Kirkpatrick's levels of evaluation[85] are also helpful in conceptualizing and framing the evaluation of effectiveness. They include:

- *Reaction* – Participants' views on the learning experience;
- *Learning* – Changes in participants' attitudes, knowledge, or skills;
- *Behavior* – Changes in participants' behavior; and
- *Results* – Changes in the organizational system, the patient, or the learner.

At a minimum, a practical and feasible evaluation should include an assessment of utility and relevance, content, and educational methods. Moreover, as evaluation is an integral part of the educational cycle, it should be conceptualized at the beginning of any program and whenever possible, should include qualitative and quantitative assessments of learning and behavior change, using a variety of methods and data sources.

Strategies to promote professionalism and professional identity formation

As noted in the different chapters of this book, strategies for teaching professionalism and supporting professional identity formation span the spectrum from large-group didactic lectures to small-group discussions, role plays and simulations, reflective essays, and independent learning. In this section, we will highlight role modeling, an oft-neglected teaching strategy highlighted in Chapter 6, as well as several other methods that have particular appeal in teaching professionalism and supporting professional identity formation (e.g., the use of case vignettes and case presentations; sentinel events and critical incidents; art and literature; narrative-based medicine; and portfolios) and that align with a constructivist paradigm. Reflection, which underpins learning from experience, has been highlighted in an earlier section in this chapter. Other pedagogical practices that can be used to promote professionalism and identity formation (e.g., immersion in community practices, supportive group processes, longitudinal curricula) have been described elsewhere.[57,86]

Role modeling

Coulehan[13] (p. 896) has said that the "first requirement for a sea change in professionalism is to increase dramatically the number of physicians who are able to role model professional virtue at every stage of medical education." Role modeling has been described as one of the most important educational methods for instilling the attitudes, behaviors, ethics, and professional values of medicine to students and residents.[87–91] However, although role modeling is at the heart of "character formation"[92] and professional identity formation,[21] students and residents have observed that many of their clinical teachers are poor role models. As educators, we also frequently undermine this powerful method of teaching and learning.

The characteristics of effective role models are described in Chapter 6. As previously articulated,[87] these include *clinical competence*, which encompasses knowledge and skills, communication with patients and staff, and sound clinical reasoning and decision making; *teaching skills*, which comprise effective communication, feedback, and opportunities for reflection that promote student-centered learning; and *personal qualities* such as compassion, honesty, and integrity as well as effective interpersonal relationships, enthusiasm for practice and teaching, and an uncompromising quest for excellence. All of these characteristics are essential to effective role modeling. The challenge is to articulate the process and make the implicit explicit. At the same time, we should be cognizant of lessons articulated by Benbassat[93] (p. S50), who argues that students and residents often learn from negative role models and need to be reflective in their assessment of preceptors' behaviors so that they can "discern those that are worth imitating."

Learning from role models occurs through observation and reflection. Figure 5.3 provides a schematic representation of the process of role modeling, a complex mix of conscious and unconscious activities.[94] While we are all aware of the conscious observation of observed behaviors, understanding the power of the unconscious component is essential to effective role modeling. As Swick[2] has cautioned, we must pay attention to the behaviors manifested by practicing physicians, not only for what it means to the patients they care for, but also for the impact it has on learners who observe them providing care.

The use of case vignettes and case presentations

The use of case vignettes and case presentations can be particularly powerful in the teaching and learning of professionalism. For example, case studies that involve clinical concepts allow students to critically evaluate specific problems by integrating and applying basic knowledge.[54] Vignettes that integrate context and conflict in medical professionalism can also be useful tools.[95] However, application to other situations may be limited. For example, Goldie et al.[96] used vignettes describing a dilemma concerning professionalism to study knowledge of professional norms. In particular, these vignettes addressed situations in which clinical clerks were confronted with suboptimal

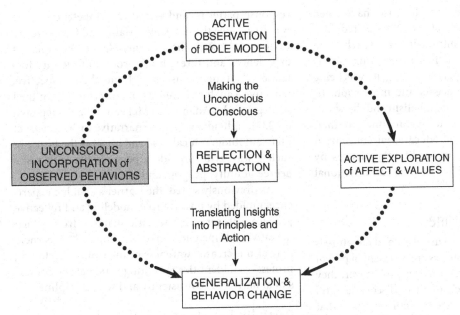

Figure 5.3. Schematic representation of the process of role modeling.[87] The process of incorporating the attributes of a role model can proceed through two different mechanisms.[94] The first, shown on the right, involves an active thought process which leads to change. Related to this, but somewhat different, is a change brought about by active reflection, often expressing ideas in abstract terms. This can convert an unconscious feeling into one which is conscious and can be actively translated into principles and action. There is also an equally powerful process, shown on the left, in which observed behaviors are unconsciously incorporated into the belief patterns and behaviors of the student. Role models should be aware of these components of observational learning.

practice as well as value clashes and personal emotions. The results of this educational intervention indicated a positive effect; however, students did not generalize their knowledge to new vignettes or clinical scenarios. At the same time, Kon[97] observed that educators should consider using both student-generated and instructor-generated cases, as the former facilitate relevance and personal interest. Irrespective of the origin, and whether they are paper based or illustrated through film, case vignettes allow for an exploration of attitudes, values, and beliefs; case presentations offer the same advantages, with the added benefit of authenticity and relevance.

Sentinel events and critical incidents

A number of authors have described the role of sentinel events in the formation of professional identities.[98–100] These events, which are usually laden with both positive and negative emotions, include the first cadaver dissection, first night on call, and first death of a patient. Critical incidents also bring emotion to the fore and emphasize participants' real-life experiences. As an example, Rademacher et al.[99] used the critical incident technique as a way of structuring the

teaching and learning of professional behaviors. As these authors stated (p. 245), "By attending to the detail and context from a learner's real-life professionalism related incident, the learner is engaged." Critically reflecting upon the meaning of an event, as well as lessons for the future, further helps to reinforce professional behaviors and shape professional identities.

The use of art and literature

Art and literature can also be useful adjuncts in teaching professionalism and promoting identity formation, especially as these media can emotionally engage students and residents and help to evoke some of the professional ideals that initially led them to choose a career in medicine. Winter and Birnberg[101] described a seminar in which residents were asked to read a selection on "Virtues and Ideals in Professional Life," view two paintings depicting different but complementary aspects of the medical profession, and discuss three video clips, to explore whether or not physicians have legitimate self-interests. As the authors stated (p. 171), it was clear that "the paintings and video clips touched the residents on an emotional level and had a much greater impact than would otherwise have been experienced from didactic lectures and isolated clinical vignettes." This multimedia approach also enabled residents to discuss their professional beliefs without feeling that their personal integrity was being threatened and fostered a deeper and more sophisticated understanding of professionalism and the work-related expectations they have for one another. Students at all levels of the educational continuum can enhance their repertoire of life experiences by exposure to the narratives of real and fictional patients and physicians.[102–106]

Narrative-based medicine

Closely tied to the educational use of art and literature is narrative medicine.[107–108] Stories are an essential part of the social *construction* of knowledge;[33] moreover, they help learners to keep track of their discoveries and provide a meaningful structure for remembering what has been uncovered. Stories have also been described as a type of "expert system" for storing, linking, and readily accessing information,[33] and, in fact, there appears to be an increasing emphasis on stories as a tool for learning, understanding, and remembering. For this and other reasons, the use of narrative-based medicine[107,108] becomes a compelling strategy in the teaching and learning of professionalism and in the acquisition of a professional identity.

Narrative competence can be understood as "the ability to acknowledge, absorb, interpret, and act on the stories and plights of others."[107] (p. 1897) Narrative medicine also provides a way of reframing the knowledge, skills, and attitudes of good doctoring under the aegis of language, symbol, story, and the cultural construction of illness,[102] as it draws upon the centrality of clinical empathy in establishing and maintaining therapeutic relationships and builds upon the broader, more imaginative empathy that allows observers to "connect with" the experience of persons not immediately known to them.[103] For example, Coulehan[13] proposed a narrative-based approach to learning professionalism to help students address the tension between self-interest and altruism. In so doing, he states that "one of the prerequisites for developing narrative-based professionalism is to provide, throughout medical school and residency, a safe venue for students and residents to share their experiences and enhance their personal awareness." (p. 896) Physicians in training need to understand their own beliefs, feelings, attitudes, and

response patterns, and narrative competence is one way to achieve this objective. Mann and Gaufberg (in Chapter 6) describe how learners "make meaning" of experiences and through the process of identity formation "author themselves." From this perspective, narrative can be viewed as a powerful educational strategy. As McAdams and McLean[109] have suggested (p. 233), individuals can use narrative to "reconstruct their 'autobiographical past' and imagine the future in such a way as to provide a person's life with some degree of unity, purpose and meaning."

As previously stated, the learner's own life experience, molded by positive role modeling and reflective practice, can serve as the basic material from which narrative competence may develop.[13,107] Learners may also increase awareness of their own developing professional identities by writing personal and professional narratives consistently and with discipline.

Portfolio learning

Portfolio learning is closely tied to reflection and a narrative-based approach to learning professionalism and acquiring a professional identity. Portfolios have been defined as "a purposeful collection of student work that demonstrates the student's efforts and progress in selected domains."[110] (p. 1066) In medicine, portfolios can encourage self-directed learning, foster reflection, and demonstrate progress toward identifiable outcomes.[111] Portfolios also have the added advantage of respecting individuality and diversity while developing life-long learning skills.

Portfolios were originally introduced in medicine to assess performance in authentic contexts and stimulate learners to reflect on their own functioning.[112–113] Their use has been extended beyond this original intent and much has been written about the role and value of portfolios, both electronic and paper based, in medical training.[57,114–116] In this context, it is important to appreciate how portfolios can enhance the teaching of professionalism and support professional identity formation, specifically as they promote critical reflection in authentic contexts. In an interesting study, Wong and Trollope-Kumar[116] identified five major themes in students' portfolios that related to professional identity formation: prior experiences; role models; patient encounters; formal and hidden curricula; and societal expectations. These findings reflect the schemata in Chapter 1 (Figures 1.4 and 1.5) and demonstrate the potential value of portfolios in supporting professional identity formation.

The culture of medicine

No discussion of educational theory, design, or strategies would be complete without also addressing the environment in which teaching and learning take place. As highlighted by many authors,[77,117,118] the environment in which our students and residents learn is sometimes "toxic" and can negate the impact of what we are trying to achieve. The academic environment may also impede learning and professional development. As Goldie et al.[119] (p. 610) reflected, "The clinical milieu should be controlled to maximize the influence of role models, and opportunities for guided reflection should be sustained"; we should also be cognizant of the hidden curriculum which can provide both opportunities and threats to learning.

Chapter 18 provides a case study of one department's attempt to change the organizational culture. As we know, medical education is carried out in an environment heavily influenced by economic, cultural, and organizational forces,[77] and many of these institutional factors can negate the impact of our "formal" educational programs.[120,121] There is also an extremely powerful informal curriculum, consisting of unscripted, unplanned, and highly interpersonal forms of teaching and learning that take place among and between faculty and students, and attention must be paid to the informal and the hidden curriculum, whose influences can be extremely positive or negative.[122] In fact, all teachers and educators must work together to change their institutional cultures and try to influence the informal and the hidden curriculum, while structuring formal teaching and learning programs. Brainard and Brislen,[118] two medical students, propose that the main barrier to the teaching and learning of professionalism is unprofessional conduct by their teachers. They also maintain that deficiencies in the learning environment, combined with the subjective nature of many evaluations, often leave students feeling persecuted or confused, and they recommend that teachers and administrators, together with learners, show a commitment to addressing the hidden curriculum openly and proactively. It would be wise to heed their recommendations.

Conclusion

Educational programs designed to promote the teaching of professionalism and the support of professional identity formation clearly need to pay attention to the academic environment in which students and residents learn. However, knowledge of a theoretical framework for teaching and learning, as well as an understanding of principles of adult learning, experiential learning, and instructional design, will strengthen the educational program and promote pedagogical excellence and coherence.

Cruess and Cruess[16] have stated that professionalism is a fundamental aspect of the process of socialization, during which individuals acquire the values, attitudes, interests, skills, and knowledge of the groups they seek to join. Situated learning, with its emphasis on cognitive apprenticeship, collaboration, reflection, practice, and articulation of skills within an authentic context, provides a useful framework for the acquisition of professional behaviors and professional identities, all of which develop in an evolving, often work-based, community of practice.

References

1. Lewin, K. *Field Theory in Social Science: Selected Theoretical Papers*. New York, NY: Harper and Row; 1951.

2. Swick, HM. Viewpoint: professionalism and humanism beyond the academic health center. *Acad Med.* 2007; **82**(11):1022–28.

3. Hodges, BD, Ginsburg, S, Cruess, R, Cruess, S, Delport, R, Hafferty, F, Ho, MJ, Holmboe, E, Holtman, M, Ohbu, S, Rees, C, Ten Cate, O, Tsugawa, Y, Van Mook, W, Wass, V, Wilkinson, T, Wade, W. Assessment of professionalism: recommendations from the Ottawa 2010 Conference. *Med Teach.* 2011; **33**(5):354–63.

4. Birden, H, Glass, N, Wilson, I, Harrison, M, Usherwood, T, Nass, D. Teaching professionalism in medical education: a Best Evidence Medical Education (BEME) systematic review. BEME Guide No. 25. *Med Teach.* 2013; **35**(7): e1252–e1266.

5. Cooke, M, Irby, DM, O'Brien, BC. *Educating Physicians: A Call for Reform of Medical School and Residency*. San Francisco, CA: Jossey Bass; 2010.

6. Cruess, RL, Cruess, SR, Boudreau, JD, Snell, L, Steinert, Y. Reframing medical education to support professional identity formation. *Acad Med.* 2014; **89**(11):1446–51.

7. Jarvis-Selinger, S, Pratt, DD, Regehr, G. Competency is not enough: integrating identity formation into the medical education discourse. *Acad Med.* 2012; **87**(9):1185–90.

8. Wald, HS. Professional identity (trans)formation in medical education: reflection, relationship, resilience. *Acad Med.* 2015; **90**(6):701–06.

9. Gordon, J. Fostering students' personal and professional development in medicine: a new framework for PPD. *Med Educ.* 2003; **37**(4):341–49.

10. Cruess, RL, Cruess, SR. Teaching medicine as a profession in the service of healing. *Acad Med.* 1997; **72**(11):941–52.

11. Cruess, SR, Cruess, RL. Professionalism must be taught. *BMJ.* 1997; **315**(7123):1674–77.

12. Swick, HM. Toward a normative definition of medical professionalism. *Acad Med.* 2000; **75**(6):612–16.

13. Coulehan, J. Viewpoint: today's professionalism: engaging the mind but not the heart. *Acad Med.* 2005; **80**(10):892–98.

14. Huddle, TS; Accreditation Council for Graduate Medical Education (ACGME). Viewpoint: teaching professionalism: is medical morality a competency? *Acad Med.* 2005; **80**(10):885–91.

15. Kinghorn, WA. Medical education as moral formation: an Aristotelian account of medical professionalism. *Perspect Biol Med.* 2010; **53**(1):87–105.

16. Cruess RL, Cruess SR. Teaching professionalism: general principles. *Med Teach.* 2006; **28**(3):205–08.

17. Erikson, EH. *Identity: Youth and Crisis.* New York, NY: WW Norton; 1968.

18. Kegan, R. *The Evolving Self: Problem and Process in Human Development.* Cambridge, MA: Harvard University Press; 1982.

19. Marcia, JE. Development and validation of ego-identity status. *J Pers Soc Psychol.* 1966; **3**(5):551–58.

20. Cruess, RL, Cruess, SR, Boudreau, JD, Snell, L, Steinert, Y. A schematic representation of the professional identity formation and socialization of medical students and residents: a guide for medical educators. *Acad Med.* 2015; **90**(6):718–25.

21. Hafferty, FW. Professionalism and the socialization of medical students. In Cruess, RL, Cruess, SR, Steinert, Y, eds. *Teaching Medical Professionalism.* New York, NY: Cambridge University Press; 2009:53–70.

22. Monrouxe, LV. Identities, identification and medical education: why should we care? *Med Educ.* 2010; **44**(1):40–49.

23. Monrouxe, LV. Identities, self and medical education. In Walsh, K, ed. *Oxford Textbook of Medical Education.* Oxford, UK: Oxford University Press; 2013:113–23.

24. *Oxford English Dictionary.* Second edition. Oxford, UK: Oxford University Press; 1989. [Accessed Nov. 27, 2007]. Available from www.oed.com/view/Entry/2004 31?redirectedFrom=theory#eid.

25. Krumboltz, JD, Nichols, CW. Integrating the social learning theory of career decision making. In Walsh, WB, Osipow, SH, eds. *Career Counseling: Contemporary Topics in Vocational Psychology.* Hillsdale, NJ: Lawrence Erlbaum Associates; 1990:159–92.

26. Adger, D. *Why Theory is Essential: The Relationship between Theory, Analysis and Data.* Southampton, UK: Centre for Languages, Linguistics and Area Studies, University of Southampton; 2002. [Accessed Nov. 27, 2007]. Available from www.llas.ac.uk/resources/gpg/ 405.

27. Bailey, KD. *Sociology and the New Systems Theory: Toward a Theoretical Synthesis.* Albany, NY: State University of New York Press; 1994.

28. Marris, L. *A Practitioner's Perspective.* Monograph on the internet. Coventry, UK: National Guidance Research Forum; 2003. [Accessed Nov. 27, 2007.] Available from www.guidance-research.org/EG/ impprac/ImpP2/ImpP2ii/ImpP2iia.

29. Bandura, A. *Social Learning Theory.* Englewood Cliffs, NJ: Prentice Hall; 1979.

30. Bandura, A. *Self-Efficacy: The Exercise of Control.* New York, NY: WH Freeman; 1997.

31. Holland, D, Lachicottw, W Jr, Skinner, D, Cain, C. *Identity and Agency in Cultural Worlds.* Cambridge, MA: Harvard University Press; 1998.

32. Brown, JS, Collins, A, Duguid, P. Situated cognition and the culture of learning. *Educ Res.* 1989; **18**(1):32–42.

33. McLellan, H, ed. *Situated Learning Perspectives.* Englewood Cliffs, NJ: Educational Technology Publications; 1996.

34. Lave, J, Wenger, E. *Situated Learning: Legitimate Peripheral Participation.* Cambridge, UK: Cambridge University Press; 1991.

35. Wenger, E. *Communities of Practice: Learning, Meaning, and Identity.* Cambridge, UK: Cambridge University Press; 1998.

36. Steffe, LP, Gale, J, eds. *Constructivism in Education.* Mahwah, NJ: Lawrence Erlbaum Associates; 1995.

37. Lincoln, YS, Guba, EG. *The Constructivist Credo.* Walnut Creek, CA: Left Coast Press; 2013.

38. Billett, S. Situating learning in the workplace – having another look at apprenticeships. *Industrial and Commercial Training.* 1994; **26**(11):9–16.

39. Billett, S. Toward a workplace pedagogy: guidance, participation, and engagement. *Adult Education Quarterly.* 2002; **53**(1):27–43.

40. Boud, D, Middleton, H. Learning from others at work: communities of practice and informal learning. *Journal of Workplace Learning.* 2003; **15**(5):194–202.

41. Eraut, M. Informal learning in the workplace. *Studies in Continuing Education.* 2004; **26**(2):247–73.

42. Maudsley, G, Strivens, J. Promoting professional knowledge, experiential learning and critical thinking for medical students. *Med Educ.* 2000; **34**(7):535–44.

43. Mann, K. Learning and teaching in professional character development. In Kenney, N, Shelton, W, eds. *Lost Virtue: Professional Character Development in Medical Education.* Oxford, UK: Elsevier; 2006:145–83.

44. Collins, A, Brown, JS, Holum, A. Cognitive apprenticeship: making thinking visible. *American Educator*. 1991; **15**(3):6–11, 38–46.

45. Choi, JI, Hannafin, M. Situated cognition and learning environments: roles, structures, and implications for design. *Educ Technol Res Dev*. 1995; **43**(2):53–69.

46. Brandt, BL, Farmer, JA Jr, Buckmaster, A. Cognitive apprenticeship approach to helping adults learn. *New Directions for Adult & Continuing Education*. 1993; **59**:69–78.

47. Harley, S. Situated learning and classroom instruction. *Educational Technology*. 1993; **33**(3):46–51.

48. Kinsella, EA. Practitioner reflection and judgement as phronesis: a continuum of reflection and considerations for phronetic judgement. In Kinsella, EA, Pitman, A, eds. *Phronesis as Professional Knowledge: Practical Wisdom in the Professions*. Rotterdam, the Netherlands: Sense Publishers; 2012:35–52.

49. Mann, K, Gordon, J, MacLeod, A. Reflection and reflective practice in health professions education: a systematic review. *Adv Health Sci Educ Theory Pract*. 2009; **14**(4):595–621.

50. Schön, DA. *The Reflective Practitioner: How Professionals Think in Action*. New York, NY: Basic Books; 1983.

51. Epstein, RM, Hundert, EM. Defining and assessing professional competence. *JAMA*. 2002; **287**(2):226–35.

52. Hewson, MG. Reflection in clinical teaching: an analysis of reflection-on-action and its implications for staffing residents. *Med Teach*. 1991; **13**(3):227–31.

53. Robertson, K. Reflection in professional practice and education. *Aust Fam Physician*. 2005; **34**(9):781–83.

54. Lachman, N, Pawlina, W. Integrating professionalism in early medical education: the theory and application of reflective practice in the anatomy curriculum. *Clin Anat*. 2006; **19**(5):456–60.

55. Boud, D, Keogh, R, Walker, D. Promoting reflection in learning: a model. In Boud, D, Keogh, R, Walker, D, eds. *Reflection: Turning Experience into Learning*. London, UK: Kogan Page; 1985:18–40.

56. Roth, RA. Preparing the reflective practitioner: transforming the apprentice through the dialectic. *J Teach Educ*. 1989; **40**(2):31–35.

57. Goldie, J. The formation of professional identity in medical students: considerations for education. *Med Teach*. 2012; **34**(9):e641–e648.

58. Sandars, J. The use of reflection in medical educators: AMEE Guide No. 44. *Med Teach*. 2009; **31**(8):685–95.

59. Graungaard, AH, Andersen, JS. Meeting real patients: a qualitative study of medical students' experiences of early patient contact. *Educ Prim Care*. 2014; **25**(3):132–39.

60. Brown, AL, Palincsar, AS. Guided, cooperative learning, and individual knowledge acquisition. In Resnick, LB, ed. *Knowing, Learning, and Instruction: Essays in Honor of Robert Glaser*. Hillsdale, NJ: Erlbaum; 1989:393–451.

61. Palincsar, AS, Ransom, K, Derber, S. Collaborative research and development of reciprocal teaching. *Educational Leadership*. 1988; **46**(4):37–40.

62. Mann, KV. Theoretical perspectives in medical education: past experience and future possibilities. *Med Educ*. 2011; **45**(1):60–68.

63. Barab, SA, Barnett, M, Squire, K. Developing an empirical account of a community of practice: characterizing the essential tensions. *Journal of the Learning Sciences*. 2002; **11**(4):489–542.

64. O'Brien, BC, Irby, DM. Enacting the Carnegie Foundation call for reform of medical school and residency. *Teach Learn Med*. 2013; **25** Suppl 1:S1–S8.

65. Wenger, E, McDermott, R, Snyder, WM. *Cultivating Communities of Practice*. Boston, MA: Harvard Business School Publishing; 2002.

66. Swanwick, T. See one, do one, then what? Faculty development in postgraduate medical education. *Postgrad Med J*. 2008; **84**(993):339–43.

67. Billett, S. Towards a model of workplace learning: the learning curriculum. *Studies in Continuing Education*. 1996; **18**(1):43–58.

68. Billett, S. Workplace participatory practices: conceptualising workplaces as learning environments. *Journal of Workplace Learning*. 2004; **16** (6): 312–24.

69. Winn, W. Some implications of cognitive theory for instructional design. *Instr Sci*. 1990; **19**(1):53–69.

70. Norman, GR. The adult learner: a mythical species. *Acad Med*. 1999; **74**(8):886–89.

71. Merriam, SB. Updating our knowledge of adult learning. *J Contin Educ Health Prof*. 1996; **16**(3):136–43.

72. Knowles, MS. *Andragogy in Action: Applying Modern Principles of Adult Learning*. San Francisco, CA: Jossey-Bass; 1984.

73. Knowles, MS. *The Modern Practice of Adult Education: From Pedagogy to Andragogy*. New York, NY: Cambridge Books; 1980.

74. Kaufman, DM, Mann, KV, Jennett, PA. *Teaching and Learning in Medical Education: How Theory Can Inform Practice*. Edinburgh, UK: Association for the Study of Medical Education; 2000.

75. Kolb, DA, Fry, R. Towards an applied theory of experiential learning. In Cooper, CL, ed. *Theories of Group Processes*. London, UK: John Wiley; 1975:33–58.

76. Hilton, SR, Slotnick, HB. Proto-professionalism: how professionalisation occurs across the continuum of medical education. *Med Educ*. 2005; **39**(1):58–65.

77. Inui, TS. *A Flag in the Wind: Educating for Professionalism in Medicine*. Washington, DC: Association of American Medical Colleges; 2003.

78. Wear, D, Castellani, B. The development of professionalism: curriculum matters. *Acad Med*. 2000; **75**(6):602–11.

79. Evans, BJ, Stanley, RO, Mestrovic, R, Rose, L. Effects of communication skills training on students' diagnostic efficiency. *Med Educ*. 1991; **25**(6):517–26.

80. Novack, DH, Dubé, C, Goldstein, MG. Teaching medical interviewing: a basic course on interviewing and the physician-patient relationship. *Arch Intern Med*. 1992; **152**(9):1814–20.

81. Burack, JH, Irby, DM, Carline, JD, Root, RK, Larson, EB. Teaching compassion and respect. Attending physicians' responses to problematic behaviors. *J Gen Intern Med*. 1999; **14**(1):49–55.

82. Epstein, RM. Assessment in medical education. *N Engl J Med*. 2007; **356**(4):387–96.

83. Popham, WJ. *Educational Evaluation*. Needham Heights, MA: Allyn and Bacon; 1993.

84. Wholey, JS, Hatry, HP, Newcomer, KE, eds. *Handbook of Practical Program Evaluation*. San Francisco, CA: Jossey-Bass; 1994.

85. Kirkpatrick, DL. *Evaluating Training Programs: The Four Levels*. San Francisco, CA: Berrett-Koehler; 1994.

86. Branch, WT. Teaching professional and humanistic values: suggestion for a practical and theoretical model. *Patient Educ Couns*. 2015; **98**(2):162–67.

87. Cruess, SR, Cruess, RL, Steinert, Y. Role modelling– making the most of a powerful teaching strategy. *BMJ*. 2008; **336**(7646):718–21.

88. Park, J, Woodrow, SI, Reznick, RK, Beales, J, MacRae, HM. Observation, reflection, and reinforcement: surgery faculty members' and residents' perceptions of how they learned professionalism. *Acad Med*. 2010; **85**(1):134–39.

89. Shuval, JT, Adler, I. The role of models in professional socialization. *Soc Sci Med*. 1980; **14A**(1):5–14.

90. Wright, S. Examining what residents look for in their role models. *Acad Med*. 1996; **71**(3):290–92.

91. Wright, S, Wong, A, Newill, C. The impact of role models on medical students. *J Gen Intern Med*. 1997; **12**(1):53–56.

92. Kenny, NP, Mann, KV, MacLeod, H. Role modeling in physicians' professional formation: reconsidering an essential but untapped educational strategy. *Acad Med*. 2003; **78**(12):1203–10.

93. Benbassat, J. Role modeling in medical education: the importance of a reflective imitation. *Acad Med*. 2014; **89**(4):550–54.

94. Epstein, RM, Cole, DR, Gawinski, BA, Piotrowski-Lee, S, Ruddy, NB. How students learn from community-based preceptors. *Arch Fam Med*. 1998; **7**(2):149–54.

95. Boenink, AD, de Jonge, P, Smal, K, Oderwald, A, van Tilburg, W. The effects of teaching medical professionalism by means of vignettes: an exploratory study. *Med Teach*. 2005; **27**(5):429–32.

96. Goldie, J, Schwartz, L, McConnachie, A, Morrison, J. The impact of three years' ethics teaching, in an integrated medical curriculum, on students' proposed behaviour on meeting ethical dilemmas. *Med Educ*. 2002; **36**(5):489–97.

97. Kon, AA. Resident-generated versus instructor-generated cases in ethics and professionalism training. *Philos Ethics Humanit Med*. 2006; **1**:10.

98. Beagan, BL. "Even if I don't know what I'm doing I can make it look like I know what I'm doing": becoming a doctor in the 1990s. *Can Rev Sociol Anthropol*. 2001; **38**(3):275–92.

99. Rademacher, R, Simpson, D, Marcdante, K. Critical incidents as a technique for teaching professionalism. *Med Teach*. 2010; **32**(3):244–49.

100. Branch, WT Jr. Use of critical incident reports in medical education. A perspective. *J Gen Intern Med*. 2005; **20**(11):1063–67.

101. Winter, RO, Birnberg, BA. Teaching professionalism artfully. *Fam Med*. 2006; **38**(3):169–71.

102. Morris, DB. Narrative, ethics, and pain: thinking with stories. *Narrative*. 2001; **9**(1):55–77.

103. Coulehan, J, Clary, P. Healing the healer: poetry in palliative care. *J Palliat Med*. 2005; **8**(2):382–89.

104. Bolton, G. Stories at work: reflective writing for practitioners. *Lancet*. 1999; **354**(9174):243–45.

105. Reynolds, R, Stone, J, eds. *On Doctoring: Stories, Poems, Essays*. New York, NY: Simon & Schuster; 2001.

106. Coles, R. Testa, R, eds. *A Life in Medicine: A Literary Anthology*. New York, NY: New Press; 2002.

107. Charon, R. Narrative medicine: a model for empathy, reflection, profession, and trust. *JAMA*. 2001; **286**(15):1897–1902.

108. Charon, R. Narrative and medicine. *N Engl J Med*. 2004; **350**(9):862–64.

109. McAdams, DP, McLean, KC. Narrative identity. *Curr Dir Psychol Sci*. 2013; **22**(3):233–38.

110. Kalet, AL, Sanger, J, Chase, J, Keller, A, Schwartz, MD, Fishman, ML, Garfall, AL, Kitay, A. Promoting professionalism through an online professional development portfolio: successes, joys and frustrations. *Acad Med*. 2007; **82**(11):1065–72.

111. Gordon, J. Assessing students' personal and professional development using portfolios and interviews. *Med Educ.* 2003; 37(4):335–40.

112. Snadden, D, Thomas, M. The use of portfolio learning in medical education. *Med Teach.* 1998; **20**(3):192–99.

113. Davis, MH, Friedman Ben-David, M, Harden, RM, Howie, P, Ker, J, McGhee, C, Pippard, MJ, Snadden, D. Portfolio assessment in medical students' final examinations. *Med Teach.* 2001; **23**(4):357–66.

114. Driessen, EW, van Tartwijk, J, Overeem, K, Vermunt, JD, van der Vleuten, CP. Conditions for successful reflective use of portfolios in undergraduate medical education. *Med Educ.* 2005; **39**(12):1230–35.

115. Wilkinson, TJ, Challis, M, Hobma, SO, Newble, DI, Parboosingh, JT, Sibbald, RG, Wakeford, R. The use of portfolios for assessment of the competence and performance of doctors in practice. *Med Educ.* 2002; **36**(10):918–24.

116. Wong, A, Trollope-Kumar, K. Reflections: an inquiry into medical students' professional identity formation. *Med Educ.* 2014; **48**(5):489–501.

117. Wear, D, Kuczewski, MG. The professionalism movement: can we pause? *Am J Bioeth.* 2004; **4**(2): 1–10.

118. Brainard, AH, Brislen, HC. Viewpoint: learning professionalism: a view from the trenches. *Acad Med.* 2007; **82**(11):1010–14.

119. Goldie, J, Dowie, A, Cotton, P, Morrison, J. Teaching professionalism in the early years of a medical curriculum: a qualitative study. *Med Educ.* 2007; **41**(6):610–17.

120. Hafferty, FW. Beyond curriculum reform: confronting medicine's hidden curriculum. *Acad Med.* 1998; **73**(4):403–07.

121. Hafferty, FW, Franks, R. The hidden curriculum, ethics teaching, and the structure of medical education. *Acad Med.* 1994; **69**(11):861–71.

122. Suchman, AL, Williamson, PR, Litzelman, DK, Frankel, RM, Mossbarger, DL, Inui, TS. Toward an informal curriculum that teaches professionalism: transforming the social environment of a medical school. *J Gen Intern Med.* 2004; **19**(5 Pt 2): 501–04.

6 Role modeling and mentoring in the formation of professional identity

Karen V. Mann and Elizabeth Gaufberg

The question for us as teachers is not whether but how we influence our students. It is a question about relationship: where are our students going and who are we for them on their journey?[1]

Introduction

Role models and mentors are frequently spoken of in the same breath. Both play important roles in helping new and "becoming" members to develop and navigate their journey into the profession. Indeed, it might be argued that the influence of role models and mentors extends from well before the time one enters professional studies, right through a practice lifetime. There are clearly articulated differences between the roles and processes of mentor and role model. However, they are related functions, and may grow from similar philosophical positions. Both processes are dynamic and reciprocal, involving interactions and adaptive changes occurring in the developing professional.

Certain assumptions inform our exploration of these two processes. First, we have chosen a constructivist approach to understand both role modeling and mentoring. Constructivism refers to the way in which individuals build their own understanding and knowledge of the world through direct experience and reflection on experience. Constructivism focuses on meaning-making, on "making sense" both individually and collectively of our world.[2] Such meaning-making is essential to our development as professionals. The processes of learning through role modeling and mentoring are not passive; in both, the learner actively forms an understanding of his or her own developing identity.

Our goals for this chapter are to:

- Explore the processes of role modeling and mentoring, to understand how they contribute to the formation of professional identity;

- Describe, based on the literature, how current understandings have evolved and how they align with understandings of how learning occurs; and
- Suggest and consider implications of the literature for educators, teachers, and learners, to enhance, support, and grow through these processes.

Two important shifts have occurred in the field of medical education, both of which highlight the importance of role modeling and mentoring. The first shift concerns what many would consider the core of our educational mission: creating the "professional" who, in addition to acquiring necessary skills and knowledge, will also adopt the values of the profession and enact them in an ethical, competent, and professional manner, based in mutually respectful interactions in the context of practice.

The ideas of professionalism and how it is best taught and learned have challenged educators – definitions of professionalism; whether it is an innate characteristic (a trait of the individual) or constructed in interaction with others; whether it can be taught or learned; and how it can be demonstrated and assessed have all been the subject of much scholarly consideration.[3] One major approach has been to link professionalism to certain observable behaviors that can be taken as indicators of underlying beliefs and values. Over the last decade, leading scholars in medical education have begun to refocus the conversation at a deeper level.[4,5] This focus emphasizes the development not of a set of behaviors but of a professional identity, "a way of *being* a physician," which embodies the desired attributes, which in turn gives rise to professional behavior.

The second significant shift concerns our understandings of how learning occurs, which have been enriched and broadened by contributions from the disciplines of sociology and anthropology. Sfard[6] has

---

Teaching Medical Professionalism, 2nd Edition, ed. Richard L. Cruess, Sylvia R. Cruess and Yvonne Steinert. Published by Cambridge University Press. © Cambridge University Press 2016.

described two metaphors for learning that illustrate that change: acquisition and participation. The *acquisition* metaphor describes learning as the acquisition of knowledge, skills, and abilities. These are seen as attributes of the individual, which can then be applied to the problems of professional practice. In the *participation* metaphor, we recognize that learning occurs not only through individual acquisition; it is also developed through active participation in the practices of the community. The *participation* metaphor reminds us that learning is always "situated" and inseparably linked to the context in which it is learned.

Of these two important influences for change, the first has led to the writing of this book. The second shift has implications for understanding the influence of role models and mentors as an integral part of the context and culture of the learning environment. We turn now to explore how role models and mentors contribute to the formation of professional identity.

Understanding the influence of role modeling and mentoring on professional identity formation

Though curricula change, whether by evolution or revolution, the influence of role models remains a central contributor to the formation of physicians. Learners at all levels, and of diverse backgrounds, report that role models play an important part in their education, and educators continue to cite role modeling as the way in which much of clinical learning occurs.[7-10] Similarly, mentors have played a consistently important role in the socialization of new professionals, guiding and advising their junior colleagues and providing a "scaffolding for the learning process."[11]

Learning from role models and mentors can be understood through various theoretical and conceptual perspectives. In keeping with our constructivist view, these can be grouped into those theories that address how individuals learn and develop as they make meaning of their experience and those that emphasize the importance of social, cultural, and environmental influences on learning and development. Jarvis-Selinger et al.[12] write of professional identity formation in medicine as an adaptive process occurring at two levels: the individual level of psychological development, which occurs largely within the person; and the collective level, whereby the individual learns through interaction in the social context

about the roles he or she may play, and how he or she may participate in the work of the community of practice (in our case the profession of medicine).

Theories of identity formation are addressed in greater depth in Chapter 3 of this book. For our purposes, we have selected theories that can both illuminate the process and also suggest implications for us as teachers.

Individual theories of learning and development

Individuals learn and make meaning of their environment through the mental structures or schemata they develop. As people learn and develop, these schemata become increasingly complex and form the bases for problem-solving, decision-making, judgment, and critical-thinking abilities.[13,14] Several important approaches to learning are informed by constructivism, including adult learning principles, reflection, and self-assessment. Development at the individual level has also been seen as a progression through a number of conceptually distinct stages.[15,16] Generally, these stages are assumed to follow each other and may require completion of one stage before moving on to the next. Each stage differs from the others in that it reflects the individual's ability to understand the world in a qualitatively different way.[12] Examples of approaches to learning, which are informed by developmental theory, might include motivation of learners, self-directed learning, and moral and ethical decision-making.

Social learning theories

Sociocultural theories of learning extend our thinking beyond the individual (see Chapter 5). Learning and identity development is seen as social, involving the interaction of the individual with society, through participation and practice. Learning happens between people rather than solely within an individual. For our purposes in this chapter, we will focus on four theoretical approaches: social cognitive theory,[17] communities of practice,[18,19] figured worlds,[20] and the hidden curriculum.[21] For each, we have briefly described the theory and illustrated its relevance to medical education.

Social cognitive theory

Social cognitive theory (SCT), as described by Bandura,[17] brings together individual learning and the influence of the environment. The process of learning includes all of the experience, beliefs, and values that the learner brings to new professional interactions and situations. SCT posits that the developing professional and his or her new environment have continuous, dynamic, *reciprocal* effects on each other. A second fundamental aspect of SCT is *vicarious* or *observational learning*, in which learning occurs powerfully, through observing the actions of others and the consequences of those actions. A third aspect of SCT is *self-efficacy*, i.e., learners' perceptions of their capability to perform the roles and tasks they observe as important in the environment. Bandura[17] describes vicarious learning as second only to personal experience in its influence on self-efficacy. Learners in medical education observe the actions of others in the learning environment (including more senior members of the profession, peers, and patients) and consider whether they might adopt those ways of acting for themselves. Attitudes and values are also learned vicariously, sometimes without the learner's awareness. Finally, through observation, learners also form judgments about their own competence as they develop as physicians.

Communities of practice theory

First described by Lave and Wenger[18] and further elaborated on by Wenger,[19] communities of practice is a second helpful conceptual framework. In this framework, learners enter a community of practice, in this case the profession of medicine, at the periphery. Beginning as newcomers, they gradually move closer to the center in the community as they gain skills and knowledge, become more competent, assume more responsibility, and develop more fully as participating members. Importantly, learning and knowledge are seen as being held not only by the individual but also collectively within and distributed across the community. Role models do not only exert influence as individuals; they also influence learners collectively through their ongoing interactions with each other and their shared values and understandings. Learning is about engaging in and contributing to the practice of the community, in increasingly complex and responsible ways.

Wenger[19] describes developing a sense of identity as one of the most important aspects of participation in the community. To Wenger, identity is fluid and continually negotiated and constructed in interaction with the community. Identity is developed through three key processes: imagination, participation, and alignment. *Imagination* involves learners imagining themselves as a member of the community; *participation* involves participating actively in the practices of the community, in this case the activities of the profession; and *alignment* involves uncovering and adopting the values of the community enacted by its members. In all of these processes, both role models and mentors figure significantly.

A second aspect of communities of practice theory can highlight the potential influence of role models and mentors further. *Paradigmatic trajectories* are visible paths that are provided by members of the community. In any one community, a variety of different career paths may be visible to learners. In the early stages of medical education, perhaps even prior to entering their professional education program, learners may distinguish different trajectories; for example, the trajectory of a surgical career will be different from that of a career in a medical specialty. These different paths shape, and are shaped, as the developing professional finds meaning within his or her community. Similarly, different trajectories can be seen within a specific discipline. Hill and Vaughn[22] have described the different trajectories that are available within the discipline of surgery, how the experience of men and women may differ in the trajectories available to them, and how this may affect their career choices.

Hill and Vaughn[22] studied medical students' experiences of surgery and described four ways in which role models influenced both aspiration and understanding: seeing, hearing, doing, and imagining. *Seeing and hearing* role models enabled newcomers to see who succeeds and what is needed or valued to do so. *Doing* also enabled an understanding of the culture and how certain roles were enacted. *Imagining* built on all of this information to stimulate learners to think about identities within that culture and whether these were identities they could imagine themselves assuming.

As Jarvis-Selinger et al.[12] note in writing about medical education, we can only know ourselves in relation to the groups with whom we interact and the roles we are given in those groups. Socialization into a community of practice can involve many models; indeed, as learners move from the classroom to the clinical setting, and as they assume increasing responsibility, peers and near-peers may provide important models for them as to how to navigate those transitions.[12] Both through their own experience and through observing others in the community, learners gain an understanding of what a community is and its values and of important aspects of practice such as teamwork and interprofessional interactions.

Figured worlds theory

Figured worlds, as theorized by Holland,[20] is a third and complementary conceptual framework. Through this lens, identity is seen as being constantly negotiated between the individual and society. Identity is fluid; it is a "process of becoming" that changes in response to our interactions as we journey through a social landscape. The individual and society meet and affect each other through interpretations and imaginings that mediate behavior. Meanings draw on history and culture as well as current experience, and they are negotiated through language. As the individual makes meanings and interpretations, the meanings can become internalized as a kind of "inner voice." Identity formation is "the meaning we make of ourselves," as we "author ourselves."

As Dornan et al.[23] describe figured worlds in medical education, they note that students may hear many different voices in their world (doctors, nurse, peers, for example); these voices speak about being a doctor in dynamically different, sometimes contradictory, ways. Learners can choose which voices and other aspects of their environment they can use to tell their own stories as they develop. Dornan shows us the rich availability of role models in the environment. In this process, learners have agency; although they may be placed in certain roles in the community, they have the power to creatively improvise and "author" their own identity. As we shall see later in this chapter, a fundamental role of the mentor can be thought of as supporting the learner in this process of self-authoring.

Hidden curriculum

Hidden curriculum, a fourth lens, illuminates another way of understanding how learning may be influenced by role models and mentors. Introduced to medical education in 1994 by Hafferty and Franks,[21] the concept of the hidden curriculum provided a way of exploring the reasons for apparent disconnects between espoused values and goals of the formal curriculum and what might be called values-in-action, as seen through the practices of institutions and the individuals who were part of them. The hidden curriculum has been defined as "a set of influences that function at the level of organizational structure and culture" and included "understandings, customs, rituals, and taken-for-granted aspects of what goes on in the life-space we call medical education."[24] (p. 404) The authors suggested that the hidden curriculum of medical education could be uncovered by examining areas such as institutional "slang," institutional policies, evaluation (assessment) practices, and resource allocation decisions of our institutions.

Scholars have examined the hidden curriculum across many contexts of medical education. More recently, Hafferty and Hafler (p. 17) have described it as "the cultural mores that are transmitted but not openly acknowledged through the formal and informal curriculum."[4] Their analysis focuses not only on the elements of the curriculum and the routines that are taken for granted: it also focuses clearly on role models as those who enact the hidden curriculum. As Bleakley et al.[10] also noted, role models enact the values of the institution. In this way, participants both shape and are shaped by their interaction within the institution or setting of their practice. Not all aspects of socialization are explicit. Indeed, as many of the elements of the hidden curriculum are unspoken, socialization through implicit messages is powerful, and individuals can have internalized some particular values and approaches without ever being aware that they have done so. The hidden curriculum may also be transmitted through the student-teacher relationships that learners experience as they are developing.[25]

Summary

In this section, we have described several conceptual lenses through which to understand learning from role models and mentors and how this learning may influence professional identity formation. While they take different perspectives, there are important congruent messages that emerge: First, learning occurs powerfully from observing others, the roles they play, and the ways in which they enact those roles. Second, through active participation, learners come to understand the values and practices of the community they wish to join, and the meaning of their experience to them as they develop. Third, role models and mentors are important figures in the world which students enter. They influence learning both individually and collectively. They are part of the social landscape, with which students interact as they negotiate their developing identity. Both can help learners to examine how their behaviors align with the emerging identities they are constructing, both at their current level of training and as they work toward developing their identity as a physician.

We turn now to review selected literature related to role models and mentors and their influence on professional identity formation.

What does the literature on role modeling and mentoring tell us?

There is a plethora of literature to inform our thinking about both role models and mentors. We have selected an approach that highlights current thinking and particularly that informs our understanding of professional identity formation.

Role modeling

Role models and their influence on learners have been studied for several decades. The process of role modeling, however, is not fully understood, and there remain some differences of opinion as to how its effect is exerted. Jochemsen-van der Leeuw et al.[26] conducted a systematic review including 17 articles in 2013. Positive role models were frequently described as excellent clinicians who were invested in the doctor-patient relationship. They inspired and taught trainees while carrying out other tasks, were patient, and had integrity. Negative role models were described as uncaring toward patients, unsupportive of trainees, cynical, and impatient. The authors suggested that these findings confirmed the implicit nature of role modeling and proposed that it would be helpful to orient students to the characteristics they should imitate.

In contrast, a systematic review by Passi et al.,[9] while acknowledging the informal and unplanned aspects of role modeling, noted other studies that have suggested that the process of learning and teaching through role modeling must be more deliberate. Specifically, surgical residents[27] perceived that effective learning from role models involved three components: observation, reflection, and reinforcement of desirable behaviors. A study by Weissmann et al.[28] of distinguished teachers identified that those teachers consistently identified the importance of being aware of oneself as a model and mindful in using role modeling as a teaching strategy. The sociology literature describes both "silent" and "articulate" models. The silent model may fulfill only part of the teaching that occurs through role modeling.[9] Passi et al.[9] suggest that being able to reflect on one's actions, and to clarify what was intended, is helpful in facilitating learners to consider various models deliberately. Benbassat[29] suggests that learners should be encouraged to reflect critically on the positive and negative attributes of the role models they have observed, to examine how these experiences fit with their developing identity and their values and goals. Lastly, Cruess et al.[30] described an active, experiential process through which learning from role models occurred.

The literature consistently reports the influence of role models on career choice.[31-33] Further, the attributes desired in a role model remain consistent across many surveys and studies over time. Generally, these attributes of desirable models fall into three groups: personal attributes, clinical competence (which includes relationships with patients), and teaching attributes.

Negative role models are less well understood; however, their impact can profoundly affect learners in the development of their professional behaviors.[9] Their influence appears most commonly to occur in the informal and hidden curriculum.[34] Learners who observe negative behaviors of more senior doctors can experience feelings of powerlessness and of conflict between what they were taught in the classroom and what they see modeled in the clinical environment.[9]

Mentoring

The literature on mentoring, while plentiful, is less robust in terms of demonstrating its effect. The literature on mentors has been explored in depth in two recent systematic reviews. In 2006, Sambunjak et al.[35] reviewed quantitative studies that focused on mentoring outcomes in academic medicine. While mentorship was reported to be perceived as an important influence on personal development, career guidance, career choice, and productivity, experimental studies were lacking. According to the available evidence, fewer than fifty percent of medical students, and in some fields fewer than twenty percent of faculty members, had a mentor. Women appeared to have more difficulty finding mentors than did men.

To gain a deeper understanding, the authors conducted a second systematic review of qualitative research on the meaning and characteristics of mentoring in academic medicine.[36] Mentoring emerged as a complex relationship grounded in mutual interests between parties, both professional and personal.

Consistent with social learning theory, the mentoring relationship was seen as "inextricably situated in a social context and shaped by institutional culture and climate."[36] (p. 77) The good mentor was sincere in his or her dealing with mentees, created a safe environment, listened actively to understand the needs of the mentees, helped the mentee to clarify feelings, motivated and fostered self-reflection, and was well established within the academic community. An engaged, active mentee was seen as important to the development of effective mentoring relationships, as was a facilitating environment at the institution. Barriers to effective mentoring included personal factors, relational problems, and structural and institutional barriers. There was inconclusive evidence on the importance of gender, race, and ethnic congruence between mentor and mentee, and the sensitivity of the mentor appeared more important than matching on any of these factors. Systems of multiple mentors were recommended as an appropriate response to the challenges of mentoring across difference. Both reviews called for more rigorous research to expand and deepen knowledge. In particular, the authors called for deeper understanding of relational and reciprocal outcomes of mentoring such as personal growth, interdependence, and connectivity.

Scholars of mentoring have recognized a disparity between the importance and utility of mentoring and a paucity of theory development for the construct.[37] One reason for this disconnect is the multifaceted nature of the construct, the lack of consensus on "what counts" as mentoring, and how it is distinguished from related functions such as teaching, precepting, and apprenticeship. Many studies fail to clearly define mentoring and instead rely on common understanding. Often a list of attributes suffices for a definition. Darling[38] somewhat poetically identified fourteen parameters of the mentor role, including model, envisioner, energizer, investor, supporter, career counselor, standard prodder, teacher, coach, feedback giver, challenger, eye opener, door opener, idea bouncer, and problem solver. Levinson[39] names five functions inherent to the mentoring relationship: teaching, sponsoring, guidance, socialization into a profession, and provision of counsel and moral support that allows the mentor to aid the mentee in the realization of dreams. The literature reveals several dualities or tensions in descriptions and discussions of mentoring, among them the following: formal–informal, career–psychosocial, hierarchical–mutual, dyadic–networked, and maintaining status quo versus critical appraisal. Each of these has some relevance to how mentoring might affect professional identity formation. We will explore each very briefly.

Formal–informal

Informal mentoring relationships arise naturally and spontaneously on the basis of shared values, interpersonal comfort, and perceived utility to meet career needs.[40] Such relationships are not structured or supported by the institution or other third party. In contrast, formal mentoring relationships are assigned by the institution, and generally involve regularly scheduled meetings and specific productivity goals. There is little evidence as to whether formal or informal mentoring differs in terms of outcomes[40] or whether a supervisor can simultaneously be an effective mentor.

Career–psychosocial

The goal of career mentoring is productivity and advancement including academic advancement, promotion, publication, and attainment of leadership positions. Psychosocial mentoring is more aligned with the construct of professional identity formation and functions to "provide a sense of competence and clarify the 'identity' of the mentee."[41] Outcomes of psychosocial mentoring align with developing and negotiating identity, and include career satisfaction, joy, and work-life balance.

Hierarchical–mutual

In most conceptions of mentoring, the mentor is a more senior person with experience and connections to share and valuable advice for the less experienced protégé. Much more is written about how to be a mentor than how to be a mentee, perhaps reflecting a historical top-down, teacher-to-learner understanding of the mentoring relationship. More recently, the importance of active engagement of the mentee and mutuality of the relationship has emerged. For example, Viggiano[42] tells us that the successful mentee takes responsibility for the mentoring relationship; engages in self-assessment, monitoring, and reflection; respects and appreciates the mentor's time and advice; and cultivates an appropriate personal relationship with the mentor and demonstrates professionalism. Zerzan et al.[43] encourage the mentee to "manage up." The possibility for reciprocity and mutual growth is gaining recognition.

Dyadic–networked

The traditional singular hierarchical dyadic relationship between a more experienced mentor and a less experienced mentee is being re-imagined with the understanding that mentees might gain perspective or advantage from having mentors at several points along the spectrum of age, status, and clinical and life experience, as well as gender, race, and cultural backgrounds. Many authors have identified the need for additional mentoring models and an "expanded vision" of mentoring.[44] Such alternative approaches include mentoring networks (which we will explore in more detail), mentoring panels, and facilitated peer mentoring. Such alternative models may also address the paucity of available women and minority mentors.

Maintaining status quo versus critical appraisal

The final duality aligns squarely with formation of professional identity. Wear and Zarconi in their work on "mentoring for fearlessness" state (p. 54) that it is a mentor's job to "forthrightly and unapologetically nurture the skills *and* values associated with self, profession and society."[45] In contrast to traditional notions of a mentor "passing down" values and standards of the profession, the mentor is obligated to encourage critical reflection on these same values and standards. A primary goal of the mentoring relationship is to help the mentee develop "moral courage."[45] Medical students, for example, at the height of the process of professional enculturation must be supported to actively resist perpetuating practices that characterize the negative aspects of medicine's hidden curriculum – arrogance, lack of empathy, distancing from emotions, and dehumanizing attitudes toward patients. This requires the mentor to model skills of critical inquiry and speaking up, to understand "emotion as a source of knowledge and a catalyst for understanding, rather than a distraction from one's academic development"[45] (p. 61), and to help the mentee explore how power operates in various domains relative to patient care and academic advancement. Wear and Zarconi's[45] paradigm compels us to transcend traditional notions of mentoring solely for career outcomes.

In this brief overview of the literature, we can see an emerging change in the way both role modeling and mentoring are seen. The literature speaks of both processes as active, deliberate, dynamic, and relating to the development of the person rather than resulting in specific outcomes. When we consider this literature in concert with various perspectives on learning, they provide a basis for a view of role modeling and mentoring in which educators and educational environments can support and optimize these processes to support the development of our learners.

Enhancing role modeling and mentoring to support professional development

We wish to highlight two important areas that are essential to support enhancement. These are reflection and reflective practice, and faculty development.

Reflection in effective role modeling and mentoring

No discussion of role modeling, mentoring, or professional identity formation would be complete without a discussion of the importance of critical reflection in optimizing the effectiveness of both processes.

For learners, the literature tells us that reflection is the essence of active learning. It is important for self-awareness in negotiating the process of identity formation; in understanding and making meaning of one's experience; in resolving gaps and uncertainties; in critically reflecting on role models and which aspects of models one might incorporate; and in examining and understanding one's values and ways of enacting them in the face of impediments.[46–48]

Reflection is equally important for our teachers who are role models and mentors. It is essential to developing "role model consciousness" and the ability to reflect on and be deliberate about modeling; it is important for being explicit about what one is intending and modeling.[49] Most importantly, in keeping with changing views, reflection can provide both mentors and role models a means to growth and transformation and personal and professional development. For mentors, reflection allows the mentor to be aware of the personal experience, goals, and expectations that he or she brings to the relationship. For role models, reflection allows the examination of one's own practice, which enables conscious change.

Reflection need not be a solitary activity. In both role modeling and in mentoring relationships, mutual reflection on the experience can build a shared understanding and a joint construction of meaning that will facilitate growth and change for both parties.

Faculty development for role modeling and mentoring

The literature suggests that faculty development to enhance role modeling in support of professional identity formation can be effective.[50] Jochemen-van der Leeuw et al.[26] reported that improved teaching was associated with improved ratings of teachers as role models; a similar finding was reported by Boereback et al.[51] Branch et al.[49] described a multi-institutional longitudinal faculty development program, conducted at five institutions. Faculty members were involved over an eighteen-month period in regular meetings of approximately one-and-one-half hours, in which they learned new teaching skills, and in alternate sessions, reflected together on their teaching experiences. The authors found that participation in long-term small communities of like-minded physician teachers – both learning new skills and having the opportunity to reflect on their experience – was associated with higher learner ratings of them as humanistic doctors, than a comparable group of faculty members who has not participated. The findings of these and other studies[52] support that role modeling may be enhanced by opportunities to examine one's own practices. In working to help our learners develop a professional identity that is humanistic and caring, these findings are important.

A similar initiative is described by Tsen et al.[53] of the development, implementation, and assessment of a faculty mentoring leadership program. The program consisted of monthly one-and-one-half-hour facilitated discussions of topics related to mentoring, using cases and issues from participants' own experiences. The program was established to help a diverse group of experienced mentors grapple together with challenging cases and to further develop their own mentoring skills. The most highly rated sessions were *Mentoring across Differences*, and *Giving and Receiving Feedback*. Emphasis was placed on the value of mentoring networks, encouraging seeking mentorship outside departmental or role "silo," and creating a supportive community of mentors who could turn to one another for consultation and support.

The studies by Branch et al.[49] and Tsen et al.[53] highlight the importance of developing a supportive community of colleagues who develop shared understanding and values and who can enhance each other's ongoing growth and improvement. Steinert[54] has identified the importance of developing communities of practice in faculty development. Such communities may be an instrument for wider institutional change.

An expanded vision of mentoring and role modeling in support of professional identity formation

In this section, we draw on the constructivist and social learning theory outlined earlier, along with the evidence available in the literature, to suggest an expanded vision of mentoring and role modeling.

A constructivist view compels faculty (and indeed all community members) to recognize that one is always modeling, whether intentionally or not. The opportunities for role models and mentors to understand that they are continually observed by learners, that they illuminate pathways or trajectories, that they are important "figures" in learners' worlds, and that they become part of learners' "imaginings" should serve to make them more self-conscious (in the best sense of the term). In addition, the appreciation that, as with their learners, role models and mentors are also in a process of professional formation, and that they themselves both shape and are shaped by the professional learning environment, should inspire in them a more reflective attitude.

As a result, we have envisioned the process of role modeling in ways that support professional identity formation. Role models might strive to:

- Develop and maintain an awareness of themselves as role models. One is always modeling, whether consciously or unconsciously.
- Recognize that the formation of professional identity is not smooth: it is marked by uncertainties and challenges. Models can assist developing physicians, both through modeling different ways to negotiate these uncertainties, and by demonstrating that there are different ways to be a physician.
- Reflect with learners on their own behavior and that of other models they are seeing, as a means to support learners to develop a critically reflective approach to choosing those models from whom they wish to learn.
- Understand that individuals will experience role models and interpret what is modeled in very different ways, in the light of their own values, goals, and experience.
- Encourage learners to critically reflect on what they observe to understand how it might align

with their own values and beliefs. Such factors as gender, ethnicity, and age may affect how learners interpret their experiences.

- Recognize that there is a plurality of ways to be a physician and to enact the values of the profession. Learners may need help to access and observe different models, and see different "figures," as they negotiate their developing identity.
- Encourage learners to reflect on many models, not just physicians, but also other health professionals, and patients.
- Recognize and utilize the value of peer models. They may be especially important as learners make their way through different stages of learning and education and as they understand the roles they fill at each of these stages.
- Understand that role models have a collective as well as an individual influence. Members of a community share the knowledge and values of a community or profession, and the collective influence may be pervasive and powerful.
- Understand that, just as models may be unaware of everything they are modeling, learners may also learn from them without being aware that they have learned.
- Understand that institutional cultures and values are transmitted by role models, and reflect on how those enacted values align with the institution's espoused values.
- Learn through reflecting on their own practices both on their own, but particularly with colleagues and other community members.

Similarly, a constructivist understanding of professional identity formation suggests the desirability of multiple mentoring relationships that map to various aspects of the individual's identity and that meet an individual's myriad needs over time. This allows for the exploration of multiple trajectories and for support in a variety of domains. As with traditional dyadic mentoring relationships, mentors within a network have a genuine interest in the mentees' learning and development and provide access to knowledge, opportunities, resources, and career guidance. The range and reach of such networked relationships can be powerful. These have the advantage of offering diverse viewpoints, experiences, and learning to the mentees more readily than a dyadic relationship that draws only on the experience of a single senior mentor.

Developmental networks can grow, change, and evolve with an individual's career trajectory and work

and life needs and should be regularly assessed and re-configured. Mapping the network can be an important tool. The group composition depends on where one is in a career trajectory and what the mentee feels he or she needs help with – for example, one might find value in having a mentor with success in a particular academic pursuit, another with expertise in negotiation skills, a third who comes from a similar cultural background, and a fourth who is particularly sensitive to the mentee's role as a mother or caregiving daughter. Such models pull for active engagement of the mentee in considering his or her identities, needs, and goals in constructing the network and for iterative consideration as these goals and needs change over time.

Wear's work on "mentoring for fearlessness"[45] has inspired us to imagine what the mentor and mentee might strive for in a relationship that is focused on supporting identity formation. What attitudes and skill set do mentors and mentees need to engage effectively with one another? The mentoring relationship is conducted through language: it involves empathy, learning, talking, and listening. How do mentors and mentees have successful conversations that lead to growth? How do they sensitively and safely explore the places in which a mentee's personal identity(ies) might be dissonant with the dominant conceptions of "appropriate" professional identity? This involves making oneself vulnerable and can be hard work both emotionally and intellectually. Engaging in such effective conversation is a skill that can be learned, and institutions may be wise to invest in such training.

We envision that functions of a mentoring relationship in support of professional identity formation might include:

- Clarifying deeply held core values and giving those values expression in the form of a meaningful career (both mentee and mentor). Working toward integration of "soul and role."[55]
- Using the mentoring relationship to openly reflect on the work and learning environment, including the impact of role models and critical appraisal of institutional values implicit in policy and practice. The alignment or misalignment of personal values, roles, and goals with institutional values and goals should be explicitly explored. Issues of power and hierarchy will come into play and need to be acknowledged.
- Cultivating effective use of nonjudgmental questions, mindful listening, and reflection as a primary medium for the mentoring conversations.

- Tuning into emotional responses to gain deeper understanding of assumptions and values (even as this runs counter to medicine's emphasis on emotional detachment and "objectivity").
- Considering professional formation to be a lifelong journey, on which the mentor and mentee are fellow travelers.
- Striving for authenticity in the relationship, which will likely involve making oneself vulnerable at times. This involves a commitment to talk about the nature and boundaries of the relationship and to navigate problems or difficulties in the relationship, as well as to come to an understanding of when the relationship might need to change or end.
- Cultivating courage, and a commitment to making positive change in the institution and profession. This may involve a critical and responsible examination of the status quo.
- Bringing into the conversation the mentee's (and mentor's) personal, cultural, religious, racial, and ethnic identities – with openness, curiosity, and acceptance – and working to foster integration of identities. Careful consideration of mentoring across differences of gender, race, ethnicity, and socioeconomic background is especially important.
- Understanding that there are multiple relational influences on professional identity formation and encouraging multiple, simultaneous mentoring relationships, group mentoring, and other forms of "mentoring within a community."

Implications and recommendations for consideration

In this chapter, we have attempted to enhance our understanding of the ways in which role modeling and mentoring influence the development of professional identity. In so doing, we have also proposed a broadened view of how both of these processes might be enhanced. We conclude the chapter with some practical implications and considerations for learners, teachers, and institutions.

Implications for teaching and learning

- Learning from both role models and mentors is an active process. Learners must be helped to understand their role in their own formation and provided explicit guidance in how they can participate and learn effectively. Such guidance

may involve practice in critical reflection and discussion of the responsibilities of mentees in creating effective relationships.
- Learners also can benefit from appreciation of the many models that are available to them as they develop their identity as a physician. Beyond faculty members, important models can be found among peers and in other members of the healthcare team.
- Faculty members can also benefit from a renewed understanding of their influence as role models. Opportunities to reflect on their own actions, values, and beliefs can enhance their awareness of themselves as role models, and lead to more intentional modeling.
- Opportunities to meet and interact with colleagues in an environment that builds trust and mutual respect can allow faculty members to learn with and from colleagues through sharing strategies and experience and to give and receive feedback that can lead to improvement.

Implications for institutions

Providing effective role modeling and mentoring for professional identity formation cannot happen without institutional support. Institutions can provide such support in a variety of ways, including:

- Identifying, recognizing, and rewarding those who commit and contribute to these processes, understanding that time and commitment are required.
- Examining and reflecting upon the culture and values of the institution, to ensure that these are congruent with the desired attributes it wishes its members to develop.
- Examining institutional structures, policies, and practices, to ensure that these are aligned with its stated culture and values.
- Providing support and mentoring for role models and mentors, to assist them in the challenges they encounter in their work with learners.
- Providing and encouraging faculty development opportunities, particularly the opportunity to join a group or community of colleagues that will allow for mutual support, reflection, and growth.
- Encouraging and supporting ongoing rigorous study of both role modeling and mentoring, to inform our continued enhancement of these processes in support of professional identity formation.

Conclusion

In this chapter, we have examined various theoretical lenses and literature that can help to understand how role models and mentors can support the processes of professional identity formation. From this background, we have proposed an active and deliberate approach to both mentoring and role modeling. Finally, we have suggested some implications for institutions.

Role modeling and mentoring are fundamentally important processes in the development and negotiation of professional identity at all stages of a professional lifetime. Just as in wider society, it behooves educators to adapt our approaches to preparing "becoming physicians" to shape and be shaped by a complex and changing world.

References

1. Daloz, LA. *Mentor: Guiding the Journey of Adult Learners*. Second edition. San Francisco, CA: Jossey-Bass; 2012.

2. Lincoln, YS, Guba, EG. *The Constructivist Credo*. Walnut Creek, CA: Left Coast Press; 2013.

3. Hodges, BD, Ginsburg, S, Cruess, R, Cruess, S, Delport, R, Hafferty, F, Ho, MJ, Holmboe, E, Holtman, M, Ohbu, S, Rees, C, Ten Cate, O, Tsugawa, Y, Van Mook, W, Wass, V, Wilkinson, T, Wade, W. Assessment of professionalism: recommendations from the Ottawa 2010 Conference. *Med Teach*. 2011; 33(5):354–63.

4. Hafferty, FW, Hafler, JP. The hidden curriculum, structural disconnects, and the socialization of new professionals. In Hafler, JP, ed. *Extraordinary Learning in the Workplace*. Dordrecht, the Netherlands: Springer; 2011:17–35.

5. Cruess, RL, Cruess, SR, Boudreau, JD, Snell, L, Steinert, Y. Reframing medical education to support professional identity formation. *Acad Med*. 2014; 89(11):1446–51.

6. Sfard, A. On two metaphors for learning and the dangers of choosing just one. *Educ Res*. 1998; 27(2): 4–13.

7. Reed, DA, Wright, SM. Role models in medicine. In Humphrey, HJ, ed. *Mentoring in Academic Medicine*. Philadelphia, PA: ACP Press; 2010:67–80.

8. Kenny, NP, Mann, KV, MacLeod, H. Role modeling in physicians' professional formation: reconsidering an essential but untapped educational strategy. *Acad Med*. 2003; 78(12):1203–10.

9. Passi, V, Johnson, S, Peile, E, Wright, S, Hafferty, F, Johnson, N. Doctor role modelling in medical education: BEME Guide No. 27. *Med Teach*. 2013; 35(9): e1422–e1436.

10. Bleakley, A, Bligh, J, Browne, J. *Medical Education for the Future: Identity, Power and Location*. Dordrecht, the Netherlands: Springer; 2011.

11. Walker, WO, Kelly, PC, Hume, RF. Mentoring for the new millennium. *Med Educ Online*. 2002; 7:15. [Accessed April 27, 2015.] Available from http://med-ed-online.net/index.php/meo/article/view/4543.

12. Jarvis-Selinger, S, Pratt, DD, Regehr, G. Competency is not enough: integrating identity formation into the medical education discourse. *Acad Med*. 2012; 87(9):1185–90.

13. Quirk, M. *Intuition and Metacognition in Medical Education: Keys to Developing Expertise*. New York, NY: Springer; 2006.

14. Schmidt, HG, Rikers, RM. How expertise develops in medicine: knowledge encapsulation and illness script formation. *Med Educ*. 2007; 41(12):1133–39.

15. Erikson, EH. *Identity and the Life Cycle*. New York, NY: WW Norton; 1980.

16. Kegan, R. *The Evolving Self: Problem and Process in Human Development*. Cambridge, MA: Harvard University Press; 1982.

17. Bandura, A. *Social Foundations of Thought and Action: A Social Cognitive Theory*. Englewood Cliffs, NJ: Prentice-Hall; 1986.

18. Lave, J, Wenger, E. *Situated Learning: Legitimate Peripheral Participation*. Cambridge, UK: Cambridge University Press; 1991.

19. Wenger, E. *Communities of Practice: Learning, Meaning, and Identity*. Cambridge, UK: Cambridge University Press; 1998.

20. Holland, D, Lachicotte, W Jr, Skinner, D, Cain, C. *Identity and Agency in Cultural Worlds*. Cambridge, MA: Harvard University Press; 1998.

21. Hafferty, FW, Franks, R. The hidden curriculum, ethics teaching, and the structure of medical education. *Acad Med*. 1994; 69(11):861–71.

22. Hill, E, Vaughn, S. The only girl in the room: how paradigmatic trajectories deter female students from surgical careers. *Med Educ*. 2013; 47(6):547–56.

23. Dornan, T, Pearson, E, Carson, P, Helmich, E, Bundy, C. Emotions and identity in the figured world of becoming a doctor. *Med Educ*. 2015; 49(2):174–85.

24. Hafferty, FW. Beyond curriculum reform: confronting medicine's hidden curriculum. *Acad Med*. 1998; 73(4):403–07.

25. Haidet, P, Stein, HF. The role of the student-teacher relationship in the formation of physicians. The hidden curriculum as process. *J Gen Intern Med*. 2006; 21(Suppl 1): S16–S20.

26. Jochemsen-van der Leeuw, HG, van Dijk, N, van Etten-Jamaludin, FS, Wieringa-de Waard, M. The attributes

of the clinical trainer as a role model: a systematic review. *Acad Med*. 2013; **88**(1): 26–34.

27. Park, J, Woodrow, SI, Reznick, RK, Beales, J, MacRae, HM. Observation, reflection, and reinforcement: surgery faculty members' and residents' perceptions of how they learned professionalism. *Acad Med*. 2010; **85**(1):134–39.

28. Weissmann, PF, Branch, WT, Gracey, CF, Haidet, P, Frankel, RM. Role modeling humanistic behaviour: learning bedside manner from the experts. *Acad Med*. 2006; **81**(7):661–67.

29. Benbassat, J. Role modeling in medical education: the importance of a reflective imitation. *Acad Med*. 2014; **89**(4):550–54.

30. Cruess, SR, Cruess, RL, Steinert, Y. Role-modelling-making the most of a powerful teaching strategy. *BMJ*. 2008; **336**(7646):718–21.

31. Wright, S, Wong, A, Newill, C. The impact of role models on medical students. *J Gen Intern Med*. 1997; **12**(1): 53–56.

32. Stahn, B, Harendza, S. Role models play the greatest role – a qualitative study on reasons for choosing postgraduate training at a university hospital. *GMS Z Med Ausbild*. 2014; **31**(4):Doc45.

33. Sternszus, R, Cruess, S, Cruess, R, Young, M, Steinert, Y. Residents as role models: impact on undergraduate trainees. *Acad Med*. 2012; **87**(9):1282–87.

34. Murakami, M, Kawabata, H, Maezawa, M. The perception of the hidden curriculum on medical education: an exploratory study. *Asia Pac Fam Med*. 2009; **8**(1): 9.

35. Sambunjak, D, Straus, SE, Marusić A. Mentoring in academic medicine: a systematic review. *JAMA*. 2006; **296**(9):1103–15.

36. Sambunjak, D, Straus, SE, Marusić, A. A systematic review of qualitative research on the meaning and characteristics of mentoring in academic medicine. *J Gen Intern Med*. 2010; **25**(1): 72–78.

37. Bozeman, B, Feeney, MK. Toward a useful theory of mentoring: a conceptual analysis and critique. *Adm Soc*. 2007; **39**(6):719–39.

38. Darling, LA. What do nurses want in a mentor? *J Nurs Adm*. 1984; **14**(10): 42–44.

39. Levinson, DJ, Darrow, CN, Klein, EB, Levinson, MH, McKee, B. *The Seasons of a Man's Life*. New York, NY: Random House; 1978.

40. Ragins, BR, Cotton, JL. Mentor functions and outcomes: a comparison of men and women in formal and informal mentoring relationships. *J Appl Psychol*. 1999; **84**(4):529–50.

41. Shollen, SL, Bland, CJ, Center, BA, Finstad, DA, Taylor, AL. Relating mentor type and mentoring behaviors to academic medicine faculty satisfaction and productivity at one medical school. *Acad Med*. 2014; **89**(9): 1267–75.

42. Viggiano, TR. Mentoring of faculty in academic medicine: a review of best practices and policies. In Humphrey, HJ, ed. *Mentoring in Academic Medicine*. Philadelphia, PA: ACP Press; 2010: 129–49.

43. Zerzan, JT, Hess, R, Schur, E, Phillips, RS, Rigotti, N. Making the most of mentors: a guide for mentees. *Acad Med*. 2009; **84**(1);140–44.

44. Pololi, L, Knight, S. Mentoring faculty in academic medicine: a new paradigm? *J Gen Intern Med*. 2005; **20**(9):866–70.

45. Wear, D, Zarconi, J. Challenging the profession: mentoring for fearlessness. In Humphrey, HJ, ed. *Mentoring in Academic Medicine*. Philadelphia: ACP Press; 2010:51–66.

46. Mann, K, Gordon, J, MacLeod, A. Reflection and reflective practice in health professions education: a systematic review. *Adv Health Sci Educ Theory Pract*. 2009; **14**(4): 595–621.

47. Sandars, J. The use of reflection in medical education: AMEE Guide No. 44. *Med Teach*. 2009; **31**(8):685–95.

48. Driessen, E, van Tartwijk, J, Dornan, T. The self critical doctor: helping students become more reflective. *BMJ*. 2008; **336**(7648):827–30.

49. Branch, WT Jr, Frankel, R, Gracey, CF, Haidet, PM, Weissmann, PF, Cantey, P, Mitchell, GA, Inui, TS. A good clinician and a caring person: longitudinal faculty development and the enhancement of the human dimensions of care. *Acad Med*. 2009; **84**(1):117–25.

50. Mann, K. Faculty development to promote role-modeling and reflective practice. In Steinert, Y, ed. *Faculty Development in the Health Professions: A Focus on Research and Practice*. Dordrecht, the Netherlands: Springer; 2014:245–64.

51. Boerebach, BC, Lombarts, KM, Keijzer, C, Heineman, MJ, Arah, OA. The teacher, the physician and the person: how faculty's teaching performance influences their role modelling. *PloS One*. 2012; **7**(3): e32089.

52. Wilkes, MS, Hoffman, JR, Usatine, R, Baillie, S. An innovative program to augment community preceptors' practice and teaching skills. *Acad Med*. 2006; **81**(4):332–41.

53. Tsen, LC, Borus, JF, Nadelson, CC, Seely, EW, Haas, A, Fuhlbrigge, AL. The development, implementation, and assessment of an innovative

faculty mentoring leadership program. *Acad Med.* 2012; **87**(12):1757–61.

54. Steinert, Y. Learning from experience: from workplace learning to communities of practice. In Steinert, Y, ed. *Faculty Development in the Health Professions: A Focus on Research and Practice.* Dordrecht, the Netherlands: Springer; 2013:141–58.

55. Palmer, PJ. *A Hidden Wholeness: The Journey Toward an Undivided Life.* San Francisco, CA: Jossey-Bass; 2004.

Experiential learning and reflection to support professionalism and professional identity formation

Thomas A. Hutchinson and Mark Smilovitch

At times I felt like a thief because I heard words, saw people and places – and used it all in my writing…. There was something deeper going on, though – the force of those encounters. I was put off guard again and again, and the result was – well, a descent into myself.[1]

When I (TAH) was a first-year resident in internal medicine, my wife and I attended a New Year's Eve party given by some English people whom we had met recently. We were new immigrants to Canada and so were they, and I suppose we were trying to assuage our mutual loneliness and longing for home. There were a lot of people at the party whom we did not know. We were standing at the edge of a room when we were approached by a man in his sixties. He was interested, interesting, and charming. He, like our hosts, was also from England but had been in Canada much longer. We felt cared for in the safe embrace of his conversation. We talked with him for over an hour and had a wonderful evening. I remember thinking after we left the party, "What a delightful man," and how much he had contributed to us that evening.

One week later, I was on call for the Cardiac/Respiratory Care Unit, receiving sign-over with my senior resident. Various patients were signed out. This one had an inferior myocardial infarction and some arrhythmias; that one had had an episode of pulmonary edema. The last patient to be signed out was a man in his 60s with COPD due to many years of smoking, recurrent episodes of pneumonia and respiratory failure, a probable problem with alcohol, and a history of psychiatric illness. He was now in with pneumonia and respiratory failure, and the clear message was not to try too hard. If we lost this one, the world would not be much worse off. I was doing my rounds that night, and when I walked into the room of this last patient, I felt like I was seeing a ghost. This was the same man that my wife and I had spoken with at the party one week earlier. There was a moment of crashing clarity – what James Joyce would have called an epiphany,[2,3] in which I saw both medicine and this gentleman in a completely new light. I realized how cruel and wrong we could be; this was an injustice not only to this patient, but to all patients we objectify and misjudge. It was also a trigger pushing me towards the professional identity we wish to promote – bringing our full selves to the practice of medicine. It was the very personal and unexpected nature of this experience that made it so powerful.

Knowledge, experience, and identity formation

In the first book of his six-volume masterpiece, *My Struggle*, Karl Ove Knausgård makes a key point about knowledge and experience.[4] Contrary to our initial expectation, he says that knowledge destroys experience. Once we feel we know something, we begin to distance ourselves from our experience and stop being fully present to what is happening. We would argue at the same time that our growth and development slows down or stops. We see the shift from a focus of teaching professionalism to promoting professional identity formation as a move from teaching our students about professionalism to directly attempting to affect their growth and formation as persons and as professionals. In that endeavor, experience is more important than knowledge.

The above observations do not mean that we stop teaching didactically or that we simply wait for students to have the kind of experience related above. A structure to teaching that gives students an authentic experience that promotes growth and professional

Teaching Medical Professionalism, 2nd Edition, ed. Richard L. Cruess, Sylvia R. Cruess and Yvonne Steinert.
Published by Cambridge University Press. © Cambridge University Press 2016.

identity formation is needed. A powerful example is contained in *The Choice is Yours*, a movie that we show to the first-year medical class at McGill. Victor Frankl, the film's protagonist, is faced with a shocking and terrifying choice – take his visa for America and leave his parents to the mercy of the Nazis, concentration camp, and probable death, or stay in Vienna and join them in the same fate.[5] Contrary to every instinct for self-preservation that the students share with him, Frankl stays. And yet, this choice responds to a deep longing that we all share to be there for those we care about and love. We find that students find it hard to remain unmoved by this movie and this choice. We have had individual students read more about Frankl, and multiple students form a group to read Frankl's book, *Man's Search for Meaning*.[6] The movie provides an experience that brilliantly combines profound yearning[7] and a difficult dilemma in a way that promotes professional identity formation and deep reflection.[8] Frankl's life[6] also illustrates to students how identity is not imposed but created by the connection and meaning we discover in our experience. In the chapter that follows, we have attempted to combine what the literature says about experience and experiential learning, with ideas and methods that have proved powerful in our lives and our core teaching of medical students.

Experience, experiential learning, and reflection

Experiential learning

What is experience and how do we learn from it? A good definition of experiential learning is "constructing knowledge and meaning from real-life experience."[9] John Dewey was the first person in modern times to address this issue in education.[10] Dewey was reacting to traditional education, which attempted to impose an accepted structure of knowledge on students. He argued that teaching should start with students' own experience. He saw experience as having two dimensions: interaction and continuity. The interaction was between the person and the environment in the moment. This interaction occurred in the context of past experience, the present, and the future experience to which it would lead. Dewey saw the need for the interaction between the student and the learning environment to have balance. The interaction needed to include enough of the students'

experience to not overwhelm him or her with dry theories or facts. Effective teaching and learning were not simply dependent on the intensity or balance of the current interaction. The final judgment of whether learning had taken place should be based on the future experience to which it would lead. Knowles,[11] who focused particularly on adult education, is in agreement with Dewey's basic structure, stressing issues of particular relevance to adults: the need to know; the learner's self-concept; the role of the learner's experience; readiness to learn; orientation to learning; and motivation. Kolb[12] sees experiential learning as a four-stage process going from concrete experience, to reflective observation, to abstract conceptualization, to active experimentation, and then back to concrete experience. The process as described by Dewey would fit Kolb's staged process very well. However, as other authors have pointed out, the real world is probably more chaotic than Kolb's simple four-stage process suggests.[13] Other writers such as Levin and Piaget have also contributed to the understanding of experiential learning, which focuses primarily on the learning, growth, and development *within the individual*.[13]

An additional perspective coming primarily from Marxist writers such as Vygotsky[13] is that of learning as a sociocultural phenomenon. From this point of view, it is not only the individual student who learns – the milieu in which he or she operates also changes; in fact, it is a two-way street – the student is changed by the environment in which he learns, and in turn changes the environment. With this realization as the primary focus, the main concern becomes how to ensure that students have an "authentic experience gained in clinical workplaces."[13] This is the objective of giving students early clinical exposure and particularly relates to the importance of clerkship in the development of students' professional identity. It is not just a question of what students are taught cognitively in this clinical environment, but how they are included and supported as participants in clinical care. There is some concern that the authentic clinical milieus in which students participate are not ideal[14] and are difficult to structure in a way that optimizes students' learning and development.[15] We have a lot to learn and probably to change in the future. It is also true that Dewey's model of experiential learning remains relevant, specifically his idea that experiential learning has an element of continuity.[10] Students' experience in the clinical milieu will be affected by their prior experience and preparation, by parallel educational activities that help them make sense of their experience, and by the future to which they see their clinical education leading. Whether viewed primarily on an individualistic basis or as a sociocultural phenomenon, the key to experiential learning is reflection.

Reflective thinking

Dewey was very much aware of the need for reflection in the kind of experiential learning he proposed. He defined reflection as "active, persistent, and careful consideration of any belief or supposed form of knowledge in the light of the grounds that support it and further conclusions to which it tends."[16] He gives three progressively more abstract examples of reflective thinking: deciding how to get to an appointment on time given different possibilities of transportation; what the purpose of a long pole projecting from the upper deck of a ferry boat is; and why bubbles appear on the outside of an upended tumbler after washing.[17] The logic and clarity of the reflective thinking outlined by Dewey is exactly the kind of thinking that leads to the increased knowledge and scientific understanding that we hope medical students and doctors will bring to solving the diagnostic and therapeutic problems with which they are faced. This is the kind of reflection that might occur in a small group studying renal function and the concept of glomerular filtration rate or in a group trying to understand the concept of length-time bias in clinical epidemiology. Such understanding is crucial in developing the scientifically sophisticated physicians that patients need; however, it is not the whole story of the kind of reflection necessary for professional practice.

Reflective doing

In 1983, Donald Schön published *The Reflective Practitioner*.[18] Schön was looking at various professions, including medicine, and focused on "how professionals think in action." He understood that a professional did not simply bring scientific data (whether derived from basic or applied research) to the problems with which he or she interacted – an approach he criticized as mistakenly positivist. He also understood that the professional was not simply trying to solve a pre-defined problem. In fact, too much focus on what appeared to be the problem could divert the professional from seeing the clients'

issue in a larger context that might suggest different problems and different solutions. Rather, he was searching for an epistemology of practice that would include the intuitive processes that professionals bring to their work when they face issues such as uncertainty, instability, uniqueness, and conflicts of values. We believe that the kind of reflection-in-action that Schön highlights is called for continuously in clinical practice and is essential for students to learn. Judgments about how seriously to take a particular patient's complaints, when to pursue a diagnosis vigorously and when to follow and to observe, and when it is safe to send a patient home from the emergency room and when it is better to keep him or her for another day are some of the myriad of such judgments that need to be made on a daily basis by doctors in practice. There is no doubt that the abilities that Schön outlines are important for medical students to learn and practitioners to use, but are they sufficient?

Reflective presence

There is another dimension to medical practice that requires reflection on the part of the practitioner – the presence of the physician in relationship to the patient. Physicians are not merely diagnosticians, therapists, or problem solvers, even in Schön's very broad definition of these words. Whereas Schön saw the primary problem as better thinking and doing, later theorists[19] would see the fundamental problem in clinical care as creating better space for the clinician to use his or her whole person to create a healing connection with patients. In their book *Presence*, published in 2004, Senge et al. focus on the space between thinking and doing.[20] They suggest that it is the depth of our presence in that gap that determines the effectiveness of our relationships and provides opportunities for outcomes that are often unanticipated at the beginning of an interaction. They give numerous examples of this process, from the work of individuals to change in organizations. We believe that we have experienced the same phenomenon in our clinical practice – the more that we can be fully present to the patient and to what emerges moment to moment, the better the process and the outcome. We have become increasingly aware that the relationship with the patient serves an important and perhaps primary role in medical care.[21] To understand this better, we need to examine the nature of medical care, the importance of the healer role, and the kind of medical professional that we wish to create.

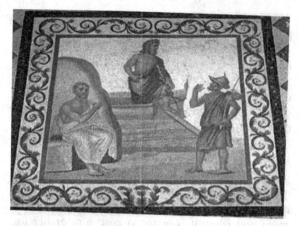

Figure 7.1. Mosaic from the island of Kos. Reprinted with permission from Springer Science+Business Media, LLC.

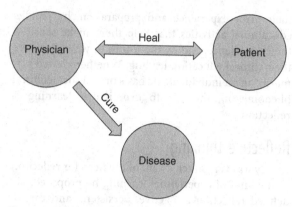

Figure 7.2. The physician's therapeutic relationships to the patient and to the disease. Reprinted with permission from Springer Science+Business Media, LLC.

What kind of medical professional?

Whole person care

Although there are many aspects to being an effective medical professional, as exemplified for instance by the CanMEDS roles,[22] we believe that one relationship – the role of a physician in relationship to a sick patient – precedes and preempts all others in the practice of medicine.[23] We also believe that in that relationship, there are two simultaneous, contrasting, and synergizing roles that practitioners need to fulfill.[24]

Figure 7.1 shows a mosaic from the Greek island of Kos, the birthplace of Hippocrates.[25] On the right of the picture is a Greek patient coming to see a physician. Actually, he is coming to see two physicians; in the centre of the diagram is Asclepius, the Greek God of *healing*, and to the left of the diagram is Hippocrates, representing the *curing* aspect of medicine. This separation of healing and curing is at least as old as the ancient Greeks and is probably much older. It continues in an unbroken line to the current day. As explained in more detail elsewhere,[25] when we make a diagnosis we separate the physician's job into two separate endeavors (see Figure 7.2). In his or her relationship to the disease, the physician's role is to cure, to fix, to control, and possibly to eradicate. In his or her relationship with patients, the job is to promote healing.

Table 7.1 shows some of the contrasts between healing and curing, from both the patient's perspective and the physician's perspective.[26] It starts with the contrast between curing and healing. Curing is an attempt to control or eradicate a disease for which the energy primarily comes from the practitioner and the medical system.[27] Healing is a move toward a greater sense of integrity or wholeness (whether or not the disease is cured), for which the energy primarily comes from the patient.[28] Still, the physician has a crucial role in supporting or facilitating this transformative healing process.[29] The table demonstrates that each characteristic that is important for curing is contrasted with a diametrically opposed process that is important for healing. This contrast is very real, and these truly are diametrically opposed processes. One cannot be replaced by the other, but they do synergize and reinforce each other. For instance, the more competence and knowledge a physician possesses in curing disease, the more open the patient is likely to be in relating to the physician in a way that facilitates healing. By contrast, the more effective the physician is in relating to the patient as a person, the more likely he or she is to join the physician in curing the disease by following advice, taking medications as prescribed, and so on. Medicine is a complicated and challenging job in which we are asked to do two diametrically opposed and synergizing jobs at the same time – a process we call whole person care.[30] How do we support the formation of a medical professional who is able to do what Scott Fitzgerald said was the test of a first-rate intelligence – "the ability to hold two opposed ideas in mind at the same time and still function"?[31]

Mindfulness

Although a great deal of attention has been given to reflective practice in the medical literature, most of

Table 7.1. Differences in the Hippocratic and Asklepian approaches. Reprinted with permission from Springer Science +Business Media, LLC.

	Hippocratic	Asklepian
Patient		
Problem	Symptoms or dysfunction	Suffering
Possibility	Being cured	Healing
Action	Holding on	Letting go
Goal	Survival	Growth
Self-image	At the effect of disease	Responsible for coping with illness
Doctor		
Focus	Disease	Person with illness
Communication	Content Digital Conscious	Relationship Analog Unconscious
Power	Power differential	Power sharing
Presence	Competent technician	Wounded healer
Epistemology	Scientific	Artistic
Management	Standardized	Individualized
Effect	Real	"Placebo"

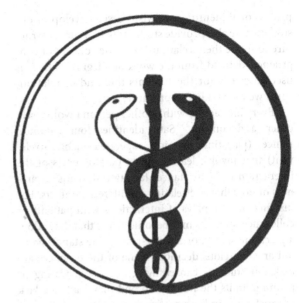

Figure 7.3. The metaphor of the two snakes. Reprinted with permission from Springer Science+Business Media, LLC.

the published studies have focused primarily on the cognitive components of reflection – how to train practitioners to think and do differently and better.[32] We would suggest that a deeper focus for reflection should be on the being or presence of the practitioner that provides the ground for his or her thoughts and actions. Mindfulness has been described by Kabat-Zinn as the awareness that arises from paying attention moment to moment nonjudgmentally.[33] This is the kind of awareness that physicians require to provide the deep presence that is necessary to promote relationships, real change, and problem resolution.[20] Mindfulness as a practice that focuses on being present was first introduced to the medical literature by Epstein[34] and is now recognized as a form of reflective practice.[35] There is evidence that mindfulness practice improves the well-being of practitioners[36] and that mindfulness itself improves quality and patient satisfaction in the clinical encounter.[37] It is also the type of awareness that will allow physicians to encompass simultaneously the two aspects of medicine,[24] the curing

face and the healing face. The caduceus is used as a metaphor, with the white snake representing curing and the black snake representing healing to symbolize this process to our students (see Figure 7.3).[26]

The story goes that one day the god Hermes came upon two warring serpents.[38] He thrust his staff between them, separating them and preventing either snake from overcoming the other, but maintaining them in a balance and tension between opposing forces. This represents the balance and tension between curing and healing in medicine. And what does the staff between the two snakes represent? The staff represents the mindful physician whose ability to be fully present allows him to identify, not with curing and not with healing, but with what is emerging in the moment-to-moment interaction with the patient. This sounds like a difficult task but it is exactly what we have experienced in our own practices. When faced with a difficult problem, we have found that what works best is not favoring the curing agenda or the healing agenda, but being open to both, focusing on moment-to-moment engagement with the patient. An example of this process in a young woman contemplating discontinuation of her dialysis treatment for her chronic renal failure is described in detail elsewhere.[30]

Congruent presence

Since it is improving their presence in their relationship with patients that is the primary goal in the professional identities we wish to see develop in our students, we also provide students with a simple structure to frame these relationships. The concept of congruence, derived from the work of Virginia Satir,[39] is used to clarify for the students the kind of relationships we are seeking to promote.

Every interaction with another person involves self, other, and context.[25] Satir identifies four common stances (placating, blaming, super-reasonable, irrelevant) that involve leaving out a part or parts of the interaction.[40,25] The stances facilitate students' awareness of how they are relating in different contexts. For instance, in role plays of interactions with patients or colleagues, students may become aware that they adopt a placating stance, or a super-reasonable stance, without any conscious decision. None of these stances are bad, but students can easily sense how placating or blaming limits the interaction and may lead to a lack of satisfaction in both parties or even to outright conflict. Once a stance is brought to awareness, the student has a choice – to stay in that stance or put back the missing part(s). Being aware and present for all parts in an interaction is what Satir would call *congruent*.[39] Students are encouraged to seek congruence in all of their relationships because this is central to the kind of professional identity formation we wish to promote – that of the competent clinician who is also a healer.

Interestingly, the mindful awareness that allows one to be present for both curing and healing is the same awareness that allows one to be congruent in our clinical interactions – present to ourselves, the patient, and the clinical context. Clinical congruence is a learned skill that takes all of our human capabilities and also requires us to address an obstacle that is very powerful in the medical context – death anxiety.

Death anxiety and professional identity formation

One self-evident aspect of medicine is that our patients die. Even with the best possible care, they die, and when they don't die, we fear (and know) that they will. Solomon et al.[41] have shown in numerous experiments that anything that makes us aware of our own mortality triggers defenses that shield us from the terror that thoughts of our own death involve – terror management theory.[42] Such triggers can be anything from passing by a funeral parlor to answering a questionnaire that mentions death. We in medicine live in a world bombarded by such triggers.

What defenses would we expect to see activated and how might they be expected to affect our professional practice? According to Pyszczynski et al.,[42] the first or proximal defenses consist in suppressing the information and attendant anxiety. This explains why most people, including physicians, deny that they think a lot about their own mortality. These proximal defenses are not very effective and the psyche seeks a more powerful solution to the problem – the distal defenses. Awareness of our own mortality (that we could disappear tomorrow, virtually without trace) is a severe blow to our self-esteem. The distal defenses drive us to bolster our self-esteem by associating with a group with whom we have some connection. Presumably, we feel better about ourselves if a group who shares our values will survive, even if we ourselves may die. More problematically, we distance ourselves from groups who do not share our values – those we consider "other." These researchers have demonstrated multiple examples of this phenomenon in controlled experiments, whether the group identities are associated with religion, ethnic origin, social class, or other factors.[43] We, and others, have posited that medical professional identity can function in exactly the same way. And the group considered "other" in this context may be patients.[41]

Controlled experiments to demonstrate this phenomenon in medicine do not yet exist (though such research would be very important), but we believe that we see this phenomenon frequently in our clinical practice. It is at the heart of why doctors tend to distance themselves from their patients and of why they tend to focus more on the curing than on the healing aspects of medicine. In a curing mode, my skills and knowledge are what distinguish me from my patients and make them appear as other. They are dying but they are not part of my group. On the other hand, in the healing mode, I need to adopt the wounded healer role (the patient and I are brothers), and no such distancing or "othering" will work.[44]

How can we envisage ways to deal with this inherent aspect of medical practice and avoid turning medical professional identity formation into a means of bolstering our own self esteem by distancing ourselves from our patients? There is no quick answer to this problem, but the solution probably lies in deliberately bringing death anxiety to consciousness. This is supported by a long tradition in Buddhist meditation in which bringing one's own mortality to consciousness is a powerful path to mindfulness.[45] We also believe that there is a lesson to be learned from the experience of the palliative care and hospice movement.[46]

Reflection on experiential learning, reflection, and identity formation

How does the focus on mindfulness and congruence fit with our previous discussion of experiential learning and reflection and with what we see as priorities in medical professional identity formation? It is important to realize that our task will never be to focus on healing at the expense of curing, or thinking and doing at the expense of being. However, we do see a gradation in terms of order and depth. Perhaps the best analogy is Satir's iceberg metaphor,[47] with actions clearly visible at the top, and deeper levels of the psyche such as thoughts, feelings, expectations, and powerful longings and yearnings at progressively lower levels. The key aspect of this vertical perspective is to realize that lower levels provide the energy for higher levels. Most of us have had the experience of the ease with which we are motivated to think and to act when we are passionate about an endeavor.[48] We want, as far as possible, to nurture students' passion for medicine, which is why our priority in both experiential learning and the reflection based on it is to put students in deep touch with why they are pursuing a medical career and what they hope to bring to their work. Our experience is that most students are very much in touch with what might be called their deepest yearnings to make contact with and make a profound difference in the lives of their patients early in their careers, and that this can become eroded as their professional identity develops. So, we see that the highest priority in experiential learning and reflection is to keep students deeply in touch with themselves and their deepest motivations.

In an excellent article on reflection and phronesis, Kinsella[49] identifies four kinds of reflection, which she names: receptive reflection; intentional reflection; embodied reflection; and reflexivity. She sees them respectively as relating to being, thinking, doing, and deconstructing and becoming. The correspondence of the first three to our categories of reflective presence, reflective thinking, and reflective doing is very clear. We see reflective presence as being primary and feeding into the other two. This is why we put such a high value on

mindfulness as a way of helping students deal with distractions, preoccupations, and their own reactivity so that they can make deep contact with themselves and with their patients in the service of both curing and healing. This also fits with Satir's model of congruence, in which the motor force for being congruent (fully present to self, others, and context) is being in touch with deep levels of our personal icebergs, and in particular, our yearnings and longings.[7]

What about the fourth kind of reflection that Kinsella calls reflexivity? We see this form of reflection as very relevant to medicine and to professional identity formation as a sociocultural phenomenon in which students are changed by, and participate, in an ongoing sociocultural change in medicine and society.[13] It is important that students become aware of the sociocultural realities that surround them in medicine and society and are able to reflect on and respond to their environment in a broad sense – reflexivity. We do not see students as only passive recipients in the process; in addition, they are agents capable of not only accepting and participating in the norms of their environment but also of "resisting" when their deepest values are threatened. In fact, as Shem and Bergman point out, resisting may be the most important act of medical students and residents to maintain their integrity and professional identity in a medical environment that is too often uncaring and dehumanized.[50] We believe that the real hope of medicine lies not in passing on current medical practices and attitudes to students as they become doctors, but in promoting a new kind of professional identity in our students that sees deep connection as the highest priority in their own lives and in their relationships with patients.

Pedagogic strategies

Orientation

In the section that follows, we illustrate some of the ways we use experiential learning and reflection to promote mindful congruence in a clinical context. All of the sessions involve reflection on the part of students, although, as Kinsella points out,[49] it is impossible to completely separate the four kinds of reflection, particularly in a live session. We attempt to keep in mind the words of T.S. Eliot from his *Choruses from "The Rock."*[51]

Where is the life we have lost in living?

Where is the wisdom we have lost in knowledge?

Where is the knowledge we have lost in information?

We follow the order suggested by Eliot, first to attempt to provide students with a powerful experience, then to tap their own and others' wisdom, and only as necessary to aid in those primary purposes to impart a cognitive framework (knowledge) and relevant supporting data (information). We believe that this is likely to have a long-term impact on our students.

Lectures

Because of the way McGill's curriculum is organized, lectures occur primarily in the first year. We seek to use our lectures to harness the students' optimism and enthusiasm in the service of a professional identity that emphasizes mindful congruence in relating to patients and commitment to both technical excellence and the facilitation of healing. Part of this is clarifying some of the cognitive frames through which we see medicine. However, lectures are also a good way of touching students' emotions, getting them engaged both cognitively and at a deeper level, and inspiring them to put their whole selves into their development as doctors.

To have this kind of effect, lectures need to become experiential, and we concur with Heath and Heath on ways to do this.[52] Their formulation of what makes teaching effective is useful. All of our teaching sessions have the following four elements: Surprise; Engagement; Emotional involvement; Stories. Let us briefly examine each of these in turn.

Surprise. Most students arrive at lectures carrying with them whatever happened earlier in the day, concerned about what more they need to do before their day is complete, with an overriding attitude of "business as usual." It is how most of us live most of our lives. It takes something unexpected to get us and them out of this mode. We attempt to use the material we are presenting to give students a surprise early in our lectures. This might be a short story with a surprising ending, an interactive exercise that raises their awareness, or anything else within the topic to be discussed that gets their attention because it is unexpected. This requires creativity on the part of the lecturer, but it is surprisingly easy once mastered and part of the joy and (for us) duty of a medical teacher.

Engagement. The objective is to get the students to work with the lecturer. There are several techniques: posing questions to the class, getting them to talk with each other about a topic before answers are provided, and frequently asking for comments and questions to which the lecturer then responds. The class should become a conversation, not a monologue. It may include doing role plays in front of the class with students playing the roles. One of the factors that we have found interferes with engagement is students who spend the whole class on their laptops or phones. We have been unwilling to outlaw this practice but have found that simply requesting that students close their electronic devices is remarkably effective.

Emotional involvement and Stories. We have found these two elements to be the most important factors in making our lectures experiential and effective. They are discussed together because it is difficult to involve students emotionally without stories, and stories have the additional benefit of tying a lecture together and making it memorable.[52] We have used performed stories in the form of movies or passages from books, but, in our experience, the most effective stories are personally experienced and emotionally charged clinical experiences that put the student in a patient's or physician's shoes. If possible, we like to have a single major story that is introduced early on and returned to for further elaboration at intervals and at the end of the lecture. For us, the success of a lecture depends more than anything on our ability to find a suitable and powerful story to involve our students emotionally and illustrate the points we are trying to get across.

Panel discussions

One effective way that we have found to engage in reflection and retain students' attention and engagement, to involve them emotionally, and to teach effectively about the impact of medical care on patients and on practitioners, are panel discussions in which patients or physicians respond to questions about their own experience.

We run these sessions with three or four panel members who consist of either patients or physicians (we usually do not mix them). We attempt to pick participants with very different experiences and backgrounds. The panel is chaired by one of us who poses the questions, reflects on the answers if appropriate, and keeps the discussion on track so that the lessons emerging are highlighted. The questions that we pose are very straightforward, focusing on a brief resumé of the person's background and story, their worst experience, their best experience, and what they learned that they wish they had known earlier or would like to pass on. It is extraordinary how effectively and movingly both patients and physicians respond to these questions. These are not questions that students normally get to ask their patients in clinical care or to pose to their mentors. For both patients and physicians, the stories and experiences they remember most vividly almost exclusively concern the relationship between patient and doctor at a human rather than technical level. In our experience, patients do remember clinical mistakes, but they primarily focus on the attitude and response of the physician(s) involved.

Often, the issue is primarily one of attitude and communication. A woman in her 50s who had been diagnosed with ovarian cancer recalled asking her doctor after the operation to remove the tumor, "Tell me whether I will survive with this disease." His response as he left the room was to say, "Ask me again in two years." She was devastated and said she spent the next two years in a state of limbo waiting for the tumor to return. It did not recur, and now, ten years later, she was doing well. She praised her doctor for his wonderful care in every other way, but the words he used that day would never be forgotten.[53] Doctors have their own failures in relationships that may stay with them for a lifetime. A senior medical subspecialist recalled that many decades ago, when he was beginning his medical practice, he had been caring for a young man with a serious but treatable disease. As it became evident that the treatments were not working and the patient was deteriorating and probably beginning the dying process, our colleague stopped visiting. He felt he did not know what to say but realized in retrospect (and to some extent at the time) that his presence could have been very important to the patient. He recounted this failure (rather than cognitive or technical failures) as the worst experience in his long and productive career. There are many other such stories that touch the students deeply and help them reflect on the values that are fundamental to medical practice. Teaching students about such values didactically is important, but hearing authentic accounts of how patients and physicians experience these values in clinical care has more impact and is likely to have a more lasting effect.

Patients and physicians also very vividly remember the good things that were done. Patients remember the doctor who took the extra time to explain a problem in detail or to reassure them; doctors remember the times they went beyond the call of duty or usual practice for a particular patient and how rewarding that was for the doctor himself or herself. Students find these sessions very motivating and inspiring. There are always many questions to the participants, and our main challenge is to bring these sessions to a close in the face of students' overwhelming curiosity and enthusiasm.

A small-group course on mindful medical practice

Despite the impactful nature of our simulation sessions described later, we realize that students may require a more prolonged exposure to these ideas and experiences to have a long-term effect. For this reason, a seven-week small-group core course aimed at helping students to be mindfully congruent in a clinical context was designed.[54] Each class includes an experiential element, an opportunity to reflect, and a clear cognitive message. The process involves brief periods of guided awareness, narrative exercises, simple role plays, dyadic sharing, and group reflection and discussion. Topics of individual classes include medical mistakes, resilience, being present to suffering and death, and challenging interviews. The aim is to prepare students for the intense clerkship experience with awareness and skills that will help them to be both more resilient and more effective in their clinical work.[55]

Essays and whole class reflection

The most significant influence on students' professional identity formation is probably not the preclinical teaching in the first two years, but the intense experience in the third- and fourth-year clerkships. As evidenced by a change in students' attitudes and values during this period, not all of the clinical exposure is supportive of the desired professional identity. To get students to reflect on their clinical experience, and at the same time to turn back the clock to their values and views before clerkship, they are asked to write an essay on a topic related to healing. To pass the course, each student must write an essay that addresses a variety of topics relating to healing that can be summarized as "Experience of the healer role at its best" or "Experience of the healer role at its worst."

Part of the benefit is in the students' reflective process in writing the essay and receiving faculty feedback. A second aspect of the learning process is that these essays are used in a recall day in which selected essays are discussed with the entire medical class. Three or four essays (including the winning essay) are selected to be read in front of the whole class. A facilitated discussion takes place that includes the students and a panel of four faculty members, each of whom are assigned a specific role in their review and reflection. The roles assigned vary slightly depending on faculty participants, but usually include the following: Dr. Healing, Dr. Ethics, Dr. Professionalism, and Dr. Physicianship. Despite the artificiality of these assignments, it has been found that the resulting multifaceted discussions that include active student participation are extremely rich and powerful. Students are interested to hear the essays of their classmates, and the essays that are chosen have proved to be excellent, provocative, and illuminating. Students appreciate a day out of their busy clinical work to reflect on their personal experience and those of their peers. We find that whatever the specifics of the essays chosen for review, there is enough common in the students' experience that they can easily relate their own experience to that recounted. The subsequent discussion allows for broadening and deepening of their reflection.

Simulation

One of the more powerful experiential strategies in promoting reflection and professional identity formation is simulation of clinical interactions, with trained actors playing the role of patients or professional colleagues. Such simulation is used at McGill to train students in taking histories and communicating, dealing with professional conflict, and being congruent and resilient in difficult and potentially abusive interactions with professional superiors and patients.[54] Although these are different sessions, some occurring in second year (before clerkship) and others in third year and fourth year (during clerkship), they share a fairly similar pattern and an overarching objective of training students in how to best relate to others in a clinical context.

The sessions that are most clearly aimed at professional identity formation are conducted in third year in groups of thirty students. They are entitled *The Physician as Healer: Resilient Responses to Difficult Clinical Interactions*. We have described these sessions in more detail elsewhere.[54] The key component is that each student participates for five minutes in a deliberately stressful clinical interaction that is then debriefed with a faculty member and the two other students in his or her group of three who have observed the interaction through a one-way mirror. Every student participates in one interaction and observes two interactions. The learning and reflection is organized in three parts: reflection in action during the scenario itself; reflection on action during the small-group debrief; and further reflection for action and the opportunity to share learning between all thirty students and all ten faculty during a large-group debrief. The other parts of the day, consisting of a pre-brief and a faculty debrief, are designed to ensure that faculty and students are well prepared and clear about the objectives of the session, and that faculty have an opportunity at the end of the day to suggest possible modifications and to communicate any concerns they have about the well-being of any students.

These simulation sessions are very powerful. We deliberately push students out of their comfort zone, something that is essential if any deep experiential learning is to occur.[56] Students vary widely in their instinctive reactions, and we use the small- and large-group debriefs to help them to hold a mirror to themselves and to see alternative ways of responding. The overall objective of these sessions is to encourage mindful congruence in clinical interactions, but rather than teach them didactically, we use the students' experience in the sessions as the basis for reflection.

Long-term perspectives

Although the individual experiential strategies named above are important in promoting identity formation, the aim of this whole process is to change medical students in a way that will profoundly affect their professional careers and their lives. The aim is to help students bring their whole persons to the practice of medicine.[26] When looked at from this perspective, additional considerations become relevant.

The complete medical school experience

Medical school should not be a disjointed series of courses, but an integrated whole that promotes individual growth and professional identity formation. One model for this is the step-wise increase in responsibility and clinical expertise that students experience as they progress in their training. However, although our students' clinical responsibility and expertise increase in a progressive fashion, their development as caring professionals does not. There is data that some of the desirable qualities of a medical professional identity can actually decline and decrease, particularly during the clinical years.[57] It is an issue that should be addressed. An appropriate model might be Campbell's *hero's journey*.[58] The key feature of this model is that before people get to a better place, they may need to spend significant time in a worse place with significant suffering – Campbell's *belly of the whale*.[58] For most students, the belly of the whale appears to come during clerkship. The question might not be how to avoid the descent, but how to use it most effectively in the students' subsequent development as a caring clinician.

These new perspectives raise questions about how to best use them in the service of our students' development as professionals. We do not have answers to these questions but some suggestions.

- Our curriculum should be regarded as an integrated whole with particular attention to important transitions[59] that affect professional development.
- Major transitions should be marked with ceremonies such as the White Coat Ceremony to prepare students for future change.[60]
- Establish ceremonies to mark half-way points or completion of key stages to acknowledge change in process or completion.
- Prepare students better for the difficult stages in their development, so that they are clear that these are merely stages along the way rather than a permanent loss or change.
- Mentorship and peer support, discussed in more detail in Chapter 6, are important throughout the educational process and represent a key element in supporting our students' reflection, growth, and development. We should make certain that our mentorship and opportunities for peer support are maximized during periods of maximal stress (and potential growth).

This is clearly a learning process, and curricula will probably change further as we focus and learn more about the professional identity formation of our students.

Palliative care and medical professional identity formation

One of the profound changes in medical practice in the twentieth and twenty-first centuries has been the palliative care movement, which has radically altered how we care for dying patients.[61] We believe that the movement has not only improved symptom control and care for the dying, but has also begun to change the practice of medicine itself.[62] It is because of the experience of palliative care that the concept of healing has begun to reenter mainstream medical discourse.[28] The deep message of palliative care is the benefit to be derived from openly facing death anxiety. As alluded to earlier, a professional identity that continually suppresses or denies the triggers to death anxiety that inevitably accompany medical practice is likely to be an identity that distances itself from patients' experience and treats them as other.[41] This is not the professional identity that will accompany patients in a deep way or facilitate healing.

The question is how the palliative care stance in relation to death and death anxiety can be brought into our students' experience and reinforced as an essential element of their professional identity. Currently at McGill, all students in first year have a palliative care visit at which they meet a physician and a dying patient. The sessions last one and a half to two hours, and there is time for students to hear about the background of palliative care, to directly hear a dying patient's story and concerns, and to ask questions of the patient and the physician. These are very moving experiences, and some students say that this is the single most important experience during medical school. They do have further exposure to palliative care, but much of this concerns symptom control and other technical aspects of palliative care. It is an open question: "How do we use the palliative care experience to help our students begin to face the death anxiety that inevitably accompanies medical practice?" We believe that an effective answer to this question could be extremely beneficial to the professional identity of our students and the care of patients that they will treat.

Evaluation

The mantra in medical education appears to be that if you do not evaluate it, students will not learn it.[63] Given the difficulty of measuring experiential learning and identity formation, this appears to leave us in a difficult bind. And yet, we wonder if the mantra is correct. In a session described earlier in which students experience difficult and stressful clinical interactions in a simulated setting, no evaluation occurs. The purpose of this evaluation-free environment is to create a safe space where students can risk putting themselves in very stressful situations without fear of failure or negative evaluation. Students engage extremely actively in these sessions and give every impression of significant learning. By their own assessment, their knowledge, skills, and comfort in dealing with difficult interactions are markedly improved after, as compared to before, the session.[54]

What role should evaluation play in experiential teaching aimed at professional identity formation, and is it essential? If evaluation is important, it is not clear what form it should take. For any evaluation to be effective, it must take into account the deep and inherently subjective nature of identity formation, as well as the fact that to observe any lasting change in identity would probably require long-term and intimate exposure to the person being evaluated. Some combination of self-evaluation, evaluation by a mentor, and peer evaluation might be effective but, as outlined in Chapter 11, the development of such methods will require further work and development.[64]

Resilience and self-care

Surprisingly, we believe that the same way of being that will make our students better physicians for their patients is also the key to their own resilience.[55] To quote a *Lancet* article, "But the patient is not the only 'Whole Person' in the consulting room. Evidence in recent years suggests physicians also suffer from the dehumanization of modern medicine. There are many signs that being a physician today is not good for your health: rates of anxiety, depression, and suicide are higher among physicians than in the general population."[65] And most of us are aware that rates of burnout are high in medical students,[66] residents in training,[67] and practicing physicians.[68]

Kearney and Weininger hypothesize that the key to avoiding compassion fatigue (primarily a result of relationships with patients) and burnout (primarily a result of relating to the work environment) is increased self-awareness and clear boundaries.[69] There is increasing evidence that experiential exercises that increase self-awareness decrease burnout in practicing physicians.[36] The hypothesis about

clear boundaries primarily comes from studies of psychotherapists treating traumatized patients.[70] Kearney and Weininger further posit that increased self-awareness and clear boundaries not only help avoid compassion fatigue and burnout, but can actually turn empathy into a *healing connection* for both doctor and patient.[69] It is perhaps the lack of these healing connections that is the real underlying source of the problems that both patients *and* doctors experience with modern medicine.

Experiential training in mindful congruence (awareness of self as a person, the patient as a person, and the context, with clarity of boundaries) is the key aspect of professional formation that will lead to better care for patients and better self-care for physicians. Our personal experience suggests that congruence is important for another reason. When one of us (TAH) took up a job with a significant research component in a major academic medical center, he was almost immediately bombarded with requests to teach and take on additional clinical duties. Luckily, his research mentor had repeatedly warned him that it was important to learn how to say no in order to fulfill both his own desires and objectives (a successful research career) and the long-term objectives of those who hired him (research productivity). Physicians are faced with many such choices in their careers, including major decisions about changes in their career path, such as switching the clinical or academic context in which they work, changing career focus to or from research, to or from teaching, to or from clinical work, or to or from administration. It is probably the congruence of these decisions and how well they fit for the person who makes them that determines more than anything else the long-term health and wellness of physicians. We need to inculcate a professional identity that promotes sufficient congruence in our students and, later, physicians to allow them to make decisions that fit well with their own goals, talents, and aspirations. In the long term, they owe it to the patients, groups, and institutions with which they will work.

Individuation and professional identity formation

The ultimate goal of professional identity formation in medical school is not the production of a standardized identity that is grafted onto the student. Rather, the process is helping the students find themselves and bring themselves fully to the practice of medicine. This means that the result will be different for every student. Perhaps Jung's term "individuation" best describes the process: "In general, it is the process by which individual beings are formed and differentiated; in particular, it is the development of the psychological individual as a being distinct from the general, collective psychology."[71] This is important to consider because, instead of the standardization of process and outcomes that we increasingly rely on in medical education,[72] we are suggesting that medical school should be an environment with significant standardized elements, with a tolerance, and even encouragement, of individual differences, goals, and unique aspirations.

Conclusion

Professional identity formation as a goal in medical education is a commitment to promoting deep change in our students.[73] For that purpose, cognitive understanding will only go so far. Our students need to change in a lasting way, a way that will persist and, we hope, continue to develop and grow throughout their professional careers. We believe that to produce such change experiences rather than knowledge is the key, which is why our curricula need to emphasize experiential learning in some of the ways outlined in this chapter.

But it is not just a question of *how* we teach but *what* we teach. We believe that in the professional identity formation of our students, the ability of a physician to relate effectively and in a healing way to a sick patient should precede and preempt all other roles. In that relationship, two learnable skills and qualities can only be taught experientially and are of paramount importance: mindfulness and congruence.

We would see the story at the beginning of this chapter as a paradigmatic example of experiential learning. A powerful and surprising experience is followed by a strong emotional reaction that triggers a clear and lasting insight that supports mindful congruence in a clinical context. It illustrates key aspects of reflection, particularly passive reflection and reflexivity,[49] that are so important in helping students connect with their individual patients and stay in touch with their own values in a complex clinical and sociocultural milieu. It also epitomizes the key elements in experiential learning that we have described earlier under the acronym SEES: Surprise; Engagement; Emotional involvement; and Stories. These elements can be used to increase the impact of our teaching in formats from large class lectures to one-on-one simulation exercises.

However, it is not just individual teaching sessions, but the whole experience of medical school, that will have a lasting effect on our students. We need to take into account the probability that identity formation is not a process of linear progression, but of highs and lows, wounding and suffering, as well as healing.[74] A model that takes this into account can help us to think more effectively about how and when to support our students through this process. Part of this support would be approaches that we already use, such as transition ceremonies and a mentorship program, but the timing, nature, and intensity of these interventions might change.

Lastly, we need to be clear about whether we are attempting to graft a uniform professional identity onto our students or discover within each student the kind of values, commitment, and independent judgment that will work effectively for them and their patients in their professional careers. The latter is a more realistic and more beneficial long-term goal[75] and also fits with recent shifts in education.[76] Experience is by its nature unique to each individual student. We need to take this individuality into account, and even promote and encourage it, as we seek to design and implement curricula that help to produce the effective, caring, and resilient doctors that patients and society need.

References

1. Williams, WC. *The Doctor Stories. Compiled with an introduction by Robert Coles M.D.* New York, NY: New Directions; 1984.

2. Riquelme, JP. Stephen Hero, Dubliners, and a portrait of the artist as a young man: styles of realism and fantasy. In Attridge, D, ed. *The Cambridge Companion to James Joyce.* Cambridge, UK: Cambridge University Press; 1990:103–30.

3. Joyce, J. The dead. In *Dubliners.* Toronto, ON: Penguin Books; 1957:173–220.

4. Knausgaard, KO. *A Death in the Family.* London, UK: Vintage Books; 2012.

5. Drazen, RY. *The Choice Is Yours.* DVD. Drazen Productions; 2001. Distributed by the American Board of Internal Medicine Foundation.

6. Frankl, VE. *Man's Search for Meaning.* Boston, MA: Beacon Press; 2006.

7. Satir, V, Banmen, J, Gerber, J, Gomori, M. The transformation process. In *The Satir Model: Family Therapy and Beyond.* Palo Alto, CA: Science and Behavior; 1991:147–74.

8. Kumagai, AK. Commentary: forks in the road: disruption and transformation in professional development. *Acad Med.* 2010; **85**(12):1819–20.

9. Yardley, S, Teunissen, PW, Dornan, T. Experiential learning: transforming theory into practice. *Med Teach.* 2012; **34**(2):161–64.

10. Dewey, J. *Experience and Education.* New York, NY: Collier; 1969.

11. Knowles, M. A Theory of adult learning: andragogy. In *The Adult Learner: A Neglected Species.* Fourth edition. Houston, TX; Gulf Publishing; 1990:27–65.

12. Kolb, DA. *Experiential Learning: Experience as the Source of Learning and Development.* Upper Saddle River, NJ: Prentice Hall; 1984.

13. Yardley, S, Teunissen, PW, Dornan, T. Experiential learning: AMEE Guide No. 63. *Med Teach.* 2012; **34**(2): e102–e115.

14. Canadian Federation of Medical Students. *Resources to Support the Learning Environment for Clinical Clerks.* Second revision. Ottawa, ON: CFMS; 2014. [Accessed June 5, 2015.] Available from www.cfms.org/attachments/article/163/Clinical%20Clerk%20Learning%20Environment%20Sept%202014.pdf.

15. Ramani, S, Leinster, S. AMEE Guide no. 34: teaching in the clinical environment. *Med Teach.* 2008; **30**(4):347–64.

16. Dewey, J. What is thinking? In *How We Think: A Restatement of the Relation of Reflective Thinking to the Educative Process.* Boston, MA: DC Heath and Company; 1933:3–16.

17. Dewey, J. Examples of interference and testing. In *How We Think: A Restatement of the Relation of Reflective Thinking to the Educative Process.* Boston, MA: DC Heath and Company; 1933:91–101.

18. Schön, DA. *The Reflective Practitioner: How Professionals Think in Action.* New York, NY: Basic Books; 1983.

19. Fricchione, GL. Implications for the mission of modern medicine. In *Compassion and Healing in Medicine and Society. On the Nature and Use of Attachment Solutions to Separation Challenges.* Baltimore, MD: Johns Hopkins University Press; 2011:409–49.

20. Senge, P, Scharmer, CO, Jaworski, J, Flowers, BS. *Presence: An Exploration of Profound Change in People, Organizations, and Society.* New York, NY: Doubleday; 2005.

21. Beach, MC, Inui, T. Relationship-centered care: a constructive reframing. *J Gen Intern Med.* 2006; **21**(Suppl 1):S3–S8.

22. Frank, JR, Snell, LS, Sherbino, J, eds. *Draft CanMEDS 2015 Physician Competency Framework – Series III.* Ottawa, ON: The Royal College of Physicians and Surgeons of Canada; 2014. [Accessed June 4, 2015.] Available from www.royalcollege.ca/portal/page/portal/rc/common/documents/canmeds/framework/canmeds2015_framework_series_III_e.pdf.

23. Cruess, RL, Cruess, SR. Teaching medicine as a profession in the service of healing. *Acad Med.* 1997; **72**(11):941–52.

24. Hutchinson, TA, Hutchinson, N, Arnaert, A. Whole person care: encompassing the two faces of medicine. *CMAJ.* 2009; **180**(8):845–46.

25. Hutchinson, TA, Brawer, JR. The challenge of medical dichotomies and the congruent physician-patient relationship in medicine. In Hutchinson, TA, ed. *Whole Person Care. A New Paradigm for the 21st Century.* New York, NY: Springer; 2011:31–44.

26. Hutchinson, TA. Whole person care: conclusions. In Hutchinson, TA, ed. *Whole Person Care. A New Paradigm for the 21st Century.* New York, NY: Springer; 2011:209–18.

27. Cassell, EJ. Prologue: a time for healing. In *The Healer's Art.* Cambridge, MA: MIT Press; 1976:13–23.

28. Mount, B, Kearney, M. Healing and palliative care: charting our way forward. *Palliat Med.* 2003; **17**(8):657–58.

29. Hutchinson, TA, Mount, BM, Kearney, M. The healing journey. In Hutchinson, TA, ed. *Whole Person Care. A New Paradigm for the 21st Century.* New York, NY: Springer; 2011:23–30.

30. Hutchinson, TA. Whole person care. In Hutchinson, TA, ed. *Whole Person Care. A New Paradigm for the 21st Century.* New York, NY: Springer; 2011:1–8.

31. Fitzgerald, FS. *The Crack-Up.* Esquire Magazine; 1936. [Accessed June 5, 2015.] Available from www.esquire.com/news-politics/a4310/the-crack-up.

32. Mann, K, Gordon, J, MacLeod, A. Reflection and reflective practice in health professions education: a systematic review. *Adv Health Sci Educ Theory Pract.* 2009; **14**(4):565–621.

33. Kabat-Zinn, J. Introduction: stress, pain, and illness: facing the wisdom of your body and mind to face stress, pain, and illness. In *Full Catastrophe Living: Using the Wisdom of your Body and Mind to Face Stress, Pain and Illness.* New York, NY: Delta; 1990:1–14.

34. Epstein, RM. Mindful practice. *JAMA.* 1999; **282**(9):833–39.

35. Hodges, BD. Sea monsters and whirlpools: navigating between examination and reflection in medical education. *Med Teach.* 2015; **37**(3):261–66.

36. Krasner, MS, Epstein, RM, Beckman, H, Suchman, AL, Chapman, B, Mooney, CJ, Quill, TE. Association of an educational program in mindful communication with burnout, empathy, and attitudes among primary care physicians. *JAMA.* 2009; **302**(12):1284–93.

37. Beach, MC, Roter, D, Korthuis, PT, Epstein, RM, Sharp, V, Ratanawongsa, N, Cohn, J, Eggly, S, Sankar, A, Moore, RD, Saha, S. A multicenter study of physician mindfulness and health care quality. *Ann Fam Med*. 2013; **11**(5):421–28.

38. Davies, R. Can a doctor be a humanist? In *The Merry Heart: Selections 1980–1995*. Toronto, ON: Penguin; 1997:90–110.

39. Satir, V, Banmen, J, Gerber, J, Gomori, M. Congruence. In *The Satir Model: Family Therapy and Beyond*. Palo Alto, CA: Science and Behavior; 1991:65–84.

40. Satir, V, Banmen, J, Gerber, J, Gomori, M. The survival stances. In *The Satir Model: Family Therapy and Beyond*. Palo Alto, CA: Science and Behavior; 1991:31–64.

41. Solomon, S, Lawlor, K. Death anxiety: the challenge and the promise of whole person care. In Hutchinson, TA, ed. *Whole Person Care. A New Paradigm for the 21st Century*. New York, NY: Springer; 2011:97–108.

42. Pyszczynski, T, Solomon, S, Greenberg, J. Terror management research: coping with conscious and unconscious death-related thoughts. In *In the Wake of 9/11: The Psychology of Terror*. Washington, DC: American Psychological Association; 2003:37–70.

43. Pyszczynski, T, Solomon, S, Greenberg, J. Terror management research: prejudice and self-esteem striving. In *In the Wake of 9/11: The Psychology of Terror*. Washington, DC: American Psychological Association; 2003:71–92.

44. Guggenbühl-Craig, A. The closing of the split through power. In *Power in the Helping Professions*. Second edition. Putnam, CT: Spring; 2004:87–92.

45. Wallace, BA. The first point: the preliminaries. In Quirolo, L, ed. *Buddhism with an Attitude: The Tibetan Seven-Point Mind-Training*. Ithaca, NY: Snow Lion; 2001:13–63.

46. Kearney, MK, Weininger, RB, Vachon, ML, Harrison, RL, Mount, BM. Self-care of physicians caring for patients at the end of life: "Being connected… a key to my survival". *JAMA*. 2009; **301**(11):1155–64.

47. Satir, V, Banmen, J, Gerber, J, Gomori, M. The primary triad. In *The Satir Model: Family Therapy and Beyond*. Palo Alto, CA: Science and Behavior; 1991:19–30.

48. Robinson, K, Aronica, L. The element. In *The Element: How Finding Your Passion Changes Everything*. New York, NY: Penguin; 2009:1–26.

49. Kinsella, EA. Practitioner reflection and judgment as phronesis: a continuum of reflection and considerations for phronetic judgement. In Kinsella, EA, Pitman, A, eds. *Phronesis as Professional Knowledge: Practical Wisdom in the Professions*. Rotterdam, the Netherlands: Sense Publishing; 2012:35–52.

50. Shem, S, Bergman, S. Resistance and healing. In Kohn, M, Donley, C, eds. *Return to the House of God: Medical Resident Education, 1978–2008*. Kent, OH: Kent State University Press; 2008:221–36.

51. Eliot, TS. Where is the life. In *Collected Poems, 1909–1962*. Boston, MA: Harcourt Brace Janovich; 1991:147.

52. Heath, C, Heath, D. *Made to Stick: Why Some Ideas Survive and Others Die*. New York, NY: Random House; 2007.

53. Bedell, SE, Graboys, TB, Bedell, E, Lown, B. Words that harm, words that heal. *Arch Intern Med*. 2004; **164**(13):1365–68.

54. Wald, HS, Anthony, D, Hutchinson, TA, Liben, S, Smilovitch, M, Donato, AA. Professional identity formation in medical education for humanistic, resilient physicians: pedagogic strategies for bridging theory to practice. *Acad Med*. 2015; **90**(6):753–60.

55. Epstein, RM, Krasner, MS. Physician resilience: what it means, why it matters, and how to promote it. *Acad Med*. 2013; **88**(3):301–03.

56. Satir, V, Banmen, J, Gerber, J, Gomori, M. The process of change. In *The Satir Model: Family Therapy and Beyond*. Palo Alto, CA: Science and Behavior; 1991: 85–119.

57. Newton, BW, Barber, L, Clardy, J, Cleveland, E, O'Sullivan, P. Is there hardening of the heart during medical school? *Acad Med*. 2008; **83**(3):244–49.

58. Campbell, J. The hero and the God. In *The Hero with a Thousand Faces*. Princeton, NJ: Princeton University Press; 1968:30–40.

59. O'Brien, BC, Poncelet, AN. Transition to clerkship courses: preparing students to enter the workplace. *Acad Med*. 2010; **85**(12):1862–69.

60. Gillon, R. White coat ceremonies for new medical students. *West J Med*. 2000; **173**(3):206–07.

61. Saunders, C. Foreword. In Doyle, D, Hanks, G, Cherny, N, Calman, K, eds. *Oxford Textbook of Palliative Medicine*. New York, NY: Oxford University Press; 2004:xvii–xx.

62. Mount, BM. Foreword. In Hutchinson, TA, ed. *Whole Person Care. A New Paradigm for the 21st Century*. New York, NY: Springer; 2011:vii–xiii.

63. McLachlan, JC. The relationship between assessment and learning. *Med Educ*. 2006; **40**(8):716–17.

64. Nofziger, AC, Naumburg, EH, Davis, BJ, Mooney, CJ, Epstein, RM. Impact of peer assessment on the professional development of medical students: a qualitative study. *Acad Med*. 2010; **85**(1):140–47.

65. Cole, TR, Carlin, N. The suffering of physicians. *Lancet*. 2009; **374**(9699):1414–15.

66. Jennings, ML. Medical student burnout: interdisciplinary exploration and analysis. *J Med Humanit*. 2009; **30**(4):253–69.

67. IsHak, WW, Lederer, S, Mandili, C, Nikravesh, R, Seligman, L, Vasa, M, Ogunyemi, D, Bernstein, CA. Burnout during residency training: a literature review. *J Grad Med Educ.* 2009; **1**(2):236–42.

68. Spickard, A Jr, Gabbe, SG, Christensen, JF. Mid-career burnout in generalist and specialist physicians. *JAMA.* 2002; **288**(12):1447–50.

69. Kearney, M, Weininger, R. Whole person self-care: self-care from the inside out. In Hutchinson, TA, ed. *Whole Person Care. A New Paradigm for the 21st Century.* New York, NY: Springer; 2011:109–26.

70. Harrison, RL, Westwood, MJ. Preventing vicarious traumatization of mental health therapists: identifying protective practices. *Psychotherapy (Chic).* 2009; **46**(2):203–19.

71. Jung, CG. Psychological types. In *The Collected Works of C. G. Jung.* Oxford, UK: Harcourt Brace; 1921:vol. **6**, par 757.

72. Connor, JTH, Farrell, GF. Cracks in the curriculum: an appreciation. *CMAJ.* 2013; **185**(12):1104.

73. Daaleman, TP, Kinghorn, WA, Newton, WP, Meador, KG. Rethinking professionalism in medical education through formation. *Fam Med.* 2011; **43**(5):325–29.

74. Allen, D, Wainwright, M, Mount, B, Hutchinson, T. The wounding path to becoming healers: medical students' apprenticeship experiences. *Med Teach.* 2008; **30**(3):260–64.

75. Palmer, PJ. Across the great divide: rejoining soul and role. In *A Hidden Wholeness: The Journey toward an Undivided Life.* San Francisco, CA, Jossey Bass; 2004:13–29.

76. Robinson, K, Aronica, L. *Creative Schools: The Grassroots Revolution that's Transforming Education.* New York, NY: Viking; 2015.

General principles for establishing programs to support professionalism and professional identity formation at the undergraduate and postgraduate levels

Sylvia R. Cruess and Richard L. Cruess

When the first edition of this book was written, there was a substantial body of information in the literature on how to design and implement programs to teach professionalism at the undergraduate and postgraduate levels. It was possible to elaborate a set of principles on the subject based on both our experience and that of others.[1–3] As we transition to recommending the addition of supporting professional identity formation as the educational objective, equivalent experience is not reflected in the medical literature. Any principles designed to assist individuals in establishing such programs must be derived from the literature on identity formation outside of medicine,[4,5] from the thoughts and recommendations of those who have studied professional identity formation in physicians,[6–11] and from the recommendations of authors who have contributed to this book.

As is emphasized repeatedly in this book, the experience gained in teaching professionalism has been enormously valuable and provides a foundation upon which educational programs on professional identity formation can be built. While some of the principles elaborated to help design programs of teaching professionalism are still useful, new principles are required for new educational objectives.

Any set of principles must be compatible with the complex nature of the medical curriculum, through which individuals become transformed from members of the lay public into skilled physicians.[12] When the teaching of professionalism was the educational objective, there was no unanimity of opinion on how best to organize the teaching, with two schools of thought being predominant. Those who emphasized the need for detailed knowledge of the subject tended to stress formal instruction, making the nature of professionalism explicit.[13–15] They defined professionalism, listed its attributes, emphasized the role of trust, and stressed its importance to medicine's relationship to society. Others believed that the teaching of professionalism should be approached primarily as a moral endeavor, emphasizing altruism and service, stressing the importance of role modeling, efforts to promote self-awareness, community service, and other methods of acquiring experiential knowledge.[1,16,17]

While it would be wrong to overemphasize the differences between these two approaches, they did exist. Establishing professional identity formation as the educational goal quite effectively brings the two groups together. As medicine is a community of practice that students and residents wish to join (see Chapters 1 and 5), the values and norms of the community must be widely known and communicated to learners. Medicine's norms are encompassed in the concept of the profession and professionalism and in the attributes of a professional. For this reason, professionalism must continue to be taught explicitly as the acquisition of knowledge about the nature of professionalism becomes a foundational element in the construction of a professional identity. However, the techniques espoused by those whose educational approach stressed the importance of ensuring that the traditional qualities of the healer were present become essential if the aim is to ensure that the medical profession is made up of individuals who "think, act, and feel like physicians."[18]

Because socialization is the means through which an individual's identity is transformed,[6,7,11] medical

Teaching Medical Professionalism, 2nd Edition, ed. Richard L. Cruess, Sylvia R. Cruess and Yvonne Steinert.
Published by Cambridge University Press. © Cambridge University Press 2016.

educators must ensure that the process is supportive of individuals as they develop their professional identities. The principles outlined below, along with the schematic representations[19] included in Chapter 1, were developed to assist those designing, implementing, and managing programs devoted to the support of professional identity formation in medicine.

Principles

Teaching the cognitive base of professionalism and professional identity formation is not difficult. Establishing an environment where the process of socialization in its most positive sense can take place is much more challenging. The following principles encompass three large areas of activity. First, faculties of medicine and their associated teaching institutions must take a series of decisions that will publicly declare their support for programs designed to assist students as they develop their professional identities. This includes the provision of sufficient resources so that the program may flourish. Second, the learning environment must welcome and support learners as they join medicine's community of practice. Third, the many factors that affect the process of socialization (see Figures 1.4 and 1.5 in Chapter 1) make up this learning environment, and each should be analyzed to ensure that its effect is positive.

In spite of the presence of a long-standing and strong consensus that medical education is a continuum that begins before students actually enter medical school and proceed to residency, and continues throughout an individual's professional life, this continuum is broken up into definable blocks that are both administered and experienced differently. When examining this continuum through the lens of professional identity formation, it is clear that some themes run throughout the continuum. The nature of the desired professional identity, the definitions that revolve around the words profession and professionalism, and the reality of medicine's social contract with society remain unchanged.[20] However, it is indisputable that undergraduate medical education, postgraduate medical education, and continuing professional development are administered separately and almost independently of each other. This separation is accentuated by the presence of separate accrediting bodies for each. Some principles will function at all levels, but many must be adapted for use at each level.

(1) Establish professional identity formation as an educational objective

Professionalism of necessity became an educational objective as it was required for both undergraduate and postgraduate accreditation. Therefore, action by faculties of medicine was required. The Carnegie Foundation report on the future of medical education[20] recommends that identity formation become an essential component of medical education. Establishing professional identity formation as an educational objective will require positive action on the part of educational institutions.[11] We agree with Merton, who stated that the objectives of medical education are to provide learners with both knowledge and skills as well as a professional identity.[18] Recognizing this duality by establishing professional identity formation as an educational objective is an essential step. It will be difficult to mobilize the energy and the resources of a faculty around this objective without such action.

It is also clear that establishing identity formation as an educational objective must occur separately at the undergraduate and postgraduate levels because the educational programs are organized differently, with their own mechanisms of accountability, including accreditation.

(2) Provide institutional support

It is difficult to mount a major change in any organization unless there is strong support from its leadership,[21–26] and educational institutions are no exception. Those directing medical schools and hospitals must first recognize the importance of professional identity formation and publicly signal their support. Financial and human resources are required, and time within the curriculum must be mobilized. Experience gained in teaching professionalism has demonstrated that the additional time required for new activities can be modest, primarily because many activities already existed in the curriculum.[21,24,25] These could be redirected toward teaching professionalism. There is little information available in the literature, but our experience gained in reorienting a program from teaching professionalism to supporting professional identity formation (see Chapter 15) indicates that although a substantial amount of planning time is required to establish educational objectives and strategies, additional time in the curriculum is not required.

The active support of the dean and associate deans for both undergraduate and postgraduate education as well as influential department chairs is key to the success of any significant curricular reform. Establishing a program on professional identity formation does constitute a major change.[23–26]

(3) Allocate responsibility

At the undergraduate level

Establishing programs to teach professionalism has highlighted the importance of allocating responsibility for the program to specific individuals or groups. The decision as to who will be responsible is of some importance, for symbolic as well as practical administrative reasons. Programs devoted to professional identity formation cross departmental and disciplinary lines and should be present throughout the continuum of medical education. An individual should be responsible for guiding the design, implementation, direction, and evaluation of these programs. This task requires a feeling for the culture and internal dynamics of the faculty, a comprehensive knowledge of professionalism and professional identity formation based on the contemporary literature, and tact and diplomacy. The individual should command respect, have easy access to senior administration, be provided with adequate resources, and have the skills and knowledge to both create and administer the program and serve as its champion.

In addition to appointing the leader–champion, most faculties choose to establish a committee or working group composed of knowledgeable individuals from the academic units where the majority of the teaching will take place, as well as local experts.[25–27] The committee's function is to advise the individuals responsible for the program, participate in planning, assist in the administration, and provide leadership in the locales where the actual teaching and learning take place.

Identity formation and socialization are complex subjects whose theoretical base has not been a part of medicine's traditional knowledge base. Much of what we do know has been contributed by social scientists with varying backgrounds who have worked within medicine and other healthcare professions. Both McGill and the University of Texas system (see Chapters 15 and 16) have found it beneficial to include such individuals in their deliberations on both identity formation and socialization.[11,27] Sociologists, psychologists, anthropologists, ethnographers, and representatives of many other disciplines have been of enormous value as programs to support professional identity formation were created. These individuals can serve as consultants or be important members of the responsible committees.

Finally, the increased emphasis on social accountability in medical education[28] has resulted in the involvement of patients and members of the lay public in the educational process. As the nature of the professional identity of practicing physicians is fundamental to meeting societal expectations, we believe that societal input into educational programs at this level is desirable.

At the postgraduate level

In spite of the fact that medical education is recognized as constituting a continuum, responsibility for undergraduate and postgraduate medical education is almost universally divided. Accountability to accrediting bodies is different and the emphasis in postgraduate education shifts to workplace learning[29] (see Chapter 17). Therefore, a separate committee for supporting professional identity formation at the postgraduate level will almost certainly be required. While we are aware of institutions that have a single "professionalism committee" responsible for both at the institutional level, this is not the norm, and the opportunities and problems posed at the postgraduate level are sufficiently different that program design and implementation must be carried out independently. Again, the committee can benefit greatly from the presence of nonmedical representatives from the social sciences and the community.

Because medical education is a continuum, the cognitive base will not change and the educational objectives will remain the same as individuals move to the postgraduate level. However, the educational strategies must change. There are two fundamental differences. First, residents are older and more mature, having already altered their identity during medical school.[6,7,9] They are in the process of layering a specialist-based identity on the identity of a generic physician while also acquiring the identity of a resident. Finally, the gradual shift to workplace learning that began during the final stages of medical school becomes complete and the strategies must thus be altered.[29] However, it is our belief that engagement at the postgraduate level remains similar to that at the undergraduate level. Residents should be challenged to examine their own identity and reflect upon the factors that have helped to develop that identity.

(4) Provide faculty development

The word professionalism was well known to the medical community as it historically represented an important aspirational goal for physicians.[13] Attracting medical teachers to workshops on professionalism was not difficult. It allowed the dissemination of the cognitive base to teachers and role models and highlighted the emphasis placed on teaching professionalism within institutions. Because the knowledge base and language of identity formation and socialization are more remote from the world of medical teachers, faculty development becomes even more important to support programs on professional identity formation.

As outlined in Chapter 9, comprehensive faculty development programs cannot focus solely on individual faculty members; they must also address the increasingly complex institutions in which teaching and learning occur.[30,31] They have the capacity to improve the knowledge and skills of faculty members and, acting through these individuals, to both improve role modeling and alter the formal and the informal curricula.

Faculty development is a powerful tool to achieve consensus and ensure that faculty have the necessary knowledge and skills to both teach and role model professional identity formation.[23,30] For role models to be effective, they must understand the identity they are modeling. This starts with faculty agreement on the norms of the community of practice that is medicine, including definitions of professionalism and its characteristics, as well as expected standards of behavior. The role to be modeled must be made explicit to the role model as well as to the learner.[32]

Well-planned faculty development programs can be beneficial in several areas that influence the support of professional identity formation. They are often instruments to effect change, leading to a revised curriculum.[23] Programs also produce a core group of knowledgeable individuals capable of not only teaching and modeling professional identity but also, through peer pressure, assisting in changing the environment.[23,30] Faculty development can be targeted at the entire faculty, bringing together individuals from various departments and disciplines to achieve a broad consensus. It can also be aimed at individual departments or academic units that have a major role in the teaching of professionalism and the support of professional identity formation. For those faculties establishing tutorial or mentorship programs as a part of their efforts to support professional identity formation, ongoing faculty development for the tutors provides invaluable support.[33]

Our original faculty development programs were constructed around several themes[23,30] (see Chapter 9). The first and most obvious was "How to Teach Professionalism." This avoided any implication that faculty members were not themselves professional. In the process of developing teaching techniques appropriate to the individual or the school, professionalism as a subject must be addressed directly. The same is true of programs addressing "How to Evaluate Professionalism in Students/ Residents/ Faculty Members" or "Role Modeling Professionalism." This allowed the institutional definition and approach to teaching to be disseminated widely. Those who have completed the programs became more knowledgeable and, hopefully, more effective role models. We believe this exerted a positive influence on the informal and hidden curriculum.

These workshops can easily be reoriented to support professional identity formation. Those activities centered on teaching professionalism can continue with some modification, as the norms of the community of practice are encompassed in the word "professionalism," and very little reorientation is required. The same is true of workshops devoted to role modeling. At the present time, evaluation of progress toward a professional identity is difficult to accomplish, and this subject may best be included in workshops devoted to identity formation and socialization.

Building on our past activities, we have added faculty development workshops on professional identity formation and socialization.[33] Faculty must understand both processes and be able to intervene directly to support students and residents as they develop their own identities. Our experience indicates that most faculty members respond very positively to the concept of identity formation, particularly if they are encouraged to think about their own personal identities and how they were formed.

(5) Develop a cognitive base

Our concept of the cognitive base is straightforward. It is the foundation of the formal curriculum, defined by Hafferty (p. 404) as "the stated, intended, and formally offered and endorsed curriculum."[34] A cognitive base should serve as the foundation for teaching and learning around professionalism and professional identity formation.[11,19]

As we shift the emphasis of medical education to supporting the development of professional identity formation, the importance of the cognitive base that was developed to teach professionalism remains essential. Knowledge of what it means to be a professional is fundamental to the development of a professional identity. For this reason, the cognitive base developed for teaching professionalism becomes incorporated into an expanded cognitive base that now includes the nature of professional identity formation and of socialization.

At the risk of being repetitious, it must be stated that medicine represents a community of practice that individuals voluntarily wish to join.[6–8,11–19] To become members of this community, they must acquire the identity expected of members of the community, a process that occurs through socialization. For this to occur, they must know the values and norms of the community that is medicine before they can accept and internalize them. These values and norms have been negotiated between medicine and society, literally over the millennia, and have been encompassed in the term "the good physician."[35] To assist those wishing to become physicians, elaborating the nature of these values and norms is essential. They are encompassed in the words "profession," "professional," and "professionalism." For this reason, the explicit teaching of professionalism remains an essential component of any program designed to support professional identity formation, and learners must understand this relationship.

One of the educational strategies used to support professional identity formation is to engage learners in the process of forming their own identity[6,8,9] (see below). It is essential that learners actually understand identity formation and socialization. These two important items must become foundational to the cognitive base. In our teaching, we use the schematic representations of identity formation and socialization (see Chapter 1, Figures 1.1, 1.4, and 1.5) that are provided to students on their first day of instruction in medical school. They are referred to throughout the four years of medical school as points of reference. Of equal importance is the inclusion in the cognitive base of the norms and values of the profession to which learners aspire. While definitions and lists are important, students and residents can also benefit from a wider comprehension of professionalism and its place

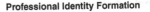

Professional Identity Formation

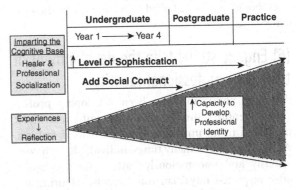

Figure 8.1. A schematic description of the relationship between the cognitive base, professional identity formation, and reflection. The cognitive base of professionalism and professional identity formation should be presented to students on a regular basis throughout the curriculum. Students, residents, and practitioners have an increasing capacity for reflection on professionalism and on their own professional identity as they gain in experiential learning. Stage-appropriate opportunities for reflection should therefore be provided.

in society.[2,36] They should understand the nature of professionalism, the profession's historical roots, its strong moral base, and the reason society supports medicine's privileged position. The obligations necessary to sustain medicine's professional status, and professionalism's relationship to medicine's social contract with society[37] are important parts of the cognitive base. Finally, as outlined in Chapter 1, definitions are important to this understanding, and the attributes of the "good doctor"[35] must be communicated (see Chapter 1, Figure 1.3).

Each institution should agree on the substance of the cognitive base that should remain consistent throughout the continuum of medical education. The definition or definitions chosen do not just dictate the nature of the desired professional identity; they determine what will be evaluated in students and residents, as well as in faculty members.

It should be noted that there is not one definition or set of values and norms for first-year students and another for those in the final year. The same is true for residents, faculty members, and practicing physicians. The cognitive base should be presented to students early in the curriculum and should be reinforced throughout the course of medical education (Figure 8.1). It is possible to present different aspects of professionalism at different stages of training, stressing definitions and attributes early and proceeding to emphasizing the social contract at a later stage. Opportunities for reflection should always be linked to instruction in the cognitive base.

(6) Engage students in the development of their own professional identity

Although physicians have been developing professional identities through the ages, until recently it happened in an unplanned and unfocused fashion. As has been stated many times, individuals both consciously and unconsciously pattern their behavior after respected physician role models.[32] During the past two decades, the requirement to teach and assess professionalism has moved professionalism into the formal curriculum, and most programs included activities aimed at ensuring that learners understood the norms and values of the medical profession.[2,3] The unstated implication was that professionalism was something that was taught by the faculty and learned by students and residents. Shifting the emphasis from teaching professionalism to supporting individuals as they develop their own professional identities represents a major change. The onus is now on individuals wishing to become physicians – joining a community of practice – to actually participate in the process of developing their own professional identities.[6–11]

It is essential that each student or resident become actively engaged in the wide variety of personal choices, activities, and social interactions that affect the process of socialization. Furthermore, they must remain engaged throughout the continuum of medical education.

The educational implications of this approach have not been explored in depth and there is very little experience documented in the literature. However, we would suggest that learners must first be attracted to the process of identity formation by making it personal.[7,8] Interest in the subject should be maintained by introducing activities at an early stage designed to maintain the level of engagement throughout the educational process. We use the schematic representations (Chapter 1, Figures 1.1, 1.4, and 1.5) beginning on the first day of instruction and employing them throughout the continuum of medical education as a means of providing continuity. Students and residents are encouraged to reflect, in a safe space, on the impact of the multiple factors that influence the development of their own identities. Our experience in engaging learners in examining

their own identities and their own progress toward a professional identity has been overwhelmingly positive.[33] This approach appears to personalize professional identity formation as a group activity.

Engagement can also be facilitated by providing opportunities for learners, along with role models or mentors, to actually trace their own progress toward their desired professional identity. Self-evaluation becomes important because how one regards oneself is fundamental to identity. Thus, simple questions asked on a regular basis such as, "What is your personal or your professional identity or identities?" or, "What factors influenced the development of your professional identity?" can serve as triggers to initiate the reflective process that maintains engagement. Simple scales are available that ask learners to rate their progress toward their professional identity – an exercise that can also lead to reflection.[37–39]

Finally, engagement can be maintained by stressing the concept of communities of practice and by both encouraging and monitoring the sense of belonging that should develop.

Experience has shown that relationships are of great importance in developing professional identities.[6–10] We have assigned many of the activities designed to engage students and maintain that sense of engagement to our mentorship program.[33] It has been shown to foster a strong sense of relationship and professional identity in both the students and the mentors. The mentors have been able to observe and support the development of their students' professional identities. Mentoring also has a profound impact on the mentors, as it forces them to examine their own professional identities, often leading to a reinforced sense of self-understanding and pride.[34]

(7) Establish membership in a community of practice as an aspirational goal

The collegial nature of medicine has long been understood. It is stressed in the earliest versions of the Hippocratic Oath, and the sense of "belonging" enjoyed by members of the medical profession has been noted by many observers.[40–42] Collegiality is thought to foster collaboration within the profession, but it can also result in unfortunate consequences, such as the protection of unethical or incompetent fellow physicians.[40] While its presence and power have been noted within the field of medical education, it has rarely been invoked in teaching, and the literature addressing it directly is sparse. In our opinion, the recent adoption of communities of practice as a description of medical practice, and of medical education as a path to joining that practice, builds on and greatly expands the concept of collegiality that has been understood for so long.

Communities of practice are described in many chapters in this book, with expanded material available in Chapters 1 and 5. Communities of practice are formed by people who engage in a process of collective learning, in a shared domain of human endeavor.[43,44] Individuals wishing to join the community move from peripheral participation in the community, which is termed "legitimate" because they have an official status. Learners gradually acquire the knowledge and skills, as well as the values and norms, of the community. In the process, they acquire the identity of the community, as well as membership in it. The process takes both time and sustained interaction for relationships within the community to develop.

The community of practice represented by healers has existed since before recorded history, and medicine's community, along with the communities of the other healing professions, can trace its origins to those times. Thus, the educational community does not have to create a community of practice – it already exists. However, the concept can be invoked as another means of engaging learners in the development of their own professional identities. Our schematic representation shown in Figure 1.1 of Chapter 1 documents this. The idea that students are moving from the periphery of the community to its center parallels the development of their professional identity, something that becomes clear as one notes that the acquisition of the identity of the community is one of the end results of joining the community.[44] As is true of professional identity formation, we present our students with the concept of communities of practice on the first day of instruction in medical school and use it, along with identity formation, as we monitor the development of their professional identity.

To our knowledge, there is nothing in the medical education literature that discusses the use of the concept of communities of practice in medical teaching. We believe that the concept has two major advantages. In the first place, it is another means of engaging students and monitoring their own progress. However, of even more significance is the fact that it

can be used to engage all members of the community – students, residents, faculty, and even other healthcare professionals – in unifying around a common concept and ideal. Furthermore, a logical consequence of this is that active means can be taken to ensure that the community is welcoming and can foster the movement of learners from the periphery toward the center.[43,44] It also offers the opportunity to ensure that this welcome is aimed at all, something that has not been true in the past.[45–47] The path to membership in medicine's community of practice must be equally available to individuals regardless of their race, religion, sexual orientation, nationality, and class.

As pointed out by Ludmerer,[29] the impact of postgraduate education on professional identity formation is probably more profound than that of undergraduate education. The sense of joining a community, be it family medicine, orthopedic surgery, psychiatry, or any other discipline, is extremely strong at both the conscious and the unconscious levels. Utilizing this concept to engage residents in participating in the development of their own identities has, in our experience, been very rewarding.

(8) Address the multiple known factors that affect professional identity formation

The schematic representations of professional identity formation and socialization[19] that are found in Figures 1.4 and 1.5 in Chapter 1 were developed from the literature in order to aid medical educators to understand the processes and to guide interventions aimed at ensuring that the impact of medical education on identity formation is more predictable and positive. We believe that each factor, or box in the diagrams, should be examined to assess its impact within each academic institution's culture at both the undergraduate and the postgraduate levels. The objective is to understand the impact of each factor and ensure that its effect on identity formation is positive.

This section will not duplicate the detailed descriptions of the processes of identity formation and socialization and the major factors found in other chapters. However, it is clear that fundamental to encouraging students to actively participate in the development of their own professional identities is reflection[6–8,46] (see Figure 8.1). Learners should be encouraged to reflect upon the nature of the identity that they wish to acquire and to recognize the process of negotiating with "self" that takes place as changes are being made to their own identities.[6,8] Role models and mentors, as well as the totality of experiences of students and residents, are factors that have a major impact. Time for guided reflection on these experiences must be provided on a regular basis. Not all experiences have a positive impact on a learner's identity formation, and these experiences must be examined and their impact discussed.[46] Every factor included in Figures 1.4 and 1.5 in Chapter 1 has the potential to promote valuable reflection at some stage in the development of a professional identity. As an example, the impact of the healthcare system will be minimal for a first- or second-year medical student, and, consequently, the potential for beneficial reflection is low. However, the closer an individual gets to full participation in medicine's community of practice, the more relevant such reflection becomes.[47] A final-year resident about to enter independent practice will inevitably reflect upon the impact of the healthcare system on his or her identity.

Another example is the role of stress, which should be examined on a regular basis throughout the educational continuum. Learners should be aware of the fact that it is difficult to change an existing identity without some stress. Reflective exercises can assist in coping with the stress.[48]

As a final example, the satisfaction and joy associated with increased competence should serve as a stimulus to reflection,[49–51] again to assist in monitoring progress toward both joining the community of practice and acquiring the professional identity of a physician.

Guided reflection is not carried out in isolation, and the impact of the reflective exercise is not limited to the learner. We have learned that it can have a profound effect on the faculty member or mentor.[33] Of necessity, mentors must examine their own identities and their own sense of commitment. The study of our mentorship program indicated a positive impact on the mentors themselves.[33]

The schematic representations have been useful at both the undergraduate and the postgraduate levels. Our experience and literature indicate that each factor is actually relevant to identity formation at both levels, but the impact varies with the educational level achieved and with the state of development of the identity of each individual student or resident.

(9) Establish an assessment program

As professional identity formation becomes a major educational objective, assessment of progress toward reaching this objective becomes essential (see Chapter 11).

While the assessment of progress toward the development of a professional identity shares some features with the assessment of professionalism, it actually requires a reorientation in our thinking. George Miller, in his classic article, proposed a four-part pyramidal structure as a framework within which the multiple levels of mastery over the art and science of medicine could be assessed.[52] Miller's triangle serves as the basis of Chapter 11. The base of the structure is an assessment of knowledge, *knows*. The next level of assessment is *knows how*, followed progressively by *shows how* and *does*. Many of the methods used to assess professionalism have been aimed at assessing the level of *does*. We believe that, given the current state of our knowledge, Miller's triangle should be expanded.[53] A fifth level, *is*, should be added to indicate that behaviors occur in individuals who have acquired a professional identity because that person must act in that way (see Figure 8.2). They have come to "think, act and feel like a physician."

The assessment of professionalism is difficult and remains a work in progress. When the educational objective was teaching professionalism and ensuring that the values and attitudes of the profession were understood, programs of assessment were developed around these objectives.[54,55] As attitudes and values are difficult to assess, the emphasis shifted to the

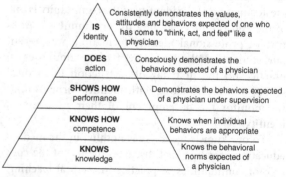

Figure 8.2. An amended version of Miller's Pyramid, with the addition of *is* and an outline of what is to be assessed at each level. This version can serve as a guide to assessment progress toward the development of a professional identity. Reprinted with permission by *Academic Medicine* © 2016.

assessment of observable behaviors that reflect these values and attitudes. To provide reliability and validity, it became clear that multiple assessors using multiple methods was required.[55] In addition, it was understood that the assessment of observable behaviors, while providing useful information, missed something, and that some form of narrative assessment by individuals familiar with students and residents was desirable. As is outlined in Chapter 11, this experience will serve as a valuable base when the educational objective is transformed to the support of a professional identity.

However, new approaches will be required, and some will rely upon the self-evaluation of students and residents. How individuals perceive and project themselves is an important component of a personal identity. Therefore, documenting an individual's perception of his or her own progress toward acquiring a professional identity becomes an invaluable tool.[6,8] This progress is nonlinear, occurs in jumps and starts, and is accelerated during times of transition; there are also times of actual regression.[6–8] Relatively uncomplicated tools have been developed to assist mentors and faculty members as they work with students to assess progress toward a professional identity. "Learning Logs,"[37] "Identity Status Interviews,"[37] "Professional Self-Identity Questionnaires,"[38] "Professional Role Orientation Inventories," and "Professional Identity Essays"[39] have been reported to be effective in tracing such progress.

It is clear that when professional identity formation is the driving force in medical education, methods of assessment of progress toward that goal that are valid, reliable, and feasible must be developed. The assessment tools that already exist represent a body of knowledge that can be expanded and built upon.

The assessment of professional and unprofessional behaviors will continue to be a priority at all levels of medical education. The impact of formative assessment on learning, including its impact on a learner's understanding of self, is powerful.[31,32] Consequently, we feel safe in predicting that the traditional assessment of professionalism will continue. In addition, medicine does have an obligation to carry out summative assessments to ensure that those entering practice are professional. It is anticipated that the assessment of progress toward the acquisition of a professional identity will take place in parallel with the assessment of professionalism, and that both systems will be compatible and congruent. A benefit of adding the concept of professional identity to assessment is that it introduces identity formation into the remediation process as is outlined in Chapter 12.

(10) Take an incremental approach

The experience of those who have instituted integrated programs on professionalism suggests that it is difficult to design and implement all aspects of the program simultaneously, and this will undoubtedly be true as the focus shifts to supporting professional identity formation. Because many steps are required to have a successful program that operates throughout the educational continuum, an incremental approach appears to be preferable.[24,26,27] The necessary steps, including naming of those responsible, educating the leaders about the nature of professionalism and professional identity formation, developing definitions and achieving buy-in from the faculty and students, promulgating this information through faculty development, and designing and introducing formal teaching and opportunities for experiential learning at all levels of instruction, take time.

Our experience[23,33] and that of the University of Texas[27] indicate that once the vision and the educational objective are present, the educational strategies can be developed and implemented in an incremental fashion.

Built into any plan to implement a major curricular innovation must be an evaluation of the impact of the program.

Conclusion

Introducing educational programs that are longitudinal, i.e., being present throughout the continuum of medical education, poses challenges. Absolute support from the leadership of the institution is required, as is collaboration and sustained efforts of individuals and academic units. Knowledge of the nature of identity formation and socialization has not, until now, been widely disseminated in the medical education community. If the shift from teaching professionalism to supporting professional identity formation is to be successful, faculty and students must understand the principles of identity formation and socialization and the norms of the community of practice that they are joining. An internally coherent and sustainable curriculum must be developed and implemented.

It is our hope that the principles elaborated in this chapter can assist those involved in medical education in accomplishing what has obviously been an unstated objective for hundreds – if not thousands – of years, to assist students as they develop their own professional identities.

References

1. Coulehan, J. Viewpoint: today's professionalism: engaging the mind but not the heart. *Acad Med*. 2005; **80**(10):892–98.

2. Cruess, RL, Cruess, SR. Teaching professionalism: general principles. *Med Teach*. 2006; **28**(3):205–08.

3. Cohen, JJ. Professionalism in medical education, an American perspective: from evidence to accountability. *Med Educ*. 2006; **40**(7):607–17.

4. Vignoles, VL, Schwartz, SJ, Luyckx, K. Introduction: toward an integrative view of identity. In Schwartz, SJ, Luyckx, K, Vignoles, VL, eds. *Handbook of Identity Theory and Research*. New York, NY: Springer; 2011:1–27.

5. Skorikov, VB, Vondracek, FW. Occupational identity. In Schwartz, SJ, Luyckx, K, Vignoles, VL, eds. *Handbook of Identity Theory and Research*. New York, NY: Springer; 2011:693–714.

6. Monrouxe, LV. Identity, identification and medical education: why should we care? *Med Educ*. 2010; **44**(1):40–49.

7. Goldie, J. The formation of professional identity in medical students: considerations for educators. *Med Teach*. 2012; **34**(9):e641–e648.

8. Jarvis-Selinger, S, Pratt, DD, Regehr, G. Competency is not enough: integrating identity formation into the medical education discourse. *Acad Med*. 2012; **87**(9):1185–90.

9. Frost, HD, Regehr, G. "I am a doctor": negotiating the discourses of standardization and diversity in professional identity construction. *Acad Med*. 2013; **88**(10):1570–77.

10. Wilson, I, Cowin, LS, Johnson, M, Young, H. Professional identity in medical students: pedagogical challenges to medical education. *Teach Learn Med*. 2013; **25**(4):369–73.

11. Cruess, RL, Cruess, SR, Boudreau, JD, Snell, L, Steinert, Y. Reframing medical education to support professional identity formation. *Acad Med*. 2014; **89**(11):1446–51.

12. Hilton, SR, Slotnick, HB. Proto-professionalism: how professionalisation occurs across the continuum of medical education. *Med Educ*. 2005; **39**(1):58–65.

13. Cruess, RL, Cruess, SR. Teaching medicine as a profession in the service of healing. *Acad Med*. 1997; **72**(11):941–52.

14. Swick, HM. Toward a normative definition of medical professionalism. *Acad Med*. 2000; **75**(6):612–16.

15. ABIM Foundation, American Board of Internal Medicine; ACP-ASIM Foundation, American College of Physicians-American Society of Internal Medicine; European Federation of Internal Medicine. Medical professionalism in the new millennium: a physician charter. *Ann Intern Med*. 2002; **136**(3):243–46.

16. Novack, DH, Epstein, RM, Paulsen, RH. Toward creating physician-healers: fostering medical students' self-awareness, personal growth, and well-being. *Acad Med*. 1999; **74**(5):516–20.

17. Branch, WT Jr, Kern, D, Haidet, P, Weissmann, P, Gracey, CF, Mitchell, G, Inui, T. The patient-physician relationship. Teaching the human dimensions of care in clinical settings. *JAMA*. 2001; **286**(9):1067–74.

18. Merton, RK. Some preliminaries to a sociology of medical education. In Merton, RK, Reader, GG, Kendall, PL, eds. *The Student Physician: Introductory Studies in the Sociology of Medical Education*. Cambridge, MA: Harvard University Press; 1957:3–79.

19. Cruess, RL, Cruess, SR, Boudreau, JD, Snell, L, Steinert, Y. A schematic representation of the professional identity formation and socialization of medical students and residents: a guide for medical educators. *Acad Med*. 2015; **90**(6):718–25.

20. Cooke, M, Irby, DM, O'Brien, BC. *Educating Physicians: A Call for Reform of Medical School and Residency*. San Francisco, CA: Jossey-Bass; 2010.

21. Inui, TS. *A Flag in the Wind: Educating for Professionalism in Medicine*. Washington, DC: Association of American Medical Colleges; 2003.

22. Kotter, JP. Leading change: why transformation efforts fail. *Harv Bus Rev*. 1995; **73**(2):59–67.

23. Steinert, Y, Cruess, RL, Cruess, SR, Boudreau, JD, Fuks, A. Faculty development as an instrument of change: a case study on teaching professionalism. *Acad Med*. 2007; **82**(11):1057–64.

24. Brater, DC. Viewpoint: infusing professionalism into a school of medicine: perspectives from the Dean. *Acad Med*. 2007; **82**(11):1094–97.

25. Wasserstein, AG, Brennan, PJ, Rubenstein, AH. Institutional leadership and faculty response: fostering professionalism at the University of Pennsylvania School Of Medicine. *Acad Med*. 2007; **82**(11):1049–56.

26. Smith, KL, Saavedra, R, Raeke, JL, O'Donell, AA. The journey to creating a campus-wide culture of professionalism. *Acad Med*. 2007; **82**(11):1015–21.

27. Holden, MD, Buck, E, Luk, J, Ambriz, F, Boisaubin, EV, Clark, MA, Mihalic, AP, Sadler, JZ, Sapire, KJ, Spike, JP, Vince, A, Dalrymple, JL. Professional identity formation: creating a longitudinal framework through TIME (Transformation In Medical Education). *Acad Med*. 2015; **90**(6):761–67.

28. Woollard, RF. Caring for a common future: medical schools' social accountability. *Med Educ.* 2006; **40**(4):301–13.

29. Ludmerer, KM. *Let Me Heal: The Opportunity to Preserve Excellence in American Medicine.* Oxford, UK: Oxford University Press; 2015.

30. Steinert, Y, Cruess, S, Cruess, R, Snell, L. Faculty development for teaching and evaluating professionalism: from programme design to curriculum change. *Med Teach.* 2005; **39**(2):127–36.

31. Wilkerson, L, Irby, DM. Strategies for improving teaching practices: a comprehensive approach to faculty development. *Acad Med.* 1998; **73**(4):387–96.

32. Kenny, NP, Mann, KV, MacLeod, H. Role modeling in physicians' professional formation: reconsidering an essential but untapped educational strategy. *Acad Med.* 2003; **78**(12):1203–10.

33. Boudreau, JD, Macdonald, ME, Steinert, Y. Affirming professional identities through an apprenticeship: insights from a four-year longitudinal case study. *Acad Med.* 2014; **89**(7):1038–45.

34. Hafferty, FW. Beyond curriculum reform: confronting medicine's hidden curriculum. *Acad Med.* 1998; **73**(4):403–07.

35. Daniels, N. *Just Health: Meeting Health Needs Fairly.* Cambridge, UK: Cambridge University Press; 2008.

36. Cruess, RL, Cruess, SR. Expectations and obligations: professionalism and medicine's social contract with society. *Perspect Biol Med.* 2008; **51**(4):579–98.

37. Niemi, PM. Medical students' professional identity: self-reflection during the preclinical years. *Med Educ.* 1997; **31**(6):408–15.

38. Crossley, J, Vivekananda-Schmidt, P. The development and evaluation of a Professional Self Identity Questionnaire to measure evolving professional self-identity in health and social care students. *Med Teach.* 2009; **31**(12):e603–e607.

39. Bebeau, MJ, Faber-Langendoen, K. Remediating lapses in professionalism. In Kalet, A, Chou, CL, eds. *Remediation in Medical Education: A Mid-Course Correction.* New York, NY: Springer;2014:103–27.

40. Ihara, CK. Collegiality as a professional virtue. In Flores, A, ed. *Professional Ideals.* Belmont, CA: Wadsworth; 1988:56–65.

41. Starr, P. *The Social Transformation of American Medicine.* New York, NY: Basic Books; 1982.

42. Krause, E. *Death of the Guilds: Professions, States, and the Advance of Capitalism, 1930 to the Present.* New Haven, CT: Yale University Press; 1996.

43. Lave, J, Wenger, E. *Situated Learning: Legitimate Peripheral Participation.* Cambridge, UK: Cambridge University Press; 1991.

44. Wenger, E. *Communities of Practice: Learning, Meaning, and Identity.* Cambridge, UK: Cambridge University Press; 1998.

45. Bleakley, A. Gender matters in medical education. *Med Educ.* 2013; **47**(1):59–70.

46. Mann, K, Gordon, J, MacLeod, A. Reflection and reflective practice in health professions education: a systematic review. *Adv Health Sci Educ Theory Pract.* 2009; **14**(4):595–621.

47. Lesser, CS, Lucey, CR, Egener, B, Braddock, CH III, Linas, SL, Levinson, W. A behavioral and systems view of professionalism. *JAMA.* 2010; **304**(24):2732–37.

48. Erikson, EH. *The Life Cycle Completed.* New York, NY: WW Norton; 1982.

49. LeBlanc, VR. The effects of acute stress on performance: implications for health professions education. *Acad Med.* 2009; **84**(10 Suppl):S25–S33.

50. Helmich, E, Dornan, T. Do you really want to be a doctor? The highs and lows of identity development. *Med Educ.* 2012; **46**(2):132–34.

51. Dornan, T, Pearson, E, Carson, P, Helmich, E, Bundy C. Emotions and identity in the figured world of becoming a doctor. *Med Educ.* 2015; **49**(2):174–185.

52. Miller, GE. The assessment of clinical skills/competence/performance. *Acad Med.* 1990; **65**(9 Suppl):S63–S67.

53. Cruess, RL, Cruess, SR, Steinert, Y. Amending Miller's pyramid to include professional identity formation. *Acad Med.* 2015. In press.

54. Wilkinson, TJ, Wade, WB, Knock, LD. A blueprint to assess professionalism: results of a systematic review. *Acad Med.* 2009; **84**(5):551–58.

55. Hodges, BD, Ginsburg, S, Cruess, R, Cruess, S, Delport, R, Hafferty, F, Ho, MJ, Holmboe, E, Holtman, M, Ohbu, S, Rees, C, Ten Cate, O, Tsugawa, Y, Van Mook, W, Wass, V, Wilkinson, T, Wade, W. Assessment of professionalism: recommendations from the Ottawa 2010 Conference. *Med Teach.* 2011; **33**(5):354–63.

Faculty development to support professionalism and professional identity formation

Yvonne Steinert

The greatest difficulty in life is to make knowledge effective, to convert it into practical wisdom.
Sir William Osler

The role of faculty development in promoting the teaching and learning of professionalism has grown substantially in the last decade, and several programs designed to enhance the knowledge, skills, and attitudes of clinical teachers and program directors in this area have been described.[1,2] At the same time, while the importance of professional identity formation has been identified by a number of authors in the field,[3,4] faculty development activities to support professional identity formation have, to date, not been described. Moreover, although there is a growing consensus regarding the importance of teaching and assessing professionalism,[5–9] many faculty members are unable to articulate either the attributes and behaviors characteristic of the physician as a professional or how they can best facilitate the process of "becoming a physician." Additionally, clinical teachers are frequently not sure how to teach this content area and support professional identity formation. As a result, faculty development is needed to ensure the successful teaching, learning, and assessment of professionalism as well as the formation of a professional identity, during both undergraduate and postgraduate training.

The goals of this chapter are to outline the principles and strategies underlying faculty development designed to facilitate the teaching and assessment of professionalism and the support of professional identity formation. In addition, we will highlight the role of faculty development in enhancing role modeling, promoting reflection, capitalizing on experiential and work-based learning, and supporting communities of practice. Several case examples, based on our own experiences, will also be provided.

Faculty development, or staff development as it is often called, refers to that broad range of activities that institutions use to *renew* or *assist* faculty in their multiple roles.[10] Moreover, although faculty development has traditionally been defined as a planned program designed to prepare institutions and faculty members for their various roles,[11] healthcare professionals engage in both *formal* and *informal* faculty development to enhance their knowledge and skills. In fact, much of their professional development is self-directed and linked to experiential and work-based learning. For the purpose of this discussion, faculty development will refer to *all* activities health professionals pursue to improve their knowledge, skills, and behaviors as teachers and educators, leaders and managers, and researchers and scholars, in both individual and group settings.[12] In multiple ways, faculty development can provide individuals with knowledge and skills about teaching and learning, curriculum design and delivery, and assessment and evaluation. It can also reinforce or alter attitudes or beliefs about teaching and learning, provide a conceptual framework for what is often performed on an intuitive basis, and introduce clinical teachers to a community of medical educators committed to the enhancement of teaching and learning for students, residents, and peers.[13]

Faculty development can also serve as a useful instrument in the promotion of organizational change.[2,14] For example, by building consensus, generating support, transmitting core content, and promoting skill acquisition, faculty development can help to facilitate curricular change. It can also influence the institutional culture by altering formal, informal, and hidden curricula,[15] setting policy, or enhancing organizational capacity.[16] As Swanwick[17] (p. 339) has said, faculty development should be "an institution-wide pursuit with the intent of professionalizing the

Teaching Medical Professionalism, 2nd Edition, ed. Richard L. Cruess, Sylvia R. Cruess and Yvonne Steinert.
Published by Cambridge University Press. © Cambridge University Press 2016.

educational activities of teachers, enhancing educational infrastructure, and building educational capacity for the future...."

Wilkerson and Irby[18] have noted that comprehensive faculty development programs should include both individual and organizational development. In the context of supporting professionalism and professional identity formation, both aspects are critical.

At the *individual* level, faculty development can:

- Address *attitudes* and beliefs that can enhance – or impede – the teaching, learning, and assessment of professionalism and the formation of a professional identity;
- Transmit *knowledge* about the core content of professionalism and the process of professional identity formation as well as effective teaching and assessment strategies; and
- Develop *skills* in teaching and assessing the behaviors that exemplify professionalism and underpin an emerging professional identity.

At the *organizational* level, faculty development can help to:

- Define a shared vision of professionalism and professional identity as well as how both will be supported and assessed;
- Create opportunities for teaching and assessing professionalism and supporting professional identity formation; and
- Address systems issues that can enhance – or impede – the teaching and assessment of professionalism as well as the acquisition of a professional identity.

Why faculty development is needed

Teaching professionalism remains a challenge for many health professionals. First, most physicians believe that they are "professional" and that teaching professionalism is intuitive. In fact, they often question why they need to learn about this content area. Second, role modeling is no longer as effective a strategy as it once was. When both society and the profession itself were reasonably homogeneous, values were shared and could be transmitted effectively through role modeling.[5,6] The increasing complexity of the practice of medicine, the ethical dilemmas faced by contemporary physicians, and the diversity of the medical profession and society make this no longer true. Faculty members must now be able to teach

professionalism *explicitly* by articulating its core concepts and by demonstrating appropriate behaviors. Third, teachers must be able to teach and assess this core competency. That is, they need to be aware of the most effective teaching and assessment strategies and realize that teaching professionalism is not an "add on"; teaching must be integrated into the clinical and classroom setting. Finally, professionalism has to be valued by the organization, and teachers must identify opportunities to recognize professionalism in their institutional culture.

The reasons outlined above also apply to supporting the acquisition of a professional identity. Although many clinical teachers will agree that one of the principal tenets of medical education is to help form a professional identity, these same individuals will often leave this formation to chance, not really understanding the nature of the identity they wish to support or the process through which this professional identity will emerge. Unaware of the factors that influence the socialization of medical students and residents, or how learners respond to this process, they may inadvertently hinder the development of a professional identity.

What are the implications of these challenges for faculty development? At an *individual level*, teachers need knowledge and skills about professionalism (and its many attributes), professional identity, the process of socialization and professional identity formation, and relevant teaching and assessment strategies; they also require a commitment to support professionalism and professional identity formation. As a result, faculty development programs need to build motivation for learning, overcome resistance, and help teachers to make the implicit explicit. At a *programmatic level*, faculty developers and educators must consider a broad range of approaches and build programs that focus on both content *and* teaching methods; they must also focus on teaching and assessing professionalism as well as professional identity formation and make learning pertinent and fun. In addition, faculty developers should assess teachers' needs, incorporate educationally useful theoretical frameworks such as situated learning[19] (discussed in Chapter 5), remain relevant and practical, and evaluate effectiveness. Faculty developers should also follow principles of adult learning and integrate faculty development to support professionalism and professional identity formation into ongoing programs. At a *systems level*, educators must address the organizational climate

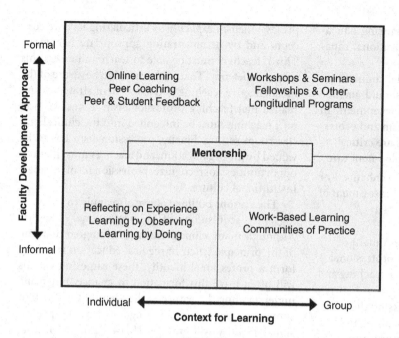

Figure 9.1. Approaches to faculty development. This figure was originally prepared for a chapter on "Becoming a Better Teacher: From Intuition to Intent."[23] Reprinted with permission by the American College of Physicians © 2010.

that impacts the socialization of students, residents, and faculty members; promote buy-in; identify opportunities for teaching, learning, and assessment; train the trainers; and facilitate dissemination.[1,13] At times, it will be more appropriate to work within the culture, responding to specific needs; at other times, organizational change will be needed.[2]

Common approaches to faculty development

Notions of professional development, which apply equally to faculty development, have changed in recent years. For example, in an interesting study of teachers' professional growth, Clarke and Hollingsworth[20] (p. 947) observed that "models of teacher professional development have not matched the complexity of the process we seek to promote." These authors also noted that it is time to shift our focus "from earlier conceptions of change as something that is done to teachers … to change as a complex process that involves learning."[20] (p. 948) A similar sentiment has been expressed by Webster-Wright,[21] who argues for a reconceptualization of professional development that moves us away from learning that occurs in "discrete, finite episodes" to a focus on continuous and authentic professional learning. More specifically, she suggests that we move toward the notion of *promoting learning* that occurs in authentic contexts rather than the *development* of colleagues, which in many ways implies a deficit model, reinforces

the notion that we "do something to" our colleagues, and ignores a critical venue for skill acquisition.

Figure 9.1 illustrates a number of ways in which health professionals learn about their multiple roles and responsibilities. Although we usually think about workshops, short courses, fellowships, and longitudinal programs as the most common approach (or strategy) for faculty development,[22] faculty members do, in fact, develop in a number of ways. As demonstrated here, health professionals can learn through both individual (independent) and group (collective) experiences while benefiting from both informal and formal approaches to teaching and learning.[23] Individual approaches to faculty development include learning from experience; learning from peers and students (at all levels of the continuum); and online learning. Group learning includes structured activities such as workshops and short courses, fellowships and other longitudinal programs, work-based learning, and learning in a community of practice. We will briefly examine what takes place in each quadrant, concluding with mentorship, because any strategy for self-improvement can benefit from "the support and challenge that an effective mentor can provide."[23] (p. 78)

Learning from experience

Health professionals often become adept at what they do by "the nature of their job responsibilities."[24]

Although this type of learning is not often viewed as a form of faculty development, it is critical to the acquisition of professionally appropriate behaviors, identity formation, self-improvement, and renewal. Learning from experience can be further divided into learning by *doing*, learning by *observing* (and through role modeling), and learning by *reflecting* on experience.[23] The challenge for faculty developers and educators is to capture the benefits of experiential learning, find ways to promote reflection in the clinical environment, and help to demonstrate that learning has occurred.

Learning from peers, residents, and students

Learning from experience can be augmented by peer feedback and learner assessments.[23] Although physicians are often reluctant to seek feedback from peers, it can be extremely beneficial to discuss an educational challenge (or critical incident) with colleagues or ask them to provide feedback after having observed a specific teaching encounter. Peer coaching, which is sometimes called co-teaching, has particular appeal for the teaching and learning of professionalism because it occurs in the practice setting, enables individualized learning, and fosters immediate application.[25] It also models many aspects of professional practice, such as the identification of individual learning goals, focused observation by colleagues, and the provision of feedback, analysis, and support,[26] all of which are critically important in learning about professionalism and the acquisition of a professional identity. Soliciting feedback from learners can be equally helpful, despite the fact that most health professionals do not actively seek out student or resident perspectives.[24] In fact, "taking the initiative to solicit [students'] observations and suggestions can be an integral part of the process of becoming a better teacher"[23] (p. 79), as an appreciative inquiry of learner assessments can help to uncover personal strengths and areas for improvement. It can also facilitate a conversation about identity formation.

Online learning

Online learning is a potentially valuable form of self-directed learning. Given that time for professional development is limited, and the technology to create interactive instructional programs is now in place, the use of online faculty development should be explored.[27] In many ways, online resources and learning programs could be considered as supplements to centrally organized faculty development programs;[28,29] they could also be used in a "staged approach," later in the development of teachers and faculty members. Importantly, online learning can allow for individualized programs targeted to specific needs, as long as educators do not lose sight of the value and importance of working in context, with colleagues.[25]

Learning from structured activities

Formal (structured) activities are the most common approaches to faculty development[22] and include workshops and short courses, fellowships and other longitudinal programs, and certificate or degree programs.

Workshops and short courses are one of the most popular approaches[30] because of their inherent flexibility and promotion of active learning through a variety of teaching methods: interactive lectures, small-group discussions and exercises, role-plays and simulations, and experiential learning.[13] Without a doubt, workshops play an important role in faculty development for the teaching and learning of professionalism;[1,2] they can also be used to learn about identity, professional identity, and socialization. Short courses have the added advantage of increased time and continuity.[22]

Fellowships, of varying duration, form another structured approach to faculty development, though their focus usually extends beyond teaching improvement to include educational leadership or scholarship. More recently, *integrated, longitudinal programs* (typified by teaching scholars programs) have been developed as an alternative to fellowship programs;[31,32] these programs allow clinicians to maintain most of their clinical, research, and administrative responsibilities while furthering their own professional development in targeted areas (e.g., the teaching and learning of professionalism). Given the need to develop curricula that focus on professionalism and professional identity formation at both undergraduate and postgraduate levels, longitudinal programs that enhance capacity in this area will be of benefit to many.

Certificate or degree programs are becoming increasingly popular in some settings, due to the "professionalization" of medical education and an increasing desire to develop pedagogical standards at a global level.[33,34] Tekian and Harris[35] recently described seventy-six masters-level programs in the health professions. As the authors suggest, an advanced degree can offer essential grounding in educational theory and practice while providing the foundation for educational research and scholarship. These programs can also "prepare leaders in the health professions who can manage change within their institutions, overcome organizational barriers, and effectively direct the future of healthcare delivery systems"[35] (p. 56), of critical importance to professionalism and the support of professional identity formation.

Work-based learning and communities of practice

A number of authors[20,21,36–37] have highlighted the role of work-based learning as integral to professional development. In fact, it is in the everyday workplace, where teachers conduct their clinical, teaching, and research activities, that learning most often takes place. It is therefore surprising that we do not currently view work-based learning as a common venue for faculty development, for by working together in a clinical or classroom setting, teachers can acquire new knowledge and refine their approaches to teaching and learning. Professional identity is also nurtured or inhibited in the workplace, and it is therefore a critical venue for learning and self-improvement. Faculty development activities have traditionally been conducted away from teachers' workplaces, requiring participants to take their "lessons learned" back to their own contexts. It is time to reverse this trend and think about how we can enhance the learning that takes place in the work environment; there is also value in rendering this learning as visible as possible so that it can be valued as an important component of faculty development.[24] A pedagogy of the workplace includes individual engagement, sequencing of activities to create pathways for learning, the provision of guidance to promote learning, environmental affordances that enable access to learning, and reflection and role modeling.[38,39] Clearly, all of these components are relevant to the acquisition of professional behaviors as well as a professional identity.

As outlined in Chapter 5, the notion of a community of practice is closely tied to that of work-based learning. Barab et al.[40] (p. 495) have defined a community of practice as a "persistent, sustaining, social network of individuals who share and develop an overlapping knowledge base, set of beliefs, values, history and experiences focused on a common practice and/or mutual enterprise." In many ways, becoming a member of a teaching community can be viewed as an approach to faculty development, and we should collectively explore ways to make this community – and the learning that it offers – more accessible to clinical teachers. We should also find ways of creating new opportunities for exchange and support, documenting the learning that takes place in the workplace, and valuing the communities of which we are a part.

Mentorship

Mentoring, a recognized component of a successful academic career,[41] is often used to promote the socialization and development of clinical faculty.[42] It is therefore surprising that mentorship is not more frequently described as a faculty development strategy,[43] for mentors can provide guidance, direction, support, or expertise to faculty members on a range of topics, in a variety of settings. Mentors can also help teachers to understand the organizational culture in which they are working and introduce them to invaluable professional networks.[44,45] Teachers often report that finding a mentor – and being mentored – is one of the most critical components to their becoming a better teacher.[46] It behooves us to recognize the value of this important strategy as an approach to faculty development, especially as it can also help to promote professional identity formation (among faculty members and learners).

Interestingly, each of the above approaches can play an integral role in developing faculty members to promote professionalism and professional identity formation; each also has its own strengths and limitations. As a result, faculty developers should consider all of these approaches in the design of comprehensive faculty development programs. However, as there is still a place for formal (more structured) activities in promoting awareness, acquiring core knowledge, developing skills, and encouraging buy-in, we offer the following guidelines for designing structured faculty development initiatives.

Guidelines for designing formal faculty development initiatives

Guidelines for designing and delivering effective faculty development programs have been outlined previously.[13,14] A brief summary of these recommendations is warranted here, as awareness of these principles is fundamental to the design of any program or activity.

Understand the institutional or organizational culture

Faculty development programs and activities take place within the context of a specific institution or organization. It is imperative to understand the culture of that institution and be responsive to its needs. Professional development programs should also capitalize on the organization's strengths and work with the leadership to ensure success. In many ways, the cultural context can be used to promote or enhance faculty development efforts. For example, it has been noted that faculty development during times of educational or curricular reform takes on added importance.[47] It is also important to assess institutional support for faculty development activities, identify available resources, and lobby effectively. Faculty development should not occur in a vacuum.

Determine appropriate goals and priorities

In designing a faculty development program or activity, it is imperative to clearly define goals and priorities. What is the program or activity trying to achieve – and why is it important to do so? It is equally important to articulate specific objectives, as they will influence the target audience (e.g., clinical teachers; program directors) as well as overall content and methodology. Determining priorities is not always easy and often involves consultations with diverse stakeholders. However, it is always essential to balance *individual* and *organizational* needs.

Conduct needs assessments to ensure relevant programming

All professional development activities should be based on the needs of the individual as well as the institution. Student needs, patient needs, and societal needs can also help to guide relevant activities. Assessing needs is required to refine goals, determine content, identify preferred learning formats, and ensure relevance. It is also a way of promoting early buy-in. Common methods for assessing needs include written questionnaires or surveys; interviews or focus groups with key informants (e.g., participants;

students; educational leaders); observations of teachers "in action"; literature reviews; and environmental scans of available programs and resources.[48,49] Whenever possible, faculty developers should try to gain information from multiple sources, distinguishing between "needs" and "wants." An individual teacher's perceived needs may clearly differ from those expressed by that teacher's learners or peers.

Target diverse stakeholders

Rubeck and Witzke[47] defined faculty development as the enhancement of faculty members' knowledge and skills so that they can make educational contributions that advance both the pedagogical program and the process of teaching and learning. For educational and curricular reform to occur, faculty development initiatives should target curriculum planners responsible for the design and delivery of educational programs focused on the teaching and assessment of professionalism as well as the support of professional identity formation; administrators responsible for medical education and clinical practice as well as the institutions in which professional behaviors are displayed; and all healthcare professionals involved in teaching and learning. The latter group might include faculty members working in a university setting, clinical teachers of diverse backgrounds in the hospital and the community, and other members of the healthcare team.

Develop different programs and activities to accommodate diverse needs

One size does not fit all. Faculty development activities should be designed to accommodate diverse goals and objectives, content areas, and needs. In this context, it is also helpful to remember that faculty *development* can include faculty orientation, recognition, and support, and different programs and activities will be needed to accommodate diverse objectives. For example, think tanks may be appropriate to promote buy-in, to develop consensus, and to design an educational blueprint.[1] Workshops may be more appropriate for knowledge or skill acquisition – or to heighten awareness and recognition of the importance of a particular topic.

Incorporate principles of adult learning and instructional design

Adults come to learning situations with a variety of motivations and expectations about teaching methods and goals. Incorporating key principles of adult learning[50] (outlined in Chapter 5) into the design of a faculty development program can enhance receptivity, relevance, and engagement. In fact, these principles should guide the development of all programs, irrespective of their focus or format, because physicians demonstrate a high degree of self-direction and possess numerous experiences that can serve as the basis for learning.

Principles of instructional design (also outlined in Chapter 5) should be followed in the design and delivery of any faculty development initiative. For example, it is important to develop clear learning goals and objectives for a specific activity, identify key content areas, design appropriate teaching and learning strategies, and create appropriate methods of evaluation – of both the learners and the curriculum. It is equally important to integrate educational theory with practice (e.g., situated learning)[19] and to ensure that the learning is perceived as relevant to the work setting and to the profession.[51] Health professionals value interactive, participatory, and experientially based learning that builds on previous learning and experience.[2,22] A positive learning environment that communicates respect and understanding of similarities and differences, as well as "equal" participation of all participants, is also essential, as is teacher readiness, buy-in, and commitment.

Offer a diversity of educational methods – in a variety of settings

In line with principles of adult learning, structured faculty development initiatives should try to offer a variety of educational methods that promote experiential learning, reflection, feedback, and immediacy of application.[22] As stated previously, common learning methods include interactive lectures, case presentations, small-group exercises and discussions, role-plays and simulations, videotape reviews, and live demonstrations. Practice with feedback is also essential, as is the opportunity to reflect on personal values and attitudes. Online modules and self-directed readings are additional methods to consider. Most importantly, whatever the method, the needs and learning preferences of the participants must be respected, and the methods should match the intended objectives. It is also helpful to remember that healthcare professionals learn best by "doing," and experiential learning should be promoted whenever possible.

Faculty development activities frequently take place in a centralized university or departmental setting. To be successful in this context, faculty development should occur where the teaching and learning of professionalism happens. Thus, some faculty development initiatives should move out of the university setting into the hospital and the community. Decentralized, site-specific activities have the added advantage of reaching individuals who might not otherwise attend faculty development activities, promoting experiential learning, and developing a departmental or program-based culture of self-improvement.[52,53]

Promote "buy-in" and market effectively

The decision to participate in a professional development program or activity is not as simple as it might at first appear. It involves the individual's reaction to a particular offering, motivation to develop or enhance a specific skill, being available at the time of the session, and overcoming the psychological barrier of admitting need.[47] Faculty developers face the challenge of overcoming reluctance and marketing their "product" in such a way that resistance becomes a resource to learning. In some settings, targeted mailings, professionally designed brochures, and product "branding" have been extremely valuable. In other contexts, continuing medical education credits, as well as free and flexible programming, help to enhance motivation and facilitate attendance. "Buy-in" involves agreement on importance, widespread support, and dedication of time and resources at both the individual and the systems level; it must also be deliberately sought in all programming initiatives.

Evaluate – and demonstrate – effectiveness

Evaluation is the final step in instructional design and of critical importance in faculty development programming. At a minimum, a practical and feasible evaluation should include an assessment of the utility and relevance of the content, teaching and learning methods, and participants' intent to change. Moreover, because evaluation is an integral part of program planning, it should be conceptualized at the beginning of any program. It should also include qualitative and quantitative assessments of learning and behavior change, using a variety of methods and data sources.

In preparing to evaluate a faculty development program or activity, educators should consider the goal of the evaluation (e.g., program planning versus decision making; policy formation versus academic inquiry), available data sources (e.g., participants; peers; students or residents), common methods of evaluation (e.g., questionnaires; focus groups; objective tests; observations), resources to support assessment (e.g., institutional support; research grants), and models of program evaluation (e.g., goal attainment; decision facilitation).[54–56] Each component requires careful planning and execution to ensure success. Kirkpatrick's hierarchy of evaluation[57] is also helpful in conceptualizing and framing the evaluation of effectiveness. This hierarchy includes the following levels:

- *Reaction* – Participants' views on the learning experience;
- *Learning* – Changes in participants' attitudes, knowledge, or skills;
- *Behavior* – Changes in participants' behavior; and
- *Results* – Changes in the organizational system, the patient, or the learner.

Although program evaluation is fundamental to the design, delivery, and improvement of faculty development activities, it also helps to ensure scholarship in the teaching and assessment of professionalism as well as professional identity formation.

Principles underlying faculty development to support professionalism and professional identity formation

Although the guidelines outlined above are all relevant to faculty development designed to support professionalism and professional identity formation, many of them are generic in nature. Based on our experience in the design and delivery of faculty development programs in teaching and learning professionalism[1,2] and supporting professional identity formation in a variety of contexts, we believe that certain principles and strategies emerge as critical to the success of programming in this area.

Teach the cognitive base

As stated at the outset, role modeling and the implicit teaching of professionalism and support of professional identity formation are no longer sufficient.

We therefore need to equip our teachers with the cognitive base underlying professionalism and professional identity formation (as outlined in Chapter 1); we also need to develop a common language so that teachers will be able to communicate their vision with colleagues and learners. In line with this thinking, faculty development efforts should include the definition of professionalism, its historical roots, and the relationship between professionalism and the ever-changing social contract between medicine and society.[5,58] Clinical teachers also need to acquire a common understanding of the attributes of professionalism and the behaviors expected of a professional. As teachers often see professionalism as a vague concept lacking a cognitive base, faculty development programs should provide teachers with operational definitions (outlined in Chapter 1) that can be taught and evaluated. Figure 1.3 in Chapter 1 outlines the core attributes of professionalism that form the norms and values of professional identity formation, and that we have used to guide teaching and learning in our setting. It is offered as an example to guide the work of others in this field. In designing faculty development initiatives to support professional identity formation, different content areas should be addressed. These include definitions of identity and professional identity; the changing nature of identity over time; the notion of multiple (and fluid) identities; the process of socialization and identity formation in medicine; the myriad of factors that influence identity formation (e.g., clinical experiences; role models; the healthcare and learning environment; peers and family members); and the role that learners play in the socialization process as well as their responses to this process (including joy and stress).[59] The schemata described in Chapter 1 (in Figures 1.1, 1.4, and 1.5) can be helpful in trying to synthesize these complex influences.

Translate core content into practice

To be effective, the attributes of professionalism must be taught and *demonstrated* in the clinical setting. Accordingly, clinicians need to translate core content into practice and see its applicability and relevance. In our own setting, we chose to promote the latter by defining professionalism and its attributes using case examples and asking faculty members to complete action plans in order to ensure implementation following a faculty development workshop.[1] With respect to identity formation, clinical teachers should be encouraged to think about their own identities (including their values, beliefs, and aspirations), their perceptions of major influences in becoming a physician (including both facilitators and barriers), and their views on how they have negotiated this process.

Start with a focus on teaching professionalism

The need to focus on teaching professionalism arises from several factors. Virtually every accrediting, licensing, and certifying body requires that professional behaviors in students and residents be assessed.[60,61] However, if professionalism is to be assessed, it must first be defined and taught. Based on our own experience in this area,[1,2] we believe strongly that a focus on teaching professionalism is less threatening to healthcare professionals than a focus on being professional. It is also easier to start with professional behaviors than with the nature of identity. We would therefore encourage colleagues to start with a focus on teaching and then examine the process of professional identity formation.

Enhance role modeling

As stated earlier (and highlighted in Chapters 1 and 6), role models – and role modeling – are critical to the acquisition of professional behaviors and the formation of a professional identity. As a result, any faculty development initiative designed to support professional identity formation must also address how clinical teachers behave as role models.[62] Cruess et al.[63] have described a number of strategies to improve role modeling at both the individual and the organizational level; these include the need to be aware of being a role model, protecting time for teaching, making the implicit explicit, and reflecting upon both positive and negative experiences. Kenny et al.[64] recommended that faculty development activities try to clarify the meaning of roles and role modeling, discuss standards and expectations, and provide safe spaces for reflection and debriefing. All of these suggestions can be integrated into a faculty development activity that focuses on professionalism and professional identity formation. Importantly, improving role modeling cannot be accomplished at the individual level alone; the institution plays a key role and needs to value teachers and teaching, as the goal is to create an environment which supports positive role modeling.[65]

Promote reflection

Reflection "in action" and "on action" has been identified as central to the teaching and learning of professionalism.[66] It is also central to the formation of a professional identity. Faculty development activities must therefore include activities that promote self-reflection, awareness, and change. If we believe that professional identity arises from "a long-term combination of experiences and reflection on experience"[67] (p. 63), and that our learners require both experience and reflection for learning to occur, then we must model these strategies when working with faculty members. The literature on reflection[68–71] has grown significantly in recent years and has highlighted the importance of a safe environment, peer support, and mentorship in promoting "mindfulness." These attributes should also characterize a robust faculty development initiative.

A number of strategies to promote reflection among health professions teachers have been suggested.[65] These include the use of written logs of teaching encounters, guided questions,[72] personal narratives, and teaching portfolios, all of which can serve as stimuli for discussion during a faculty development activity. The review of critical incidents can be another way to promote reflection. Rademacher et al.[73] described the use of critical incidents as a faculty development strategy to explore faculty members' professionalism. More specifically, they used teachers' personal experiences to identify challenges, discuss potential solutions, and highlight areas for further development. Although this approach is not commonly used, the analysis of critical incidents can be an innovative way in which to enhance experiential learning and reflective practice, key components of identity formation.

Capitalize on experiential and work-based learning

As stated earlier, much of faculty members' learning takes place through experience and in the workplace. This is especially true when thinking about their acquisition of professional behaviors as well as their professional identities. It is therefore important to think about how faculty development can maximize experiential learning (often augmented by guided reflection) and promote work-based learning, which is characterized by observation, participation, and expert guidance in an authentic environment.[38] In considering the use of work-based learning as a faculty development strategy, educators should question whether we have created a false dichotomy between work and learning, how we can guide participation while performing authentic activities, and how we can make workplace learning more visible.

Support communities of practice

As stated earlier, communities of practice play a critical role in developing faculty members' knowledge, attitudes, and skills, both in general[23] and in learning about professionalism and professional identity formation.[3] For these reasons, helping faculty members to become aware of the communities of practice to which they belong, and working with them to strengthen their communities, is an invaluable faculty development objective. As described in Chapter 5, communities of practice are characterized by common goals and shared values, sustained mutual relationships, a common language, a sense of membership that results from the experiences of working together, and the existence of common practices, stories, and rituals.[74] Knowledge of these features can help to identify the existence of a community of practice and highlight areas for further development. Individuals also belong to communities of practice for a variety of reasons, which include the ability to nurture personal connections, enhance problem-solving and innovation, and improve individual and organizational capacity. Awareness of these motivators can help to sustain community building. Wenger[74] has articulated a number of ways in which communities of practice can be cultivated. Cognizance of these principles (which include an open dialogue between inside and outside perspectives, inviting different levels of participation, developing both public and private community spaces, and creating a rhythm for the community) can play a critical role in the formation and maintenance of such communities.

Address the organizational culture

As mentioned previously, faculty development programs or activities should not be designed or delivered in isolation from other factors, including the institutional culture and organizational goals and priorities. At the same time, faculty development can serve as a useful instrument in the process of change.[2] For example, students and residents are always learning from faculty members, be it in elevators, corridors, or social settings, and faculty development activities must address these informal interactions as well as those which are considered more formal.

A case study

Faculty development to promote the teaching and assessment of professionalism

In our own setting, we have been involved in the design and delivery of faculty development to support the teaching and learning of professionalism for more than fifteen years. In this section, we will briefly describe the process that we used to promote consensus and buy-in.

When we first began our work in this area, we had expected some resistance to the concept of professionalism and its core attributes, as consensus on its importance, values, and definitions had not been established. We therefore chose a systematic approach, consisting of think tanks and workshops as key educational methods, to promote buy-in. Both methods allowed participants to explore their values and beliefs, acquire core content and skills, and begin to take ownership of this content area.

The following steps, which have been described previously,[1] were used in the development of our faculty development initiative. We hope that some of our "lessons learned" will be helpful to others interested in mounting faculty development programs in this area.

"Think tank" on teaching professionalism

To initiate the discussion, the dean of our medical school invited twenty-five educational leaders to a half-day "think tank," to highlight the importance of professionalism, develop consensus, and discuss outreach to faculty members. This session started with a brief overview of the core content of professionalism and proceeded to examine how professionalism was being taught at all levels of the curriculum. At the end of the session, a plan for a faculty development workshop had been developed. Other outcomes included a consensus on the importance of teaching professionalism, a review of how professionalism was being taught, and agreement on core content. Most importantly, this session was fundamental to the success of our faculty development endeavor.

Invitational workshop on teaching professionalism

Following the think tank, all departmental chairs and program directors were invited by the dean to a half-day workshop on *The Teaching of Professionalism*.

This workshop was limited to thirty-five participants so that we could "test" the working definitions of the attributes of professionalism, examine the strengths and weaknesses of diverse teaching methods, and receive immediate feedback. The workshop was organized into three parts: the "core content" of professionalism; personal views and beliefs; and strategies for teaching. Participants were also asked to discuss a number of case vignettes, identify attributes of professionalism, and match teaching methods to the different attributes. The workshop concluded with the completion of an action plan for each department. By the end of the workshop, we had broadened consensus regarding the importance of professionalism and its core content, developed a plan for a faculty-wide workshop, and prepared a cohort of small-group facilitators for future workshops and teaching sessions. At the same time, two key messages emerged from this workshop: (1) the importance of *role modeling*, and (2) the need to make the teaching of professionalism *explicit*.

Faculty-wide workshop on teaching professionalism

Following the invitational workshop, a faculty-wide workshop welcomed sixty-five participants, representing all major specialties. The workshop's goals were to highlight the importance of teaching professionalism in the Faculty of Medicine and to improve the teaching of this content area by transmitting core content, discussing key teaching strategies, and developing an action plan for each setting. The outcome of this workshop was increased buy-in among faculty members, new content experts, and an array of educational resources that could be used for teaching purposes.

Think tank on assessing professionalism

We realized at the outset that, for teaching to be successful, professionalism would need to be assessed in a more systematic manner. Although aspects of professionalism were being assessed on in-training evaluations, improvement was needed. We therefore held another think tank with twenty educational leaders and content experts, to examine methods for evaluating professionalism and develop the content and method of a workshop in this area. We also realized that the attributes of a physician as professional and healer had to be integrated in order for assessments to be comprehensive. Accordingly, definitions of healing attributes were developed (e.g.,

caring and compassion; openness and insight). The outcome of this session was a detailed plan for a faculty-wide workshop.

Faculty-wide workshop on evaluating the physician as healer and professional

The goal of this workshop, which welcomed ninety-five faculty members, was to develop methods for evaluating professionalism at the undergraduate and postgraduate levels. To accomplish this objective, we examined different approaches to assessing professionalism,[75–78] analyzed the benefits and limitations of different assessment methods (e.g., global rating scales; portfolios; critical incidents), and defined specific, measurable behaviors for each attribute. The latter activity highlighted the importance of behavior specificity and yielded a bank of behaviors that could be used in the development of assessment tools. By the end of the workshop, we had developed consensus on the need to improve our assessment of professionalism, identified behaviors that demonstrated the attributes, and developed a series of recommendations that were presented to the Faculty of Medicine.

Our experience in designing faculty development activities for teaching and evaluating professionalism highlighted the value of the following principles:

- Define core content and develop a "common language"
- Provide conceptual frameworks to guide thinking and learning
- Enable experiential learning and promote application to personal settings
- Work to promote buy-in
- Emphasize the *teaching* of the competency
- Build on participants' strengths
- Incorporate follow-up tasks and activities

We also noted that our faculty development program played a major role in promoting change at the undergraduate and postgraduate levels.[2] Some of these changes have included renewal of our undergraduate curriculum to include an emphasis on the physician as healer and professional;[79] increased teaching of this core competency to residents and faculty members; a renewed focus on the assessment of professionalism, which led to the validation of an instrument to assess professionalism among students and residents[80] as well as faculty members;[81] faculty development programs in other areas (e.g., interprofessional education and practice) based on the model used in teaching and learning professionalism; and a new focus on professional identity formation.

Faculty development to promote professional identity formation

In the past five years, we have conducted a number of workshops on professional identity formation, both locally and at national and international meetings. Our very first workshops were held to test our thinking about professional identity formation (and the schemata[59] described in Chapter 1). More recently, they have been designed to help colleagues support the professional identity formation of students and residents. We outline below the workshop goals, key content and underlying principles, and methods used, in the hope that this description will be helpful to others interested in more formally addressing this important content area with faculty members.

Workshop goals

Although the goals of each workshop vary according to the participants and the setting, the following are core to all:

- To define identity, professional identity, and professional identity formation;
- To encourage reflection on personal and professional identities – and their formation;
- To describe the processes of socialization and professional identity formation;
- To identify the key factors (both positive and negative) that influence socialization processes; and
- To discuss and design educational strategies that can positively influence these factors and support professional identity formation.

Key content and underlying principles

The workshop content reflects these goals and the core concepts described in Chapter 1. In addition, we also highlight the following important principles:

- The teaching of medical professionalism is not an end in itself, but a means to an end. In fact, the educational objective is to ensure that everyone entering practice has acquired a professional identity so that they "think, act, and feel like a physician."[82]
- Professional identity formation takes place through the process of socialization throughout medical education *and* practice.

- The process of professional identity formation can be enhanced by understanding the nature of identity formation, the professional identity to be created, and the process of socialization; awareness of the latter can help to create a curriculum and an educational environment that support professional identity formation.
- Adults approach each new phase of their lives (medical school, residency, practice) with pre-established identities; the transformation from being a member of the lay public to a skilled professional is a gradual process, represents a move from the periphery to the center of the group, and leads to an altered identity.
- Individuals voluntarily enter medicine and residency and they are ready for a changed identity. However, although they wish to become members of the "in-group," they are often tense and anxious as they enter a setting of ambiguity.
- Medical practice requires a professional presence that is best grounded in "what one is rather than what one does."[83] (p. 54)

Workshop modules

Following an interactive plenary in which we review the core content described above (e.g., identity formation; socialization), participants engage in a number of small group discussions which include the following topics:

What is your identity?

We first ask participants to think about their own personal and professional identities and to write them down. Importantly, we emphasize the notion of *identities*, as we believe that each individual has more than one. In addition, we highlight that identity is a complex concept, that it represents who we are at any one time, and that identities can change across situations and over time. We also ask participants to think about their personal *and* professional identities, for both overlap and build upon the other. Once participants have written down their perceptions of their identities, we ask them to share one aspect of their identities with a colleague, following which they are asked to share their insights on having engaged in this exercise with the whole group. During this process, participants often recount how their identities are intertwined (or not); how their identities have evolved over time and how some aspects (but not all) are enduring; how they value certain aspects of their identities more than others; and how their professional identity can be linked (quite strongly at times) to the organizational identity. Many participants also remark that they do not often engage in this type of reflection, and that they believe an exercise like this would be helpful for their students and residents. The multiplicity and fluidity of their identities emerge from this discussion.

Factors influencing identity formation

Following a definition and overview of the process of socialization (as described in Chapter 1), we ask participants to think about the factors (both positive and negative) that have influenced their own professional identity formation and might influence that of their learners. Some of the factors that they describe include role models (who can be positive or negative) and mentors; their clinical experiences and the learning environment; feedback from teachers and colleagues; relationships with peers, family, and friends; their own successes and sense of self-efficacy; sheer hard work; and an oft-perceived dissonance between their aspirational goals and what they may perceive as a negative culture (e.g., belonging to a culture of "shame and blame"). We conclude this session by showing participants the schemata in Chapter 1 (see Figures 1.1, 1.4, and 1.5) and indicating how their experiences reflect what the literature has shown.[59]

How students learn through socialization

When time permits, we ask participants to think about how students and residents learn through the process of socialization and how they respond to it. This includes the challenge of learning to play "the role," understanding the medical hierarchy and perceived power dynamics, and learning to live with ambiguity. We also ask participants to use their own experiences as they think about their responses to the process of becoming a professional, which may include anxiety, stress, or self-doubt, or with increasing competence, self-affirmation, joy, or pride.[59] This activity heightens their awareness and empowers them to be of help to their learners, many of whom report an incongruence between what they learn and what they see in the clinical setting.

Institutional and personal actions

We conclude each workshop by asking participants to identify personal and institutional actions that they can pursue to help support professional identity formation in their own settings, as well as possible barriers and facilitators. At an individual level, teachers frequently suggest that they would like to involve students in the process, define and redefine professionalism, and explicitly talk about identity and how it is formed. At an institutional level, they report that they would like to pay greater attention to the organizational culture and identity, the importance of role modeling, and the value of anticipatory guidance. The workshop concludes with a brief session on educational principles that are relevant to all teachers and educators. These include the importance of making identity formation and socialization explicit educational objectives for learners and faculty; enhancing role modeling and ensuring protected time for guided reflection on identity formation; engaging learners as active participants in the development of their own professional identities; identifying barriers to identity formation as well as strategies to overcome negative factors; and ensuring regular activities to enhance a "sense of belonging" for learners and faculty members alike.

Clearly, a three- or four-hour workshop cannot do justice to this important topic. However, based on our experience to date, this introductory workshop does attain its objectives of increased awareness, reflection, and understanding of the role of the teacher and the organization in supporting professional identity formation. It also underscores the importance of making this conversation – and the support of professional identity formation – explicit. Additional topics, such as guided reflection, role modeling, and narrative-based medicine, could also be included.

Conclusion

In summary, faculty development is a critical component in the teaching and learning of professionalism as well as the acquisition of a professional identity. As we collectively move forward, we should strive to bring about change at the *individual* and the *organizational* level, target diverse stakeholders, and secure agreement on the definitions, attributes, and behaviors of professionalism as well as the professional identity that is to be formed. We should also ensure that faculty development takes place in a variety of settings, using diverse formats and educational strategies, and that we evaluate the impact of all activities to ascertain that predetermined goals and objectives are being met.

As we have stated previously, faculty development can help to build consensus, generate support and enthusiasm, and implement a change initiative. Faculty development can also help to prepare teachers for their multiple roles and change the culture within the institution by altering the formal, informal, and hidden curriculum. The true test of faculty development, however, is in the improvement of teaching and learning across the educational continuum, and ultimately, in patient care.

References

1. Steinert, Y, Cruess, S, Cruess, R, Snell, L. Faculty development for teaching and evaluating professionalism: from programme design to curriculum change. *Med Educ*. 2005; **39**(2):127–36.

2. Steinert, Y, Cruess, RL, Cruess, SR, Boudreau, JD, Fuks, A. Faculty development as an instrument of change: a case study on teaching professionalism. *Acad Med*. 2007; **82**(11):1057–64.

3. Cruess, RL, Cruess, SR, Boudreau, JD, Snell, L, Steinert, Y. Reframing medical education to support professional identity formation. *Acad Med*. 2014; **89**(11):1446–51.

4. Jarvis-Selinger, S, Pratt, DD, Regehr, G. Competency is not enough: integrating identity formation into the medical education discourse. *Acad Med*. 2012; **87**(9):1185–90.

5. Cruess, RL, Cruess, SR. Teaching medicine as a profession in the service of healing. *Acad Med*. 1997; **72**(11):941–52.

6. Cruess, SR, Cruess, RL. Professionalism must be taught. *BMJ*. 1997; **315**(7123):1674–77.

7. Whitcomb, ME. Professionalism in medicine. *Acad Med*. 2007; **82**(11):1009.

8. Hodges, BD, Ginsburg, S, Cruess, R, Cruess, S, Delport, R, Hafferty, F, Ho, MJ, Holmboe, E, Holtman, M, Ohbu, S, Rees, C, Ten Cate, O, Tsugawa, Y, Van Mook, W, Wass, V, Wilkinson, T, Wade, W. Assessment of professionalism: recommendations from the Ottawa 2010 Conference. *Med Teach*. 2011; **33**(5):354–63.

9. Birden, H, Glass, N, Wilson, I, Harrison, M, Usherwood, T, Nass, D. Teaching professionalism in medical education: a Best Evidence Medical Education (BEME) systematic review. BEME Guide No. 25. *Med Teach*. 2013; **35**(7):e1252–e1266.

10. Centra, JA. Types of faculty development programs. *J Higher Educ*. 1978; **49**(2):151–62.

11. Bland, CJ, Schmitz, CC, Stritter, FT, Henry, RC, Aluise, JJ. *Successful Faculty in Academic Medicine: Essential Skills and How to Acquire Them*. New York, NY: Springer-Verlag; 1990.

12. Steinert, Y, ed. *Faculty Development in the Health Professions: A Focus on Research and Practice*. Dordrecht, the Netherlands: Springer; 2014.

13. Steinert, Y. Staff development. In Dent, J, Harden, R, eds. *A Practical Guide for Medical Teachers*. Third edition. Edinburgh, UK: Elsevier Churchill Livingstone; 2009:391–97.

14. Steinert, Y. Faculty development in the new millennium: key challenges and future directions. *Med Teach*. 2000; **22**(1):44–50.

15. Hafferty, FW. Beyond curriculum reform: confronting medicine's hidden curriculum. *Acad Med*. 1998; **73**(4):403–07.

16. Bligh, J. Faculty development. *Med Educ*. 2005; **39**(2):120–21.

17. Swanwick, T. See one, do one, then what? Faculty development in postgraduate medical education. *Postgrad Med J*. 2008; **84**(993):339–43.

18. Wilkerson, L, Irby, DM. Strategies for improving teaching practices: a comprehensive approach to faculty development. *Acad Med*. 1998; **73**(4):387–96.

19. McLellan, H, ed. *Situated Learning Perspectives*. Englewood Cliffs, NJ: Educational Technology; 1996.

20. Clarke, D, Hollingsworth, H. Elaborating a model of teacher professional growth. *Teaching and Teacher Education*. 2002; **18**(8):947–67.

21. Webster-Wright, A. Reframing professional development through understanding authentic professional learning. *Rev Educ Res*. 2009; **79**(2):702–39.

22. Steinert, Y, Mann, K, Centeno, A, Dolmans, D, Spencer, J, Gelula, M, Prideaux, D. A systematic review of faculty development initiatives designed to improve teaching effectiveness in medical education: BEME Guide No. 8. *Med Teach*. 2006; **28**(6):497–526.

23. Steinert, Y. Becoming a better teacher: from intuition to intent. In Ende, J, ed. *Theory and Practice of Teaching Medicine*. Philadelphia, PA: American College of Physicians; 2010:73–93.

24. Steinert, Y. Faculty development for teaching improvement: from individual to organizational change. In Walsh, K, ed. *The Oxford Textbook of Medical Education*. Oxford, UK: Oxford University Press; 2013:711–21.

25. Steinert, Y. Learning together to teach together: interprofessional education and faculty development. *J Interprof Care*. 2005; **19**(Suppl 1):60–75.

26. Flynn, SP, Bedinghaus, J, Snyder, C, Hekelman, F. Peer coaching in clinical teaching: a case report. *Fam Med*. 1994; **26**(9):569–70.

27. Beasley, BW, Kallail, KJ, Walling, AD, Davis, N, Hudson, L. Maximizing the use of a Web-based teaching skills curriculum for community-based

volunteer faculty. *J Contin Educ Health Prof.* 2001; **21**(3):158–61.

28. Cook, DA. Faculty development online. In Steinert, Y, ed. *Faculty Development in the Health Professions: A Focus on Research and Practice.* Dordrecht, the Netherlands: Springer; 2014:217–41.

29. Cook, DA, Steinert, Y. Online learning for faculty development: a review of the literature. *Med Teach.* 2013; **35**(11):930–37.

30. Ulian, JA, Stritter, FT. Faculty development in medical education, with implications for continuing medical education. *J Contin Educ Health Prof.* 1996; **16**:181–90.

31. Gruppen, LD, Simpson, D, Searle, NS, Robins, L, Irby, DM, Mullan, PB. Educational fellowship programs: common themes and overarching issues. *Acad Med.* 2006; **81**(11):990–94.

32. Steinert, Y, McLeod, PJ. From novice to informed educator: the teaching scholars program for educators in the health sciences. *Acad Med.* 2006; **81**(11):969–74.

33. Eitel, F, Kanz, KG, Tesche, A. Training and certification of teachers and trainers: the professionalization of medical education. *Med Teach.* 2000; **22**(5):517–26.

34. Purcell, N, Lloyd-Jones, G. Standards for medical educators. *Med Educ.* 2003; **37**(2): 149–54.

35. Tekian, A, Harris, I. Preparing health professions education leaders worldwide: a description of masters-level programs. *Med Teach.* 2012; **34**(1):52–58.

36. Billett, S. Workplace learning: its potential and limitations. *Education and Training.* 1995; **37**(5):20–27.

37. Eraut, M. Informal learning in the workplace: evidence on the real value of work-based learning (WBL). *Development and Learning in Organizations: An International Journal.* 2011; **25**(5):8–12.

38. Billett, S. Situating learning in the workplace – having another look at apprenticeships. *Industrial and Commercial Training.* 1994; **26**(11):9–16.

39. Billett, S. Towards a model of workplace learning: the learning curriculum. *Studies in Continuing Education.* 1996; **18**(1):43–58.

40. Barab, SA, Barnett, M, Squire, K. Developing an empirical account of a community of practice: characterizing the essential tensions. *Journal of the Learning Sciences.* 2002; **11**(4):489–542.

41. Farrell, SE, Digioia, NM, Broderick, KB, Coates, WC. Mentoring for clinician-educators. *Acad Emerg Med.* 2004; **11**(12):1346–50.

42. Bligh, J. Mentoring: an invisible support network. *Med Educ.* 1999; **33**(1):2–3.

43. Morzinski, JA, Diehr, S, Bower, DJ, Simpson, DE. A descriptive, cross-sectional study of formal mentoring for faculty. *Fam Med.* 1996; **28**(6):434–38.

44. Schor, NF, Guillet, R, McAnarney, ER. Anticipatory guidance as a principle of faculty development: managing transition and change. *Acad Med.* 2011; **86**(10):1235–40.

45. Walker, WO, Kelly, PC, Hume, RF Jr. Mentoring for the new millennium. *Med Educ Online.* 2002; 7:15. [Accessed May 25, 2015.] Available from www.med-ed-online.org/f0000038.htm.

46. Steinert, Y. Developing medical educators: a journey, not a destination. In Swanwick, T, ed. *Understanding Medical Education: Evidence, Theory and Practice.* Edinburgh, UK: Association for the Study of Medical Education; 2010:403–18.

47. Rubeck, RF, Witzke, DB. Faculty development: a field of dreams. *Acad Med.* 1998; **73**(9 Suppl):S32–S37.

48. Grant, J. Learning needs assessment: assessing the need. *BMJ.* 2002; **324**:156–59.

49. Lockyer, J. Needs assessment: lessons learned. *J Contin Educ Health Prof.* 1998; **18**(3):190–92.

50. Knowles, MS. *The Modern Practice of Adult Education: From Pedagogy to Andragogy.* New York, NY: Cambridge Books; 1980.

51. Kaufman, DM, Mann, K, Jennett, PA. *Teaching and Learning in Medical Education: How Theory Can Inform Practice.* Edinburgh, UK: Association for the Study of Medical Education; 2000.

52. DeWitt, TG, Goldberg, RL, Roberts, KB. Developing community faculty. Principles, practice, and evaluation. *Am J Dis Child.* 1993; **147**(1):49–53.

53. Langlois, JP, Thach, SB. Bringing faculty development to community-based preceptors. *Acad Med.* 2003; **78**(2):150–55.

54. Stufflebeam, DL. Alternative approaches to educational evaluation: a self-study guide for educators. In Popham, WJ, ed. *Evaluation in Education: Current Applications.* Berkley, CA: McCutchan Publishing; 1974:95–144.

55. Popham, WJ. *Educational Evaluation.* Boston, MA: Allyn and Bacon; 1993.

56. Wholey, JS, Hatry, HP, Newcomer, KE, eds. *Handbook of Practical Program Evaluation.* San Francisco, CA: Jossey-Bass; 1994.

57. Kirkpatrick, DL. *Evaluating Training Programs: The Four Levels.* San Francisco, CA: Berrett-Koehler; 1994.

58. Swick, HM. Toward a normative definition of medical professionalism. *Acad Med.* 2000; **75**(6):612–16.

59. Cruess, RL, Cruess, SR, Boudreau, JD, Snell, L, Steinert, Y. A schematic representation of the professional identity formation and socialization of medical students and residents: a guide for medical educators. *Acad Med.* 2015; **90**(6):718–25.

60. American Board of Internal Medicine. *Project Professionalism* (revised). Philadelphia, PA: ABIM;

1999. [Accessed June 4, 2015]. Available from www.abimfoundation.org/~/media/Foundation/Professionalism/Project%20professionalism.

61. Royal College of Physicians and Surgeons of Canada. *CanMEDS 2000 Project – Skills for the New Millennium: Report of the Societal Needs Working Group*. Ottawa, ON; RCPSC; 1996. [Accessed June 4, 2015]. Available from www.surgeons.org/media/301671/canmeds_e.pdf.

62. Quaintance, JL, Arnold, L, Thompson, GS. What students learn about professionalism from faculty stories: an "appreciative inquiry" approach. *Acad Med*. 2010; **85**(1):118–23.

63. Cruess, SR, Cruess, RL, Steinert, Y. Role modelling–making the most of a powerful teaching strategy. *BMJ*. 2008; **336**(7646):718–21.

64. Kenny, NP, Mann, KV, MacLeod, H. Role modeling in physicians' professional formation: reconsidering an essential but untapped educational strategy. *Acad Med*. 2003; **78**(12):1203–10.

65. Mann, KV. Faculty development to promote role-modeling and reflective practice. In Steinert, Y, ed. *Faculty Development in the Health Professions: A Focus on Research and Practice*. Dordrecht, the Netherlands: Springer; 2014:245–64.

66. Cruess, RL, Cruess, SR. Teaching professionalism: general principles. *Med Teach*. 2006; **28**(3):205–08.

67. Hilton, SR, Slotnick, HB. Proto-professionalism: how professionalisation occurs across the continuum of medical education. *Med Educ*. 2005; **39**(1):58–65.

68. Epstein, RM. Mindful practice. *JAMA*. 1999; **282**(9):833–39.

69. Novack, DH, Epstein, RM, Paulsen, RH. Toward creating physician-healers: fostering medical students' self-awareness, personal growth, and well-being. *Acad Med*. 1999; **74**(5):516–20.

70. Maudsley, G, Strivens, J. Promoting professional knowledge, experiential learning and critical thinking for medical students. *Med Educ*. 2000; **34**(7):535–44.

71. Mamede, S, Schmidt, HG. The structure of reflective practice in medicine. *Med Educ*. 2004; **38**(12):1302–08.

72. Graffam, B, Bowers, L, Keene, KN. Using observations of clinicians' teaching practices to build a model of clinical instruction. *Acad Med*. 2008; **83**(8):768–74.

73. Rademacher, R, Simpson, D, Marcdante, K. Critical incidents as a technique for teaching professionalism. *Med Teach*. 2010; **32**(3):244–49.

74. Wenger, E, McDermott, R, Snyder, WM. *Cultivating Communities of Practice: A Guide to Managing Knowledge*. Boston, MA: Harvard Business School Press; 2002.

75. Arnold, L. Assessing professional behaviors: yesterday, today, and tomorrow. *Acad Med*. 2002; **77**(6):502–15.

76. Ginsburg, S, Regehr, G, Hatala, R, McNaughton, N, Frohna, A, Hodges, B, Lingard, L, Stern, D. Context, conflict, and resolution: a new conceptual framework for evaluating professionalism. *Acad Med*. 2000; **75**(10 Suppl):S6–S11.

77. Papadakis, MA, Osborn, EH, Cooke, M, Healy, K. A strategy for the detection and evaluation of unprofessional behavior in medical students. *Acad Med*. 1999; **74**(9):980–90.

78. Van Luijk, SJ, Smeets, JGE, Smits, J, Wolfhagen, I, Perquin, MLF. Assessing professional behaviour and the role of academic advice at the Maastricht Medical School. *Med Teach*. 2000; **22**(2):168–77.

79. Boudreau, JD, Cassell, EJ, Fuks, A. A healing curriculum. *Med Educ*. 2007; **41**(12):1193–1201.

80. Cruess, R, McIlroy, JH, Cruess, S, Ginsburg, S, Steinert, Y. The Professionalism Mini-Evaluation Exercise: a preliminary investigation. *Acad Med*. 2006; **81**(10 Suppl):S74–S78.

81. Young, ME, Cruess, SR, Cruess, RL, Steinert, Y. The Professionalism Assessment of Clinical Teachers (PACT): the reliability and validity of a novel tool to evaluate professional and clinical teaching behaviors. *Adv Health Sci Educ Theory Pract*. 2014; **19**(1):99–113.

82. Merton, RK. Some preliminaries to a sociology of medical education. In Merton, RK, Reader, LG, Kendall, PL, eds. *The Student Physician: Introductory Studies in the Sociology of Medical Education*. Cambridge, MA: Harvard University Press; 1957:3–79.

83. Hafferty, FW. Professionalism and the socialization of medical students. In Cruess, RL, Cruess, SR, Steinert, Y, eds. *Teaching Medical Professionalism*. New York, NY: Cambridge University Press; 2009:53–71.

Chapter 10

Becoming interprofessional: professional identity formation in the health professions

Jill E. Thistlethwaite, Koshila Kumar, and Christopher Roberts

Introduction

Professional programs in higher education, such as healthcare, aim to prepare students for practice through the acquisition of appropriate and relevant knowledge, skills, attitudes, and values. They should also focus on students' integration into the profession: their becoming professionals and subsequently being professionals.[1] However, as professional identity formation has been conceptualized as "an on-going process of interpretation and re-interpretation of experiences,"[2] one could argue that an individual can never *be* but is always *becoming* a professional. There is, however, a frequently held assumption of one profession, one identity, although a professional is acknowledged as having multiple roles. In this chapter, we question what happens to professional identity in the context of modern healthcare and contemporary education of the health professions, which is increasingly characterized by teamwork and collaborative practice, and accordingly, whether healthcare professionals also need to nurture and sustain an interprofessional identity. The question then follows as to whether their interprofessional identity subsumes the uniprofessional or whether an individual may move between the two identities depending on context and inclination. Are health professionals plural actors as the French sociologist Lahire suggests? "And so we are plural, different in the different situations of ordinary life, foreign to other parts of ourselves when we are engaged in this or that domain of social existence."[3] Daily living involves circulation through different roles: employee, researcher, parent, partner, teacher, and practitioner. But in these roles, are people mainly demonstrating differences in behavior depending on context rather than identity? Are healthcare professionals and students *doing* rather than *being* or *becoming*? As

Hafferty has suggested in relation to medical students, the act of developing a "professional presence" is "best grounded in what one is rather than what one does."[4]

"Being interprofessional" has been described as consisting of three aspects: knowing what to do (thinking about what action is needed and why); having the skills to do what needs to be done (being competent and practicing correctly); and conducting oneself in the right way during performance (including appropriate attitudes and values).[5] However, these three aspects can just as easily be applied to "being professional" or being "uniprofessional." By debating and defining interprofessional competencies and their translation into behavior in the workplace, health professional educators may gain a greater sense of the additional attributes that constitute being interprofessional. Lists of such competencies frequently include the following: values and ethics, understanding roles and responsibilities of other healthcare professionals, interprofessional communication, and teamwork and collaborative practice (see, for example, the Interprofessional Education Collaborative [IPEC] of the United States core competencies document).[6] Very broad competencies are not particularly helpful as many of these are abstract, socially constructed, and difficult to translate into observable and assessable behaviors.[7] Moreover, being competent is not evidence of professional identity, just as behavior is not necessarily evidence of how people think, what they believe, and what their values are.

D'Amour and Oandasan have defined interprofessionality as "the development of a cohesive practice between professionals from different disciplines."[8] In addition, Brooks and Thistlethwaite have proposed that interprofessionality is characterized by "the transformation in practice which may result from

Teaching Medical Professionalism, 2nd Edition, ed. Richard L. Cruess, Sylvia R. Cruess and Yvonne Steinert. Published by Cambridge University Press. © Cambridge University Press 2016.

combining and blending specialist knowledge and expertise."[9] They have also posed some critical questions about the transformation in identity that is associated with working and learning across professional boundaries, such as in the context of interprofessionality, and the synergy and possible disjunctions between multiple identities.[9] We note that the term "interprofessionalism" is also found in the literature and has all the nuances and controversies associated with professionalism. IPEC defines "interprofessional professionalism" as a "consistent demonstration of core values evidenced by professionals working together, aspiring to and wisely applying principles of altruism, excellence, caring, ethics, respect, communication, [and] accountability to achieve optimal health and wellness in individuals and communities."[6]

Helping students to achieve interprofessional competencies to ultimately improve patient care is one of the functions of interprofessional education (IPE). Another, although not always as explicitly stated, is the development of an interprofessional or "collective" identity.[6] There is ongoing debate in relation to IPE as to the best time to facilitate health professional students to "learn from, with and about each other."[10] The question is informed by work on professional identity formation and professional stereotyping. Proponents of the early introduction of interprofessional learning activities feel that such interaction reduces the likelihood of one profession forming negative opinions of the others, while other educators believe that students should be confident with their own profession's identity before learning more about their future colleagues. However, no one so far has convincingly shown that the timing of IPE helps or hinders either uniprofessional identity formation or the development of an interprofessional persona. The majority of the evaluations of IPE initiatives at the pre-qualification (pre-licensure) level are short-term explorations of whether learning outcomes have been met and competencies mastered, and frequently they focus solely on learner satisfaction.[11] While change in attitudes to interprofessional learning and working may be measured before and after the learning activities (commonly through the use of *RIPLS* – the Readiness for Interprofessional Learning Scale,[12] and the *IEPS* – the Interdisciplinary Education Perception Scale)[13], such measurement says little about the process of professional identity formation. Outcomes-based evaluations focus on product rather than process and ignore the "personal

transformation" process that underlies professional socialization.[4]

In this chapter, we reengage with these important questions. In particular, we ask if "being interprofessional" is an identity in its own right in a changing and complex healthcare context characterized by teamwork and collaborative practice and, if so, whether this interprofessional identity coexists with or subsumes the uniprofessional identity. We discuss the implications for health professions education arising from our critical reflection on these questions at the end of each main section and at the end of the chapter.

Learning to be a (uni)professional

In becoming and subsequently being a healthcare professional, students and trainees develop a range of beliefs, attitudes, values, and expectations about the profession they have entered. Thus, a professional identity is forged and encompasses the norms, beliefs, values, and world views of that particular group or community.[14]

Shulman suggests that novice professionals are taught about three fundamental dimensions of professional work: "to think, to perform and to act with integrity."[15] (Note the similarity here to Hammick et al.'s three aspects of being interprofessional discussed above.[5]) Each profession tries to achieve this learning through "signature pedagogies," which acknowledge that education and training are not simply about knowledge transmission but also about preparation for a professional role.[15] While there are some similarities across the health professions in that experiential learning in clinical settings is common to most, the type of tutor or supervisor, the style of group work, and the use of simulation and skills laboratories vary. The rituals of learning in medical school, for example, include ward rounds, bedside teaching, students being asked to "clerk" patients and report back (mostly without being observed), simulated patients, and the practice of clinical skills on mannequins and plastic limbs. The predominantly siloed education of the health professions ensures that one type of student is unaware of the curriculum and signature pedagogies of another. This results in a lack of understanding of roles and responsibilities when the professions come together to attempt to work together. As Shulman writes, "Signature pedagogies are important precisely because they are pervasive.... [T]hey define the functions of expertise in a field, the locus of authority, and the privileges of rank and standing."[15]

During their prequalification programs, students are socialized into their profession and professional role and undergo a critical period of professional identity formation.[16] Role acquisition occurs through learning and teaching: didactic and interactive, social and clinical. Role models and formal, informal, and hidden curricula influence how a novice professional develops a sense of (uni)professional self.[17] Health professions education is still delivered predominantly by members of the same profession, either by faculty academics, who might no longer practice clinically, or by clinical tutors or supervisors in clinical settings. While basic scientists and specialist educators may also be involved, it is the professionals who reinforce their professional culture, values, beliefs, and practices[5] as both teachers and role models. The literature is extensive on this topic, and examples are found in individual professional and interprofessional journals. Socialization into one profession is frequently thought to preclude the ability to collaborate across professional lines, as students assimilate the culture, values, jargon, and working practices of their developing new identity.[16] IPE is seen as a way of helping individuals understand the attributes of other professions to facilitate future collaborative practice. However, other studies have shown that developing a professional identity serves an important preparatory function for interprofessional familiarization,[18] with IPE then aimed at introducing students to other professions so they may develop an understanding of their roles and responsibilities within healthcare teams and the wider health system.

Implications

Health professions education requires an appropriate mix of uniprofessional and interprofessional activities chosen to help students meet appropriate learning outcomes as defined by their professional accreditation bodies and their institutions. Learning outcomes should be assessable and cover "knowing what to do," "having the skills to do what needs to be done," and "conducting oneself in the right way during performance."[5] Learning focuses on an understanding of the nature of professionalism, professional identity, one's own professional role, and the roles of other professionals involved in healthcare delivery. Competency frameworks, such as that of IPEC,[6] are helpful in developing outcomes.

Theories of identity formation from an interprofessional perspective

While the literature is abundant with examples of identity development within (uni)professional contexts (as demonstrated in this book), there has been less discussion about professional identity formation from an interprofessional perspective. In this regard, Whittington's chapter on "Interprofessional education and identity,"[19] published by the Higher Education Academy (UK) in 2005, neatly summarized some of the most commonly applied theories of identity formation at that time. Whittington noted that identity theories are many and remain controversial, while there is no consensus on the meaning of "identity" itself. The chapter outlined three perspectives, with both similarities and differences among the three. The first of these, the social identity approach, is cited frequently in the interprofessional literature and has been the subject of empirical studies; it is grounded in social psychology. The second theory takes a constructionist viewpoint, with a focus on discourse and narrative. The last combines many elements, including social structuralism and constructionism, with psychological insights, to probe the concept of self-identity in the twenty-first century. Such theories try to make sense of what some have called the "tribes of the health professions,"[20] with their attendant tribal boundaries and conflicts that focus mainly on difference and competition.

In the sections below, we delve deeper into these three theoretical fields from an interprofessional perspective, updating Whittington's exposition with more recent work. We begin with the social identity approach by revisiting the work of Allport, the American psychologist who introduced the term "in-group" and the contact hypothesis.

Social identity theory: Allport's contribution

Allport's seminal work on prejudice was published in 1954. Its language is of its time, with his work being influenced by the prevalent social conditions and attitudes to ethnicity and race in that decade.[21] He coined the term "in-group" in relation to a person's place in society, proposing that the in-group to which one belonged depended on one's "race, stock, family tradition, religion, caste and occupational status."[21] His contact hypothesis provided a framework for considering intergroup attitudes and postulated that positive outcomes are only possible if different groups pursue common goals and, at the same time, if the environment is supportive of their working together. There are four stages of contact, which Allport described as a *peaceful progression*. In the first, *sheer contact*, different groups come into proximal contact. This may lead to *competition*, but also, over time, to *accommodation*: people from specific in-groups relax and become at ease with one another while still respecting and valuing their differences. The fourth stage is *assimilation*. Not all groups go through all four stages; groups may resist assimilation and want to hold onto what makes them distinct. In some cases, this resistance may revert to further competition or even to overt conflict.[21] Relating this to health professions education, IPE is an opportunity for health professional students to meet through contact and to accommodate over time, but it is not generally considered to be aimed at facilitating assimilation, because the professions, while frequently overlapping in scopes of practice, remain distinct.

We believe that "third culture personality,"[22] derived from intercultural work, is a better term than assimilation: ideally, professionals such as nurses with their own professional identities (first culture), come into contact with other professionals, such as physical therapists, physician assistants, and doctors (second culture), and learn together to work together within a collaborative culture of healthcare (third culture).[23]

Social identity theory: beyond Allport

Social identity theory is an amalgamation of two related theories: social identity and self-categorization. It derives in part from the work of Allport and focuses on intergroup relations.[24] While acknowledging the existence of personal identities, the hypothesis is that some of us define ourselves based on our membership in groups and the derived shared social identity. Social identity theory encompasses how individuals from one profession or community compare and differentiate themselves from other professional groups and deal with issues of rivalry, stereotyping, discrimination, and status. Tajfel and Turner appropriated the term in-group and contrasted this with "out-group," stating that there is pressure "to evaluate one's own group positively through in-group/out-group comparisons," which "lead social groups to attempt to differentiate themselves from each other."[25] Through identification with our own social group (or profession), we may form biases and become prejudiced against other groups. Furthermore, we may stereotype out-group members and make unfavorable comparisons of their attributes with our own in-group's, thus establishing our sense of self and boosting our self-esteem: the process of intergroup differentiation.[25] As Whittington succinctly states, "Social identity theory deals with the implications of distinctions between 'us' and 'them'."[19]

Self-categorization theory suggests that there are three levels that can define the self: personal identity (the individual); social identity (one's in-group); and interspecies (the self as a human being – human identity).[26] When an individual privileges group identity over self, depersonalization occurs and one's perception of group homogeneity is enhanced. Group membership is seen as prescriptive and defines what attitudes, values, and behaviors are appropriate for each situation and setting (in our context, such definition is at the core of professionalism). This process facilitates collective behavior and a move from thinking about "I and me" to "we and us."[19]

Of course, groups have status differences within any society. A group's position in the hierarchy confers varying amounts of power and influence. If one is unhappy with one's in-group's prestige, there are a number of options: leaving the group; taking the necessary steps to become part of another group (through, for example, additional qualifications or marriage); making unflattering comments about relevant out-groups; and engaging in activities to promote equity among groups. The in-group hypothesis has similarities to the thinking of Bourdieu and his conceptualization of habitus, field, and capital.[27] Habitus refers to the socialized norms or tendencies that guide behavior and thinking through one's upbringing and place in society (i.e., one's in-group), and through the influence of what have been referred to as norm circles.[28] It is not necessarily static and can be changed, as can one's membership in a group or profession through the accrual of capital – economic, social, symbolic, and cultural. Cultural capital, for example, is what you know, including professional qualifications. It has a major role in defining how much power one has in a given "field." One's field is the environment or arenas in which an individual lives and works. Position in a given field depends on the amount and quality of capital accrued and may be the result of competition with others in the same field but in a different in-group.

Taken together, the social identity approach has challenged traditional assumptions about stereotyping. Allport defined a stereotype as "an exaggerated belief associated with a category. Its function is to justify (rationalize) our conduct in relation to that category"[21] (category meaning generalization). Previously, stereotypes had been thought of as fixed mental representations, resistant to change. Now they are thought to be amenable to alteration depending on context and familiarity with alternative viewpoints.[29] This is of importance to IPE, which aims to reduce and challenge the formation of stereotyping across the health and social care professions.[30] (We discuss stereotypes in more detail below.) These theories, though nearly forty years old, are still applied in the interprofessional literature, possibly because "the social identity approach is a rare beast; a meta-theory that is ambitious in scope but ultimately rests on simple, elegant, testable and usable principles."[31]

Discourse and narrative

Whittington's second perspective focuses on discourse and narrative.[19] Many social theorists argue that discourse shapes our social world, drawing on the work of Foucault[32] and of other social constructionists. Social constructionism holds that social phenomena are understood as "the outcome of discursive interaction rather than as extra-discursive phenomena in their own right."[33] While "discourse" has many meanings, the underlying premise is that how we collectively think and communicate about the world affects the way the world is;[28] in other words, we construct meaning in interaction with others, using language as the primary medium.[19] What is important is the content of this communication, rather than the linguistic norms and the language that are used.[28]

Thus, from this perspective, identities are not given, but are continually being constructed and reconstructed through dialogue and interaction with others. Identities are affected by the age, gender, culture, values, ethnicity, sexuality, status, profession, and even health[33] of the people interacting. In relation to identity, a "narrative" approach offers a promising avenue for exploring the stories that people tell about how they make sense of their identity. A "narrative" approach to identity elaborates the account of how identity is constructed. Individuals use narrative to reconstruct their "autobiographical past" and ponder on the future so that their lives gain a degree of purpose, meaning, and usefulness.[34] Narratives can

be highly interactional and conversational.[35] The result is a coherent story of their identity over time.[35]

Self-identity in the twenty-first century

Under this third heading, Whittington[19] references the work of Giddens[36] and discusses contemporary life, with its global reach, profound changes, and technological advances that are leading people to challenge tradition and ways of behaving. Of course, Whittington was writing after the development of the Internet, but before the explosion of social media, smart phones, and interconnectivity, with their opposing features of collectivity and isolation. People no longer need to meet in the same geographical location but can still be "face-to-face." People (or at least those with access to the right technology) expect to be able to access anything at any time: instant gratification. Health professionals are able to become members of diverse virtual communities, frequently hiding their real identities behind avatars and pseudonyms, expressing opinions and feelings in postings that others may describe as "unprofessional."

Giddens[36] suggested that the self has become a reflexive project. The notion is articulated through the leading question of "Is everything alright?" as a central motif.[36] Here, self-identity refers to the "self as reflexively understood by the person"[36] and *reflexivity* means the human capacity to turn the attention of consciousness back upon itself: we are aware of being aware, of thinking about thinking, and are able to provide accounts about ourselves.[37] However, the explosion of knowledge and doubt about its veracity have led to uncertainty and a sense of risk, which can erode trust in authority and tradition, and anxiety about one's identity and place in the "system."[19]

Implications

Simply combining healthcare students for shared learning (i.e., learning the same content side by side) is not sufficient to reduce intergroup prejudice or improve intergroup attitudes and, indeed, may have deleterious effects. To reduce intergroup tensions, it is important to develop strategies that will create a positive and interactive learning environment where two or more professions learn together.[38] The experience of "us" and "them" in poorly constructed IPE can be elicited simply as an in-group consisting of students of the same discipline as the teacher and an out-group of students from another discipline, giving a sense of discrimination by the in-group against the out-group.[38]

IPE in the early stages of health professional education should frequently involve small-group work during which the students talk about their profession and its roles and responsibilities (as they understand them at the time) and tell stories about how they came to be students and the influences on that choice. Patients' stories are often interwoven into these sessions with narratives of how different members of the team collaborate to ensure the optimal outcome. Experienced clinicians may tell stories of their work. Thus, IPE, as evidenced by a UK-based audit, is being delivered through "expository, student-centered, interactive and conversational practice-based methods where the learners actively constructed knowledge for themselves from an array of experiences, rather than concentrated on knowledge-based subject matter communicated from the teacher to the taught."[39] Students learn to become reflective practitioners.

As students gain more clinical experience, interprofessional small-group work should consider the discourses of the different professions and how these might affect collaboration and power relationships; for example, what are the issues arising from identifying those who receive healthcare as patients, clients, or service users?

Threats to professional identity

We now consider the following threats to professional identity: conflict, fault lines, and stereotyping.

Conflict

In the field of healthcare delivery, conflict has been described as occurring when "behavior is intended to obstruct the achievement of some other person's goals."[40] That interprofessional practice and collaboration may engender conflict among the healthcare professions is highlighted by the inclusion of competencies related to negotiation and conflict resolution in a number of educational frameworks. For example, the Interprofessional Education Collaborative (USA) includes the following under "communication": "Use respectful language appropriate for a given difficult situation, crucial conversation, or interprofessional conflict; contributes to conflict resolution,"[6] while the National Interprofessional Competency Framework of the Canadian Interprofessional Health Collaborative

(CIHC) has interprofessional conflict resolution as the last of its six competencies: "Learners/practitioners actively engage self and others, including the patient/ client/ family, in dealing effectively with interprofessional conflict."[41] Despite the inclusion of conflict in these competency frameworks, it is rarely covered well or even at all in health professional curricula.[42]

Conflict has been linked to the hierarchy and subsequent differential treatment across professional groups that threaten professional identity.[43] While medicine may claim to be one of the oldest professions, other areas of healthcare have professionalized over the decades, with the attendant specialized body of knowledge and skills, code of conduct, and self-regulatory bodies that constitute a "profession."[44] The "newer" professions have members who develop a specific professional identity commensurate with their role. Professions, as they mature, challenge the older examples and begin to encroach on the traditional boundaries of the competition.[45] Professional boundaries and identities are interlinked; they are constructed and maintained by professionals themselves while varying over time, as the professions themselves are not static. The healthcare professions are viewed as different, with diverse approaches to patient care and varying professional jargon in spite of being united in the provision of optimal patient care. Practice is constructed from different perspectives.[46] Alongside this differentiation, each profession may hold stereotypical views of others and define their identities in contrast rather than in common.

Fault lines

McNeil et al.[43] extended the typology of Chobrot-Mason et al.[47] to explore the triggers that cause "fault lines" to appear within interprofessional teams and how these relate to conflicts of professional identity. Such fault lines, similar to geological faults in the Earth's surface, are explicit or hidden fractures that cause friction, displacement, and collisions, and have the potential to lead to dysfunctionality within teams. Chobrot-Mason et al.[47] based their typology on field data from two studies involving 11 different countries and more than 150 people, across a range of organizations, such as financial services, education, and manufacturing. Analysis was framed by social identity theory and the notion of intergroup anxiety, which has a historical basis depending on prior conflicts between groups, such as different professions, as well as current conditions. They found that conflict was escalated by anxiety related to what was happening in society in general, as well as differential treatment, conflicting values, expectation of or reluctance for assimilation (at odds with Allport's "peaceful progression"),[21] and insulting or humiliating action. When intergroup anxiety was particularly high, even simple contact could lead to polarization and adverse outcomes: "Dominant and non-dominant group members interpret differential treatment very differently.... [I]n addition to promotions, pay, disciplinary actions and allocation of developmental opportunities served as the foci of the differential treatment. All of these distribution decisions have the potential to activate employee feelings of being undervalued and underappreciated."[47]

Extrapolating the triggers to health professional identity conflicts, McNeil et al.[43] highlight the dominance of the medical profession, even in interprofessional teams when medical supervision is often deemed necessary during "collaborative care." Medicine is powerful compared to the other professions, and seeks to retain its power in many countries, restricting the autonomy of other health professionals and their scope of practice. In relation to the specific triggers of fault lines, McNeil et al.[43] provide examples from the literature such as higher pay for doctors (differential treatment), divergent views about the quality of life (different values), the medical profession arguing against independent nurse practitioners (assimilation), and offensive language being used about other professions (insult or humiliating behavior). However, they could not find examples of conflict arising from simple contact.[43]

Stereotyping

Stereotypes serve as justifying devices, which fall into three types.[48] *Ego-justification* occurs when individuals feel better about themselves through the denigration of others. *Group-justification* rationalizes discrimination against other groups and helps members feel positive about their own group and its membership. *System-justification* legitimates institutional forms of prejudice and discrimination while promoting hierarchical structures. Low-status groups tend to be referred to in more communal, socio-emotional terms, while high-status groups are described in action and achievement-orientated terms.[48] For example, in relation to their relative positions in the hierarchy of the health professions, nurses are caring; doctors are diagnosticians.[23]

Implications

Learners need to be introduced to the possibility and nature of conflict arising in and between healthcare teams, both inter- and intraprofessionally. However, this should be after they have had experience of working collaboratively with peers and have an understanding of how teams function. Formal and informal professionalism discussions should be facilitated to help identify and acknowledge conflict and its etiology and effects, while providing activities for senior students to develop skills in negotiation, shared decision-making, and values-based practice.[49,50] The fact that we form stereotypes through early experience[48] provides a strong rationale for IPE to begin early before stereotypes form, though frequently students arrive at university with preconceived ideas about the health professions through their own experiences of healthcare and media portrayal.

Boundary crossing and interprofessional identity

A professional boundary is found at the point where one health profession's role and scope of practice ends and another's begins. How boundaries are perceived as either fixed or permeable may help or hinder interprofessional practice. Boundaries may be viewed as sociocultural differences, which cause discontinuities in practice or interaction.[51] As professions mature, such boundaries may become contested spheres of practice, while collaborative practice allows for some overlapping of roles, which requires negotiation and reconstruction.[52] Boundary crossing leads to learning at a horizontal level, a form of expansive learning that is transformational and co-configured.[53] If the professions attempt to stay within their traditionally defined boundaries, the potential for interprofessional learning is lost as the professions defend their territory and reduce dialogue.

If we consider the goal of interprofessional practice is to deliver patient-centered collaborative healthcare, then barriers to achieving this goal include the factors discussed above: organizational structuralism, power relationships between the professions (and between professionals and their clients), role socialization, and differences in professional values.[50] Values "operate as standards by which our actions are selected."[55] A profession that appears homogeneous may consist of individuals with very different values.[50] There is frequently an assumption that coworkers, team members, and members of our own profession have similar values to our own[50] and therefore, we may not think of exploring these before or while working together.

A further approach to conceptualizing traversing professional boundaries has emerged from preliminary work exploring health professional education in longitudinal integrated clinical placements. Daly et al.[56] explored a setting, in which up to thirty students from different professions were placed at any one time in a rural community, from the perspective of the medical students.[56] It was the informal curriculum,[57] with multiple encounters between students, patients and their families, and clinical teachers and other health staff, that played an important role in supporting and extending student learning. Learning in a longitudinal placement and the development of professional identity as a rural practitioner took place through a process of socialization, alluding to the socially constructed and situated nature of learning. Learning can be conceptualized as a social phenomenon that reflects "our own deeply social nature as human beings capable of knowing."[58] Wenger proposed a social learning system as a way of framing learning as a social process underpinned by a dynamic interplay between "social competence and personal experience."[59] It involves communities of practice, boundary processes, and identity formation. A community of practice[58] is the basic unit of analysis within a social learning system and is defined as a "group of people who share a concern or a passion for something they do and learn how to do it better as they interact regularly." Communities of practice (CoP) can be understood as the "containers" or learning spaces, in which competence is developed within a social learning system. Individual learners participate in multiple CoPs, negotiate the boundaries between them in different ways, and so develop their personal and social identities.[60] This raises the question of whether the notion of a social learning system can be usefully applied to understand the elements and processes affecting interprofessional learning within a longitudinal integrated placement program.

Implications

We acknowledge that many of the clinical environments through which students rotate might not, or appear not to, have a strong ethos of team-based care delivery or interprofessional collaborative practice. If students only learn "with, from and about"[10] other health professionals during their formal IPE sessions, they may consider that "all this learning-about–the-other must not be so important… a null curriculum operating at full steam."[61] However, the emerging evidence of the utility of longitudinal integrated clinical placements in facilitating the acquisition of teamwork competencies[62] suggests that such placements are one way of promoting the development of interprofessionalism, providing that students from two or more professions are co-located.

The transformation of the barriers discussed earlier into facilitators may be carried out in four phases of activity: *sensitization, exploration, implementation,* and *evaluation.*

The specific actions within each phase are the following:

- Sensitization: awareness of power imbalance and professional socialization;
- Exploration: clarification of roles and values;
- Implementation: developing trust and sharing power; and
- Evaluation: team building and teamwork, team member satisfaction, client outcomes.[54]

Identity dissonance as a theoretical lens

We propose that identity dissonance[63] provides a framework for understanding and explaining potential conflicts and dilemmas related to identity. The term "dissonance" was first coined to describe how possessing conflicting cognitions could engender feelings of discomfort and unease for individuals[64] and has since been linked to emotions,[65] values,[66] and identity.[63] Dissonance is likely to occur when there is greater discrepancy in values and opinions related to a significant issue or when norms are "unclear, unspecified or inconsistently applied."[66] Much of the substantive theorizing regarding identity dissonance has been undertaken by Costello in an ethnographic study of students' experiences in higher education.[63] Drawing on extensive data from more than 300 students in their first year in the professional schools of law and social work, she suggested that students' academic and professional success or failure was dependent on the extent of alignment between their personal or self-identity, representing an individual's "assumptions and world views, taste, postures and gestures, and emotional orientations"[63] and their emerging professional identity, encompassing the values, beliefs, attitudes, world views, practices, expectations, and demands of the emerging professional role.

Dissonance has been shown to exert a strong motivational influence to reconcile conflicting cognitions, emotions, values, and identity. Festinger showed that individuals tried to reconcile their conflicted cognitions by attempting to reduce the relative importance of a conflicting belief, acquire new beliefs, or entirely remove a conflicting belief.[64] Other dissonance management strategies noted in the literature include altering internal ideals to align with external expectations and demands (reconciliation) or dismissal of external values and ideals and maintenance of internal ideals (preservation);[67] regulating emotional responses;[65] physically relocating;[68] or engaging in deliberative reflection and revision of one's understandings of everyday activity or fundamental interpretations of self.[69-71] Costello also distinguished between types of identity dissonance based on the management strategies used by participants in her study.[63] Those who attempted to minimize conflict in identities by altering or shedding their personal values and identity so these no longer conflicted with their emerging professional identity were categorized as positively identity dissonant. Participants who attempted to reconcile identity dissonance by resisting or distancing themselves from the demands and expectations of their emerging professional role were labeled as being negatively identity dissonant. Negative identity dissonance was an overwhelmingly traumatic experience associated with feelings of alienation, isolation, anxiety, doubt, frustration, low self-worth, poor academic performance, and a low likelihood of professional success.[63]

Applying the lens of identity dissonance enabled us to empirically illustrate the dilemmas and contradictions in identity experienced by researchers engaged in interdisciplinary health research (IDHR) in the higher education setting.[68] We illustrated that participants' conflicted experience of IDHR was underpinned by a disharmonious relationship between their institution-identity and affinity-identity.[68] The former is discipline-based, organizationally legitimated, and more socially valued, while the latter reflected their personal values and preferences for working across discipline boundaries and interdisciplinary conceptions of self. As a result of dissonance in identity, a specific and critical challenge for many of our study participants was defining and positioning their work and their sense of self in the higher education institution and sector. In this study, positively identity dissonant participants responded to the conflict between their affinity and institution identities by altering fundamental aspects of self and attempting to align with discipline-based values and norms of identity that were institutionally valued. This was a natural and easier option for those who had strong allegiances with and orientation to a particular academic discipline or health profession and enabled them to achieve a sense of fit and belonging within a traditional academic model. However, it was also associated with feelings of emotional vulnerability and a sense of loss associated with letting go of their personal values and preferences for interdisciplinarity.

In contrast, negatively identity dissonant health researchers responded by distancing themselves from or rejecting dominant institutional narratives of identity, which were defined in relation to a discipline. Some attempted to actively contort their self-image by drawing on multiple and flexible identity labels resonating with the notion of performative strategies[72] depending on the research context and requirements of the role. Although this strategy enabled participants to establish their credibility, competence, and legitimacy in line with normative expectations, managing the complex demands and expectations associated with multiple identities was tiring and difficult. Others questioned and challenged disciplinary-based approaches to knowledge production, research inquiry, and identity and actively affirmed their values and affinity for IDHR. For these participants, conceptualizing the boundaries between disciplines as being in flux and constant negotiation provided a more suitable framework to think about their identity, resonating with the existing literature.[73] However, they did so with the awareness that the legitimacy and credibility of this identity would be contested within the normative discipline-based higher-education sector. In contrast to Costello, who proposed that negative identity dissonance was an overwhelmingly unpleasant experience,[63] our study showed that negative identity dissonance could also be associated with positive outcomes such as enhanced self-confidence and self-efficacy, which contributed to health researchers' feelings of empowerment.[68] The notion of protecting the self also emerged as a key driver in the face of limited options to reconcile contradictions in identities, with some negatively identity dissonant participants disassociating themselves from a particular team, workplace, or institutional setting that may have been the setting for contested identities and work practices.

In summary, applying identity dissonance[63] as an analytical lens enabled us to empirically illustrate that IDHR can be essentially understood as a lived space within which researchers' identities are contested and negotiated in different ways. This notion of managing multiple and conflicting identities in different ways is echoed in the organizational identity literature, which illustrates that individuals use a number of strategies and activities to craft a more positively valued and coherent sense of self.[74] Termed "identity work," this is seen as a process that is ongoing or continuous with an emphasis on *becoming* rather than *being*[75] and that can be active and conscious or "comparatively unselfconscious."[76]

Based on our findings, we suggest that applying identity dissonance as an analytical lens can help to illustrate the identity dilemmas and contradictions that can be experienced by healthcare and social care students, trainees, and practitioners in the context of interprofessionality as they engage in working and learning across professional and discipline boundaries.

Implications

We propose that more research is required not just for exploring and describing how an interprofessional identity is developed, but also to gain a greater understanding of the possible dissonance between personal, professional, and organizational identities and how dimensions of identity can interrelate "in complex and important ways"[77] and may be accepted, contested, or negotiated in terms of which one dominates within a particular context for a particular person. We also suggest that greater understanding needs to be given to consideration of the different types of dissonance management strategies used by learners in the context of interprofessional education and practice. Such strategies help them manage and negotiate conflicting identities, and may affect their personal and professional well-being.

Becoming interprofessional

So, "what does an interprofessional identity look like?" Do student health professionals behave as if they have more than one identity at any particular time? And is being interprofessional a single identity or a way of behaving with others in certain defined contexts? From a sociological perspective, professional identity is a binary concept (i.e., one profession, one identity or the other), and is a product of uniprofessional socialization practices and traditionally separate and siloed approaches to health professions education and training.[14,78] However, such thinking is at odds with the experience of many people who move from one identity to another given their roles, responsibilities, and preferences in modern life.

In the context of exploring what an interprofessional identity looks like, Sims focused on the experiences of practitioners who had undertaken a joint training program (also referred to in the literature as interdisciplinary studies) in learning disability nursing and social work.[79] His findings illustrated that individuals who have been formally socialized into the knowledge, world views, and beliefs of two professions (referred to as *dual socialization*) described their identity as fluid but also dissonant. Fluidity was reflected on a continuum from having an identity that was context or role based to not having a fixed identity. Dissonance was reflected in the conflict between participants' personal preferences and expectations related to joint practice and socially valued and accepted identities as conferred via their job title and role description, for example, which were defined in relation to a single profession.[79] This study illustrates the value of using identity dissonance as a theoretical lens, raises interesting questions about the "meaning of professionalism and professional identity when professional boundaries become more flexible,"[79] and draws attention to the interplay of identities. Similarly, in the context of undergraduate interprofessional learning and peer facilitation, Clouder et al.[80] illustrated that there was an emergence of an interprofessional self, which appeared to coexist with uniprofessional identity. The authors suggest that a secure uniprofessional identity provided the foundation for interprofessional engagement and coined the term "perforate boundaries"[80] to reflect the movement between uniprofessional and interprofessional identities.

The process involved in developing a dual identity – encompassing both a professional and an interprofessional identity – is outlined in the interprofessional socialization model proposed by Khalili et al.[81] Stage one involves challenging notions of uniprofessional identity, including stereotypes and misconceptions about other professional groups, and enhancing learners' responsiveness for engaging in interprofessional learning. During stage two, learners are immersed in interprofessional learning and collaboration, through which they develop an interprofessional world view incorporating multiple perspectives, and accepting or encouraging the contributions of other professions. The outcome of stage two is a learner who is ready for developing an interprofessional identity.[81] These two stages can be compared to the exposure and immersion levels proposed by Charles et al. in their developmental model of interprofessional education.[82] In stage three of Khalili et al.'s[81] model, learners develop a dual identity encompassing a sense of belonging to their own profession, as well as to a broader interprofessional community.[81] Although these authors have illustrated how interprofessional socialization can facilitate the development of a dual or interprofessional identity, what they have not adequately addressed is how this interprofessional identity may coexist with or potentially destabilize the uniprofessional identity.[9]

To add to the complexity, a recent U.S. qualitative study explored professional identity development within the context of postgraduate education in primary care in which nurse practitioners and medical residents were learning and working together over one year. The authors analyzed data from twenty-eight interviews using an exploratory and constant comparative grounded theory approach. They concluded that while both sets of health professionals enhanced their uniprofessional identities, they also went through a dynamic process of group identity development. This process informed interprofessional collaboration through trust and mutual understanding of roles and responsibilities.[83] Positive factors for group identity formation, which may be compared to the IPEC's collective identity[6] mentioned above, appear to be continuity and longitudinal interaction between professionals and patients.

Overall, the studies described have reinforced that there are identity-related transformations beyond profession or discipline-specific boundaries; individuals can have multiple identities, which can interrelate in complex ways.[77] However, although it is acknowledged that there is a definite interplay between identities, the identity dilemmas (or what Sims terms the "inner conflict")[79] experienced in the context of interprofessionality, including the synergy and possible disjunctions between (uni)professional and interprofessional identities, or individual and collective identities, have not been adequately illustrated.

Implications for developing interprofessional identities

Students need to be better oriented to the "disorienting dilemmas,"[84] which may challenge and prompt questioning of their fundamental beliefs, values, world views, assumptions about others, and interpretations of self (i.e., identity). They need to be appropriately guided to articulate and critically reflect on their personal values and affinities for particular ways of working, learning, or thinking, to compare this with the norms, ethos, and expectations of their professional or organizational role and how these may align or not. These activities will need to involve mutual dialogue and active interaction with members from other health professions. In this regard, clinical educators and supervisors are charged with providing healthcare students, trainees, and other staff with the time, space, and guidance necessary for facilitating conversations about "identity" conflicts and ambiguities experienced in the context of interprofessional education and collaborative practice. Such facilitation can be through small-group work during clinical rotations similar to that which has been described for learning and debriefing about (uni)professionalism.[85] These sessions need to be student centered and involve interactive and conversational practice-based methods. Such sessions should be seen as safe and confidential so that students can talk about any issues with conflicted identities, values, and uncertainty about roles.

Conclusion

We have considered the concept and theorization of interprofessional identity formation and compared such an identity to a (uni)professional one. As twenty-first century healthcare is frequently delivered through a team-based or wider collaboration approach due to the aging of the global population and the rising incidence of chronic and complex disease, IPE has been advocated as a means of helping health professionals learn together in order to work together.[86] As shown in this chapter, and in the book as a whole, the literature has much to say about professional socialization and professional identity formation, yet there remains much more to be done in terms of developing the theoretical underpinnings of IPE to embrace this literature.

We have outlined the common theories espoused in terms of identity formation and their application in

IPE. Many more mature health professionals, whose education and training was siloed and profession specific, remember their transition to clinical practice after qualification (licensure or certification) as a time of stress and survival, having to learn an overwhelming amount of organizational knowledge and know-how in a short space of time. The existence of other health professionals was of course known to these novices, but the correct channels of communication, protocol, and hierarchy were new territory. While IPE is more common now, we are still researching its impact on both patients and professionals. Which models of IPE best reduce the sense of being overpowered and ease the transition at least in terms of understanding the roles, responsibilities, and values of other health professionals?

There are a number of implications arising from this chapter for those involved in health professions education, as outlined in the different sections. We advocate for the inclusion of assessable interprofessional learning outcomes within all health professions' accreditation standards and curricula and appropriate learning activities for students to meet these. Health professions educators need to be aware that identity dissonance can manifest particularly strongly for two groups of healthcare students, trainees, or practitioners: those expressing a personal identity or affinity for interprofessionality (but who are learning and practicing in traditional uniprofessional contexts and organizational settings), and those with strong uniprofessional allegiances and orientations (who might be learning or working in organizational settings where there is an explicit interprofessional ethos). In this regard, identity dissonance as a framework provides insights into identifying and supporting individuals who are most at risk of a negative sense of self in interprofessional settings, for example, those who have compromised their personal values and preferences for interprofessionality by conforming with professionally, organizationally, or socially sanctioned identities that relate to disciplinary or professional boundaries.

Interprofessional role models are important; we would hope that facilitators of interprofessional learning exhibit interprofessional behavior. However, such facilitation requires institutional support and training. Interprofessional facilitation requires knowledge and skills in relation to the sociology of the professions, power dimensions within a group, and the clinical environment and how to recognize and deal with potential professional differences and conflict,[87] as well as "standard" learning and teaching competencies. There are a number of established models for facilitators to enact, for example, the four phases of sensitization, exploration, implementation, and evaluation as outlined above.[54]

In this chapter, we raised three broad questions as a means of critically reflecting on contemporary theories of interprofessional identity formation. What happens to professional identity in the context of modern healthcare and contemporary education of the health professions? In what ways do healthcare professionals need to nurture and sustain an interprofessional identity? To what extent does the interprofessional identity subsume the uniprofessional, or may an individual move between the two identities depending on context and inclination?

We suggest that many health professionals have multiple interplaying identities that build on the professional identity they develop during their education. An interprofessional identity is one of these, and it helps individuals as they work in teams or wider collaborations become part of a "group" or "collective" identity, with agreed goals for the delivery of optimum patient care. However, in considering the question of interprofessionalism and professional identity formation, there remains a clear imperative for much more research to determine what a functioning interprofessional identity looks like and what the practical implications are in terms of learning and working. While it is our experience that some health professionals are more comfortable and proficient at interprofessional collaborative practice than others, there is much more to be learned about how and why this should be so.

References

1. Dall'Alba, G. Learning professional ways of being: ambiguities of becoming. *Educational Philosophy and Theory.* 2009; **41**(1):34–45.

2. Clarke, M, Hyde, A, Drennan, J. Professional identity in higher education. In Kehm, BM, Teichler, U, eds. The Academic Profession in Europe: New Tasks and New Challenges. *Dordrecht,* the Netherlands: Springer; 2013:7–21.

3. Lahire, B. *The Plural Actor.* Cambridge, UK: Polity Press; 2011.

4. Hafferty, FW. Professionalism and the socialization of medical students. In Cruess, RL, Cruess, SR, Steinert, Y, eds. *Teaching Medical Professionalism.* New York, NY: Cambridge University Press; 2009:53–70.

5. Hammick, M, Freeth, D, Copperman, J, Goodsman, D. *Being Interprofessional*. Cambridge, UK: Polity Press; 2009.

6. Interprofessional Education Collaborative Expert Panel. *Core Competencies for Interprofessional Collaborative Practice: Report of an Expert Panel*. Washington, DC; Interprofessional Education Collaborative; 2011. [Accessed Jan. 3, 2015.] Available from www.aacn.nche.edu/education-resources/ipecreport.pdf.

7. Lurie, SJ. History and practice of competency-based assessment. *Med Educ*. 2012; **46**(1):49–57.

8. D'Amour, D, Oandasan, I. Interprofessionality as the field of interprofessional practice and interprofessional education: an emerging concept. *J Interprof Care*. 2005; **19** Suppl 1:8–20.

9. Brooks, V, Thistlethwaite, J. Working and learning across professional boundaries. *British Journal of Educational Studies*. 2012; **60**(4):403–420.

10. Centre for the Advancement of Interprofessional Education. Fareham, UK: 2002. [Accessed Jan. 3, 2015.] Available from www.CAIPE.org.uk.

11. Thistlethwaite, J, Kumar, K, Moran, M, Saunders, R, Carr, S. An exploratory review of pre-qualification interprofessional education evaluations. *J Interprof Care*. 2015; **29**(4):292–97.

12. Parsell, G, Bligh, J. The development of a questionnaire to assess the readiness of health care students for interprofessional learning (RIPLS). *Med Educ*. 1999; **33**(2):95–100.

13. Luecht, RM, Madsen, MK, Taugher, MP, Petterson, BJ. Assessing professional perceptions: design and validation of an Interdisciplinary Education Perception Scale. *J Allied Health*. 1990; **19**(2):181–91.

14. Clouder, L. Becoming professional: exploring the complexities of professional socialization in health and social care. *Learning in Health and Social Care*. 2003; **2**(4):213–22.

15. Shulman, LS. Signature pedagogies in the professions. *Daedalus*. 2005; **134**(3):52–59.

16. Curran, V, Sharpe, D. Professional socialization and interprofessional education. In Kitto, S, Chesters, J, Thistlethwaite, J, Reeves, S, eds. *Sociology of Interprofessional Health Care Practice: Critical Reflections and Concrete Solutions*. New York, NY: Nova; 2011:69–85.

17. Cruess, RL, Cruess, S. Professionalism, professional identity, and the hidden curriculum: do as we say and as we do. In Hafferty, FW, O'Donnell, JF, eds. *The Hidden Curriculum in Health Professional Education*. Lebanon, NH: Dartmouth College Press; 2014:171–81.

18. Arndt, J, King, S, Suter, E, Mazonde, J, Taylor, E, Arthur, N. Socialization in health education: encouraging an integrated interprofessional socialization process. *J Allied Health*. 2009; **38**(1):18–23.

19. Whittington, C. Interprofessional education and identity. In Colyer, H, Helme, M, Jones, I, eds. *The Theory-Practice Relationship in Interprofessional Education*. London, UK: The Higher Education Academy: Health Sciences and Practice; 2005:42–48.

20. Beattie, A. War and peace among the health tribes. In Soothill, K, Mackay, L, Webb, C, eds. *Interprofessional Relations in Health Care*. London, UK: Edward Arnold; 1995:11–26.

21. Allport, GW. *The Nature of Prejudice: 25th Anniversary Edition*. Cambridge, MA: Perseus Books; 1979.

22. Benson, J. *Third Culture Personalities and the Integration of Refugees into the Community: Some Reflections from General Practice*. Australasian Transcultural Mental Health Network: Synergy No. **2**; 2003.

23. Thistlethwaite, J. Hidden amongst us: the language of inter- and outer-professional identity and collaboration. In Hafferty, FW, O'Donnell, JF, eds. *The Hidden Curriculum in Health Professional Education*. Lebanon, NH: Dartmouth College Press; 2014:158–68.

24. Tajfel, H, Turner, JC. *An integrative theory of intergroup conflict*. In Austin, WG, Worchel, S, eds. *The Social Psychology of Intergroup Relations*. Monterey, CA: Brooks/Cole Publishing Company; 1979:33–47.

25. Turner, JC. Towards a cognitive redefinition of the social group. In Tajfel, H, ed. *Social Identity and Intergroup Relations*. Cambridge, UK: Cambridge University Press; 1982:15–40.

26. Oakes, PJ, Haslam, SA, Turner, JC. *Stereotyping and Social Reality*. Oxford, UK: Blackwell; 1994.

27. Swartz, D. *Culture and Power: The Sociology of Pierre Bourdieu*. Chicago, IL: University of Chicago Press; 1997.

28. Elder-Vass, D. *The Reality of Social Construction*. New York, NY: Cambridge University Press; 2012.

29. Haslam, SA, Turner, JC, Oakes, PJ, McGarty, C, Hayes, BK. Context-dependent variation in social stereotyping 1: the effects of intergroup relations as mediated by social change and frame of reference. *Eur J Soc Psychol*. 1992; **22**(1):3–20.

30. Bainbridge, L, Purkis, ME. The history and sociology of the health professions: do they provide the key to new models for interprofessional collaboration? In Kitto, S, Chesters, J, Thistlethwaite, J, Reeves, S, eds. *Sociology of Interprofessional Health Care Practice: Critical Reflections and Concrete Solutions*. New York, NY: Nova; 2011:23–37.

31. Hornsey, MJ. Social identity theory and self-categorization theory: a historical review. *Soc Personal Psychol Compass*. 2008; **2**(1):204–22.

32. Foucault, M. *The Archaeology of Knowledge*. London, UK: Routledge; 2002.

33. McKinlay, A, McVittie, C. *Identities in Context: Individuals and Discourse in Action*. Chichester, UK: Wiley-Blackwell; 2011.

34. McAdams, DP, McLean, KC. Narrative identity. *Curr Dir Psychol Sci*. 2013; 22(3):233–38.

35. Bamberg, M. Narrative discourse and identities. In Meister, JC, Kindt, T, Schernus, W, eds. *Narratology beyond Literary Criticism: Mediality, Disciplinarity*. Berlin, DE: Walter de Gruyter; 2005:213–38.

36. Giddens, A. *Modernity and Self-Identity: Self and Society in the Late Modern Age*. Cambridge, UK: Polity Press; 1991.

37. Jackson, RL II, Hogg, MA, eds. *Encyclopedia of Identity*. London, UK: SAGE Publications; 2010.

38. Ajjawi, R, Hyde, S, Roberts, C, Nisbet, G. Marginalisation of dental students in a shared medical and dental education programme. *Med Educ*. 2009; 43(3):238–45.

39. Barr, H, Helme, M, D'Avray, L. *Review of Interprofessional Education in the United Kingdom 1997–2013*. London, UK; CAIPE: 2014. [Accessed March 12, 2015.] Available from http://caipe.org.uk/silo/files/iperg-review-15-4-14-with-links-pdf.pdf

40. NHS Institute for Innovation and Improvement. *Managing Conflict*. Leeds, UK; NHS Institute for Innovation and Improvement; 2008. [Accessed Dec. 1, 2014.] Available from www.institute.nhs.uk/quality_and_service_improvement_tools/quality_and_service_improvement_tools/human_dimensions_-_managing_conflict.html.

41. Canadian Interprofessional Health Collaborative. *A National Interprofessional Competency Framework*. Vancouver, BC: CIHC; 2010. [Accessed Dec. 1, 2014.] Available from www.cihc.ca/files/CIHC_IPCompetencies_Feb1210.pdf.

42. The Interprofessional Curriculum Renewal Consortium, Australia. *Curriculum Renewal for Interprofessional Education in Health*. Sydney, AU: University of Technology; 2013. [Accessed Dec. 1, 2014.] Available from http://caipe.org.uk/silo/files/ipecurriculum-renewal-20141.pdf.

43. McNeil, KA, Mitchell, RJ, Parker V. Interprofessional practice and professional identity threat. *Health Sociol Rev*. 2013; 22(3):291–307.

44. Johnson, TJ. *Professions and Power*. London, UK: Macmillan; 1972.

45. McCallin, A. Interdisciplinary practice–a matter of teamwork: an integrated literature review. *J Clin Nurs*. 2001; 10(4):419–28.

46. Eraut, M. *Developing Professional Knowledge and Competence*. London, UK: Falmer: 1994.

47. Chrobot-Mason, D, Ruderman, MN, Weber, TJ, Ernst, C. The challenge of leading on unstable ground: triggers that activate social identity faultlines. *Hum Relat*. 2009; 62(11):1763–94.

48. Jost, JT, Hamilton, DL. Stereotypes in our culture. In Dovidio, JF, Glick, P, Rudman, LA, eds. *On the Nature of Prejudice: Fifty Years after Allport*. Malden, MA: Blackwell; 2005:208–24.

49. Thistlethwaite, JE, Jackson, A. Conflict in practice-based settings: nature, resolution and education. *International Journal of Practice-based Learning in Health and Social Care*. 2014; 2(2):2–13.

50. Thistlethwaite, JE. *Values-Based Interprofessional Collaborative Practice*. Cambridge, UK: Cambridge University Press; 2012.

51. Akkerman, SF, Bakker, A. Boundary crossing and boundary objects. *Rev Educ Res*. 2011; 81(2):132–69.

52. MacNaughton, K, Chreim, S, Bourgeault, IL. Role construction and boundaries in interprofessional primary health care teams: a qualitative study. *BMC Health Serv Res*. 2013; 13:486.

53. Engeström, Y, Engeström, R, Kärkkäinen, M. Polycontextuality and boundary crossing in expert cognition: learning and problem solving in complex work activities. *Learning and Instruction*. 1995; 5(4):319–36.

54. Orchard, CA, Curran, V, Kabene, S. Creating a culture for interdisciplinary collaborative professional practice. *Med Educ Online*. 2005; 10:11. [Accessed March 13, 2015.] Available from http://med-ed-online.net/index.php/meo/article/view/4387/4569.

55. Mason, T, Hinman, P, Sadik, R, Collyer, D, Hosker, N, Keen, A. Values of reductionism and values of holism. In McCarthy, J, Rose, P, eds. *Values-Based Health and Social Care: Beyond Evidence-Based Practice*. London, UK: SAGE Publications; 2010:70–96.

56. Daly, M, Roberts, C, Kumar, K, Perkins, D. Longitudinal integrated rural placements: a social learning systems perspective. *Med Educ*. 2013; 47(4):352–61.

57. Hafferty, FW, Levinson, D. Moving beyond nostalgia and motives: towards a complexity science view of medical professionalism. *Perspect Biol Med*. 2008; 51(4):599–615.

58. Wenger, E. *Communities of Practice: Learning, Meaning, and Identity*. Cambridge, UK: Cambridge University Press; 1998.

59. Wenger, E. Communities of practice and social learning systems. *Organization*. 2000; 7(2):225–46.

60. Wenger, E. Conceptual tools for CoPs as social learning systems: boundaries, identity, trajectories and participation. In Blackmore, C, ed. *Social Learning Systems and Communities of Practice*. London, UK: Springer; 2010:125–44.

61. Hafferty, FW, O'Donnell, JF. The next generation of work on the hidden curriculum: concluding thoughts. In Hafferty, FW, O'Donnell, JF, eds. *The Hidden Curriculum in Health Professional Education*. Lebanon, NH: Dartmouth College Press; 2014; 233–63.

62. Thistlethwaite, JE, Bartle, E, Chong, AA, Dick, ML, King, D, Mahoney, S, Papinczak, T, Tucker, G. A review of longitudinal community and hospital placements in medical education: BEME Guide No. 26. *Med Teach*. 2013; 35(8):e1340–e1364.

63. Costello, CY. *Professional Identity Crisis: Race, Class, Gender, and Success at Professional Schools*. Nashville, TN: Vanderbilt University Press; 2005.

64. Festinger, L. *A Theory of Cognitive Dissonance*. Stanford, CA: Stanford University Press; 1957.

65. Jansz, J, Timmers, M. Emotional dissonance: when the experience of an emotion jeopardizes an individual's identity. *Theory Psychol*. 2002; 12(1):79–95.

66. Bruhn, JG. Value dissonance and ethics failure in academia: a causal connection? *J Acad Ethics*. 2008; 6(1):17–32.

67. Thompson, BM, Teal, CR, Rogers, JC, Paterniti, DA, Haidet, P. Ideals, activities, dissonance, and processing: a conceptual model to guide educators' efforts to stimulate student reflection. *Acad Med*. 2010; 85(5):902–08.

68. Kumar, K. *Interdisciplinary Health Research (IDHR): An Analysis of the Lived Experience from the Theoretical Perspective of Identity*. Ph.D. thesis. Sydney, AU: University of Sydney; 2012. [Accessed March 13, 2015.] Available from http://hdl.handle.net/2123/8858.

69. Kezar, A. The importance of pilot studies: beginning the hermeneutic circle. *Res High Educ*. 2000; 41(3):385–400.

70. McManus Holroyd, AE. Interpretive hermeneutic phenomenology: clarifying understanding. *Indo-Pacific Journal of Phenomenology*. 2007; 7(2):1–12.

71. Knipfer, K, Kump, B, Wessel, D, Cress, U. Reflection as a catalyst for organisational learning. *Studies in Continuing Education*. 2012; 35(1):30–48.

72. Collinson, DL. Identities and insecurities: selves at work. *Organization*. 2003; 10(3):527–47.

73. Brew, A. Disciplinary and interdisciplinary affiliations of experienced researchers. *High Educ*. 2008; 56(4):423–38.

74. Alvesson, M. Self-doubters, strugglers, storytellers, surfers and others: images of self-identities in organization studies. *Hum Relat*. 2010; 63:193–218.

75. Alvesson, M, Ashcraft, KL, Thomas, R. Identity matters: reflections on the construction of identity scholarship in organization studies. *Organization*. 2008; 15(1):5–28.

76. Alvesson, M, Willmott, H. Identity regulation as organizational control: producing the appropriate individual. *Journal of Management Studies*. 2002; 39(5):619–42.

77. Gee, JP. Identity as an analytic lens for research in education. *Review of Research in Education*. 2000; 25:99–125.

78. du Toit, D. A sociological analysis of the extent and influence of professional socialization on the development of a nursing identity among nursing students at two universities in Brisbane, Australia. *J Adv Nurs*. 1995; 21(1):164–71.

79. Sims, D. Reconstructing professional identity for professional and interprofessional practice: a mixed methods study of joint training programmes in learning disability nursing and social work. *J Interprof Care*. 2011; 25(4):265–71.

80. Clouder, DL, Davies, B, Sams, M, McFarland, L. "Understanding where you're coming from": discovering an [inter]professional identity through becoming a peer facilitator. *J Interprof Care*. 2012; 26(6):459–64.

81. Khalili, H, Orchard, C, Laschinger, HK, Farah, R. An interprofessional socialization framework for developing an interprofessional identity among health professions students. *J Interprof Care*. 2013; 27(6):448–53.

82. Charles, G, Bainbridge, L, Gilbert, J. The University of British Columbia model of interprofessional education. *J Interprof Care*. 2010; 24(1):9–18.

83. Meyer, EM, Zapatka, S, Brienza, RS. The development of professional identity and the formation of teams in the Veteran Affairs Connecticut healthcare system's Center of Excellence in Primary Care Education program (CoEPCE). *Acad Med*. 2015; 90(6):802–09.

84. Mezirow, J. Transformative learning: theory to practice. *New Directions for Adult and Continuing Education*. 1997; 74:5–12.

85. Rees, CE, Monrouxe, LV, McDonald, LA. Narrative, emotion and action: analysing 'most memorable' professionalism dilemmas. *Med Educ*. 2013; 47(1):80–96.

86. Thistlethwaite, J. Interprofessional education: a review of context, learning and the research agenda. *Med Educ*. 2012; 46(1):58–70.

87. Bray, J. Interprofessional facilitation skills and knowledge: evidence from a Delphi research survey. In Howkins, E, Bray, J, eds. *Preparing for Interprofessional Teaching*. Oxon, UK: Radcliffe; 2008:27–39.

Assessment of professionalism and progress in the development of a professional identity

John J. Norcini and Judy A. Shea

Introduction

Over the past few decades, the focus on professionalism has increased dramatically throughout the continuum of medical education. It is now considered an essential component of competence in a variety of countries including Canada (CanMEDS roles), India (Medical Council of India Regulations on Graduate Medical Education, 2012), the United Kingdom (Good Medical Practice), and the United States (ACGME competencies).[1-4] The emphasis on competencies such as professionalism reflects a shift to a model that starts with the desired educational outcomes and works backward to define the educational process.

Assessment is central to outcomes-based education. It constitutes the means by which stakeholders are assured that learners have achieved the competencies necessary to meet the needs of the community. For students, it offers guidance regarding milestones in their development.[5] In addition, there is a growing appreciation of the critical role of formative assessment and feedback in both learning and identity formation.[6] This chapter will address the assessment of professionalism by (1) outlining the challenges, (2) citing reasons for assessing it, (3) using Miller's pyramid as a framework for describing some of the methods of assessing professionalism and the research that supports them, and (4) suggesting some principles for developing an assessment system for professionalism. We conclude with brief consideration of lessons learned and future directions.

At the outset we note that many chapters in this book are focused on professional identity formation, rather than professionalism. Identity formation as a process has been studied for decades.[7,8] Recently, the literature has explicitly addressed the question of how the process of medical education supports and enhances professional and clinical identity formation.[9-11] We see professionalism and professional identity formation as two largely overlapping bodies of work. Because our task in this chapter is to address assessment, and there is a rich literature in the area, we chose that body of work for our focus. The goals and methods of assessment generally align with how students perform – as of yet they are not well developed (and perhaps they should not be?) for judging what a person *is*. Nevertheless, many of the tools and processes we review and the ideas behind them are readily adaptable to the concerns underlying professional identity formation, such as reflections, attitudes, and behaviors.

Challenges in assessing professionalism and professional identity

The assessment of professionalism is challenging for a number of reasons, but four are particularly salient.[12] First, as noted elsewhere in this book, professionalism can be difficult to define. The lack of a single, well-accepted conceptualization and definition creates a significant challenge since good formative or summative assessment starts with a clear understanding of what is to be measured. Hodges et al.,[13] in generating a consensus statement for the Ottawa Conference, identified three separate discourses for professionalism, each of which resulted in a somewhat different set of recommendations for its assessment. Clearly, some accommodations among these discourses must be made before developing an assessment system for professionalism.

Second, given a shared definition, actual opportunities to observe professionalism might be relatively rare. Certainly, some of them can be created in the

Teaching Medical Professionalism, 2nd Edition, ed. Richard L. Cruess, Sylvia R. Cruess and Yvonne Steinert.
Published by Cambridge University Press. © Cambridge University Press 2016.

form of test material for written exams or simulations. However, learners are on their best behavior under these conditions and, especially in an area like professionalism, social desirability will play a significant role. Of course, if examinees cannot behave well in circumstances when they know they are being assessed, there is little chance that they can behave well when unobserved. Regardless, creating and finding opportunities to make judgments about professionalism will be a significant challenge in the development of an assessment system.

Third, even when the definition is clear and relevant observations are made, assessors might operationalize the definition in different ways. They might not agree about whether particular behaviors signify a lapse in professionalism or whether they are appropriate for a specific point along the developmental course of a professional identity. In addition to the need for faculty development, this implies that it will be essential to involve multiple observers or assessors over multiple occasions for each learner.

Fourth, the current reconceptualization of professionalism within an identity formation framework offers a powerful way to support both the teaching and the learning of this competency. At its highest level, this identity is composed of values, attributes, and behaviors, and multiple identities are to be reinforced. This poses particular challenges for assessment and requires a system that draws on multiple assessment methods and is capable of capturing change over time. It also implies the need to develop new methods that offer different perspectives on this competency.

Reasons for assessing professionalism

There are at least four reasons to assess professionalism. First, it is widely accepted that assessment drives learning, and that including professionalism as part of high-stakes decisions signals a message of value. It motivates learners to prepare in order to be successful and it indicates to all stakeholders that professionalism is important.

Second, assessing professionalism supports the development of professional identity. Formative assessment, in particular, offers feedback intended to direct and catalyze learning. Properly done, this form of assessment will help students discover who they are and will offer guidance on how they can become who they want and need to be.

Third, it is an essential element of a quality improvement cycle. Assessment is needed at the start of such a cycle to recognize strengths and identify weaknesses that must be addressed as part of the planning phase. It is also needed at the end of the cycle to determine whether the educational interventions that have been implemented were successful.

Fourth, the assessment of professionalism is critical to the identification and remediation of learners whose performance may endanger patients; they have not yet incorporated into their professional identities the values and behaviors that support optimal patient care. This function is essential to protect patients and to improve the safety and quality of care rendered by healthcare systems. In doing this, assessment also establishes the accountability of the institution and the profession.

Methods of assessing professionalism

As with other competencies, there are a number of different ways of assessing professionalism and, like the assessment of other competencies, they all have strengths and weaknesses. Consequently, it is important to develop a system of assessment, composed of different methods, at different times, and for different contexts. The system needs to be responsive to the developmental needs of the learner, establish the accountability of the institution, and protect patients and the profession.

A useful way to think about the individual methods of assessment is through the lens of the traditional version of Miller's pyramid.[14] Miller developed the pyramid to classify methods of assessment based on what they require of the learner. The pyramid is composed of four levels: the lowest level is *knows*, followed upward by *knows how*, *shows how*, and *does*. Each level builds on the lower levels. For instance, learners need to *know* before they can *know how*, *show how*, and *do*. Similarly, learners must *know*, *know how*, and *show how* before they can *do*. The fact that Miller arranged the levels in a pyramid is not meant to imply that those methods at the top are better or more valued than those at the bottom. It depends on the purpose of assessment and if, for example, the purpose of the assessment is to ensure knowledge, methods higher than *knows* on the pyramid will generally be less appropriate and less efficient.

Our use of the traditional pyramid is not inconsistent with the identity formation perspective of this book. We do recognize that the focus of professional identity is on *is* rather than any of Miller's four levels.

In fact, in a recent paper,[15] the editors of this volume argued that Miller's pyramid should be modified to have a fifth level of *is*. We agree that this adaptation might be beneficial to education-focused endeavors. However, when the lens is on assessment, identity is a composite of attitudes, values, and behaviors that can best be assessed in the context of a system composed of several different methods consistent with Miller's original pyramid.

Knows

Assessing knowledge is a common endeavor at all levels of professional education. Indeed, the bulk of assessment that we have done historically fits squarely into the *knows* level of the pyramid. Traditional assessments of knowledge focused on recall and recognition of basic science facts and topics such as abnormal and normal physiology and pathology. In the 1980s, there was a strong movement to require higher cognitive skills of test-takers, including the ability to synthesize information and exercise appropriate judgment.[16] In addition, the content of these assessments was expanded to include topics such as basic biostatistics, epidemiology, public health, professionalism, and ethics.

While there is widespread consensus that the bulk of the assessment of professionalism should focus on what a person does and his or her attitudes and values, a good case can be made that there is also a body of core knowledge a physician must possess.[17] For example, many of the attributes of professionalism outlined by Veloski[18] such as ethics, multiculturalism, and confidentiality of patient data, can efficiently be measured by knowledge assessments. Kao[19] outlines the interplay between ethics, law, and professionalism, and discusses topics such as securing informed consent, protecting patient confidentiality, disclosing difficult information, and withholding or withdrawing care. In each of these areas, there are ethical principles that can be assessed; these principles are the foundation for required certifications for clinical investigators such as the widely subscribed Collaborative Institutional Training Initiative (CITI) program.[20] In each area, there are also legal standards. Healthcare professionals should be aware of the standards, and such awareness is well-suited to assessment by traditional multiple-choice examinations. Naturally, there are also instances when the ethical principle does not align with the legal standard. In these cases, it is important for a provider to know what to do. Patient scenarios and standardized patients are well-suited to these types of assessments (though, admittedly, when the prompt is *what would or should you do* rather than *what is the best thing to do*, the former questions slide into the levels of *knows how* and *shows how*).

For any assessment of knowledge, it would be desirable to follow standard procedures for instrument development, including a blueprint that specifies the content of the examination, good item-development practices, and pilot testing. After administration, score reliability should be calculated and evidence for validity should be gathered following procedures such as those outlined by Nunnally and Bernstein[21] and Streiner and Norman.[22] Each of the examples below shows strengths in some of these areas. While none of the instruments are widely used yet, each has utility as a model in prescribed circumstances.

Barry Challenges to Professionalism questionnaire

This tool is a survey comprised of six patient-based multiple-choice items, each providing four options.[23] The item topics cover the domains of conflict of interest, confidentiality, physician impairment, sexual harassment, honesty, and acceptance of gifts. These topics were chosen because they represent common issues that learners at all levels might encounter; three were adapted from the American Board of Internal Medicine Project Professionalism.[24] Candidate items were reviewed by a multidisciplinary panel of experts. Importantly, these panel members agreed that each of the six scenarios had a "best answer" and five of the six had a second "acceptable" answer.

In the initial tool development, participants were all student and postgraduate trainees at a large medical center and a random sample of physicians in the state. Item-level responses to the questions were within a reasonable range, and scores varied in expected ways across different levels of experience. Thus, this tool might be used as a brief assessment of professionalism knowledge for multiple domains and multiple levels of learners.

Test of Residents' Ethics Knowledge for Pediatrics (TREK-P)

The TREK-P is a relatively new tool that has promise as a means to assess ethical knowledge.[25] Although it is specialty-specific and thus content would need to be adapted for other specialties, the processes followed in its development might serve as a model for other domains. Content for the tool was derived from earlier work on ethical challenges supplemented by the ACGME definition of professionalism. The initial list was cross-validated against statements endorsed by the American Academy of Pediatrics. The first version of the TREK-P consisted of thirty-six knowledge questions testing professionalism, adolescent medicine, genetic testing and diagnosis, neonatology, end-of-life decisions, and decision-making for minors. American Academy of Pediatric guidelines were used to establish the correct response for each item. Each question was asked as a true or false statement and items were developed and reviewed by experts in education and ethics.

The first version of the TREK-P was given to novices (first-year medical students), third-year pediatric residents (the population of interest), and experts (pediatric clinical ethicists).[25] The investigators removed thirteen poorly performing items. The resulting twenty-three-item TREK-P had reasonable reliability. Importantly, scores improved with increasing experience: sixty-five percent for students, eighty-three percent for residents, and ninety-six percent for ethicists. Future use might focus on smaller sets of items that generalize across specialties or conversely, on developing parallel forms across specialties.

Matriculating medical students' knowledge of professionalism

A study by Blue et al.[26] aimed to examine three classes of matriculating students' knowledge and attitudes toward professionalism at two different medical schools. The investigators relied on the Swick[27] definition of professionalism and targeted five dimensions believed to be important and appropriate for medical students: subordinating self-interest, ethics and moral values, humanistic values, accountability, and self-reflection. All dimensions are clearly also a part of professional identity. Specific to the current discussion, knowledge was assessed with two instruments: medical vignettes and multiple-choice questions.

Analysis of the data revealed that there were five factors underlying the scores that are consistent with definitions of professionalism and professional identity: (1) subordinating self-interest, (2) professional responsibility, (3) managing complexity and uncertainty, (4) professional commitment, and (5) humanism. The highest knowledge score was for the attribute of humanism, followed by professional responsibility,

subordinating self-interest, managing complexity and uncertainty, and professional commitment.

Reflection/critical incident technique

The critical incident technique (CIT) is widely used in the education and assessment of healthcare providers. In general, CIT begins by asking participants to reflect on an incident – often related to professionalism or professional identity – that they observed or participated in, and write a brief summary.[28] For example, Niemi asked first-year medical trainees to keep a learning log after each visit to a primary care health center during the first year of medical school. The purpose was to record thoughts, feelings, and emotions, and to provide "a forum to reflect and wonder about your experiences." Some users of the CIT give more explicit instructions such as directing students to use a prescribed format for guided reflection.[29] Then, if aimed at professionalism, there is an analysis and often group discussion of what tenets of professionalism were involved. When formally graded, this instrument does provide an assessment of a student's knowledge and understanding of professionalism.[29] In this context, CIT fits well under *knows*.

Knows how

Knows how is the second level of Miller's pyramid and is comprised of a heterogeneous group of methods, usually written, that attempt to predict how the learner will act in situations that reflect professional values and identities. Some of these methods focus on measuring the attitudes and values of the learner; thus, they are important parts of a system of assessment aimed at identity formation. A systematic review identified many such methods[30] and the attitudes they assessed fell into several categories including professionalism as a whole, ethical issues, personal values, physician-patient relationships, sociocultural issues, and interprofessional relationships. Some investigators have argued that the development of a profile of attitudes has the advantage of providing detailed information that supports the provision of feedback.[31] Other investigators believe strongly that there is a need for a single global measure of attitudes that captures an overall viewpoint.[32] In either instance, there are many different instruments with acceptable characteristics.

Another set of methods seeks to understand whether the learner can reason in a sophisticated fashion about ways to behave in particular situations.

As such, these methods are often predicated on a developmental model, and they paint a scenario to which the examinee must respond. Some of the methods have grown out of the moral judgment literature. Included are the Moral Judgment Interview (MJI), a semi-structured interview with complex scoring, the Sociomoral Reasoning Measure, which is a paper version of the MJI with simplified scoring, and the Defining Issues Test (DIT), which is an MCQ-based version of the MJI.[33–35] Some of these instruments have been built on refinements to the growth of epistemic cognition, and others, such as the Situational Judgment Test, eschew the focus on development and come out of an industrial–organizational psychology tradition.

As a group, the *knows how* methods are of particular importance within the discourse of professionalism as an interpersonal process or effect.[13] Professional behavior grows out of the interaction of individuals' attitudes and problem-solving skills within particular learning and practice contexts. Consequently, great stress is placed on understanding and developing attitudes and thinking in a variety of situations. This can also be said for identity formation. However, within a few broad categories there are so many of these scales, and the differences among them are so minor, that future work should be focused on refining what is available rather than developing new assessment methods. Additional focus on qualitative methods, such as the MJI or those proposed by Rees and Knight,[36] might also be of interest for supporting the formative parts of a system of assessment aimed at identity formation.

The Jefferson scales

Educators at Jefferson Medical College have created a series of instruments designed to assess attitudes toward empathy, teamwork, and lifelong learning.[37–39] All of these constructs have been identified as important aspects of professionalism, and all of the instruments are similar in that they are composed of a series of questions for which the respondent supplies a rating.[32]

These instruments were developed in a similar and careful fashion. Starting from a definition and previous work in the area, a content outline and a pool of questions were developed. These went through an iterative process in which the questions were reviewed and edited by groups of faculty experts. This process resulted in the creation of one or more forms, some of which were tailored to specific populations. For example, there was a version of the empathy scale made especially for students, and one made especially for healthcare professionals. These scales were field tested and refined further.

Extensive research has been done with the Jefferson scales and they performed well.[32] Factor analyses have produced meaningful results, and measures of internal consistency have been high. More importantly, the scales have reasonable relationships with a variety of criterion measures. For example, a cross-cultural study showed that nurses and physicians from countries with a complementary model of professional roles had more positive attitudes toward collaboration.[40]

Moral Judgment Interview (MJI) and the Defining Issues Test (DIT)

In the 1950s, Kohlberg refined the work of Piaget and developed a six-stage model of the development of moral judgment.[41,42] To assess development through these stages, he created the MJI.[43] In this method, an interviewer presents the student with a number of moral dilemmas and the student is asked to resolve them. Each dilemma is followed by a series of open-ended questions that probe the reasoning of the student. The session is recorded and transcribed; the performances are assigned scores that are associated with the stages of moral development.

The DIT was developed by Rest[41] and is similar to the MJI in that students are presented moral dilemmas to which they must respond. Instead of open-ended questions, however, the students are offered a series of multiple-choice questions that they must answer. Their answers are scored as the percentage of responses from each stage of development. Because of its MCQ format, the DIT can more easily be administered in a variety of settings.

Baldwin and Self[44] point out that there are hundreds of studies supporting the use of both the MJI and the DIT as valid and reliable measures of moral reasoning. They also indicate that these assessments are related to many of the attributes of professionalism. Consequently, they suggest that these measures can be a useful component of an evaluation system for professionalism. It is not a stretch to argue that tools are also relevant to assessment of professional identity.

Situational Judgment Test (SJT)

The SJT is predicated on the idea that there is more to doing a job well than simply knowing what to do.

Regardless of profession, there is a need to interact well with other people, solve problems, work in teams, organize and plan, cope with pressure, and so on. The SJT offers realistic scenarios that are ideally based on "critical incidents," typically presented in a paper-and-pencil or video format, and followed by a series of potential responses. Respondents are asked to select the best of these or rank them.

As reported by McDaniel et al.,[45] assessments of situational judgment date back nearly a century. Through the late 1940s, they were criticized as measures of general intelligence and not unique assessments of social intelligence. Starting in the 1950s, they were used to assess the potential to supervise and to predict managerial success. They were studied extensively during this period; the data provided modest support for the method and it continues to be used and studied across a variety of occupations.

By the early 1990s, the SJT found its way into medicine. Of particular note is its use in admissions settings, where it is now being used as one basis for selection in a variety of countries (e.g., United Kingdom, Belgium, Canada, Australia). This is justified by specific studies indicating incremental validity over cognitive measures.[46]

Groningen Reflection Ability Scales

In a different type of assessment, Aukes et al.[47] developed a scale to measure personal reflection ability, the Groningen Reflection Ability Scales (GRAS). The GRAS assesses skills related to self-reflection, empathetic reflection, and reflective communication. Review of the item content suggests this scale falls somewhere between *knows* and *knows how*; for example, "I can see an experience from different standpoints" is an example of the former, whereas "I test my own judgments against those of others" is an example of the latter.

Professional self-identity questionnaire

Consistent with the notion of identity formation, this questionnaire was developed to monitor how curricula contribute to identity development across a range of healthcare professions.[48] Crossley and Vivekananda-Schmidt conducted a content analysis of curricula in several fields to develop the initial content for a questionnaire. The resulting nine-item form was tested in ten professional groups, refined, and then given to a group of student doctors. Those who had more experience in healthcare or social care roles had higher scores than their peers. In addition, the scores increased in conjunction with clinical experiences.

Shows how

The third level of the pyramid focuses on how the learner actually performs when being observed, and it incorporates a variety of simulation and workplace-based methods of assessment. Many of these are predicated on the fact that the encounter between the healthcare provider and the patient or another healthcare provider is one of the critical situations in which professionalism manifests itself. Both workplace-based assessments and simulations have strengths and weaknesses, and neither offers an assessment of all aspects of professionalism. In the following paragraphs, the relative strengths of each class of methods are reviewed, followed by discussion of a commonly used simulation method – standardized patients, and a commonly used workplace method – mini-CEX.

In workplace-based assessment, learners are observed in real encounters with patients or colleagues. The observer makes judgments about the quality of the performance. In simulation, real patients or colleagues are replaced with realistic but artificial experiences. The person being assessed interacts with the recreations and judgments are made about his or her performance. The methods can be stratified by how faithful they are to reality, with some having very high fidelity (e.g., human-patient simulators, virtual reality, standardized patients).

There is a significant research literature indicating that, regardless of method, performance is case or patient specific. How one interacts with one patient or team is not necessarily related to interactions with the next patient or team. Consequently, good assessment requires broad sampling across different encounters. For simulation, this is usually accomplished by creating a test composed of several different encounters through which learners rotate. For workplace-based assessment, different encounters are observed over a period of time, often weeks or months.[49,50] Simulation provides good fidelity and good content coverage and has the advantage of allowing the assessment of unusual circumstances. It also ensures that no harm comes to patients – this is especially relevant when learners are near the beginning of their training. Workplace methods have excellent fidelity and excellent content coverage. In addition, they allow difficult-to-simulate encounters to be included in assessment.

For examinations in which it is important to compare learners, simulation has a distinct advantage. Different examinees can be given the same cases and assessors and, when different forms of the test must be administered (e.g., over time), statistical techniques can be used to adjust the scores and make it, 'as if' all students took exactly the same test.[50] In contrast, variability due to different encounters and assessors can be reduced to some degree in workplace-based methods but it cannot be eliminated. In high-stakes settings, security is a concern for simulation but not workplace methods.

Where there are significant resource constraints, workplace methods have an advantage. Faculty development is required and the logistics can sometimes be challenging but these methods can be feasibly implemented, even in the setting of relatively small training programs. Simulation, on the other hand, often requires access to considerable amounts of space, equipment, and personnel. In addition, the development of test material requires significant resources.[49]

Standardized patients (SPs)

SPs are actors who have been trained to play the role of a patient.[51] They are given scripts and expected to perform the same each time they play the role (within the confines of the actions of the person being assessed). A string of encounters, often ten to twenty-five minutes each, is typically administered in round-robin format to as many examinees as there are SPs. A score is developed across all stations.[5]

SPs cannot assess all aspects of professionalism, but they can get at the attributes associated with it, as well as professional identity. Van Zanten et al.[53] lined up the competencies measured by an SP-based examination with the definitions of professionalism offered by the American Board of Internal Medicine and the Medical School Objectives Project (MSOP). They found overlap in areas such as honor, integrity, abuse of power, respect for patients, and so on. Similarly, Klamen and Williams[54] argued that the core professional values of compassion, responsibility, and integrity could all be demonstrated through communication skills, and assessment of these skills is a strength of SPs.

In testing a large group of international medical graduates, Van Zanten et al.[53] found that SPs offered a reliable and valid means of assessing certain aspects of professionalism. Incorporating a much broader group of studies, Klamen and Williams reached a similar conclusion – SPs provide a valid and reliable measure

of communication skills among a variety of different examinees (e.g., medical students, postgraduates, practicing doctors both individually and in teams).[54]

Mini-CEX and the Professionalism-Mini Clinical Evaluation Exercise (P-MEX)

The mini-CEX can be used to assess whether examinees behave in a professional manner.[55] The trainee conducts a brief, observed clinical encounter in any one of a number of different clinical settings. At the end of the encounter, the observer completes a rating form and offers the trainee feedback and a plan for improvement. A number of different rating forms have been developed, but the original form asked for an assessment of humanistic qualities and professionalism on a nine-point scale.

The mini-CEX captures some information on professionalism but is not solely focused on it. Consequently, Cruess et al.[56] developed a variation on the mini-CEX called the Professionalism Mini-Evaluation Exercise. At a workshop, the authors identified 142 observable behaviors that were reflective of professionalism. A subset of these was converted into a rating form that was designed for use in a variety of different settings. As in the mini-CEX, this instrument is used in the context of an observed clinical encounter.

There is extensive research concerning the mini-CEX, with several reviews of the literature having been published. For example, Kogan et al.[57] concluded that among the methods of direct observation, the mini-CEX had the strongest validity evidence. Likewise, Ansari and Donnon[58] conclude that the validity of the mini-CEX is supported by small to large effect sizes. Using Kane's framework for validity, Hawkins et al.[59] found that the scoring component yielded the most concerns but that evidence for other aspects of validity (i.e., generalization and extrapolation) was supportive.

Although less work has been done with the P-MEX, that which has been done is supportive of the measure. Cruess et al.[56] found evidence of construct and content validity as well as reasonable reliability with multiple encounters. A multi-center trial in Japan replicated these findings across cultures.[60] And of course, the findings associated with the mini-CEX are relevant to the P-MEX as well.

Does

Despite widespread agreement that how a person acts is ultimately a reflection of professional identity, assessment of professional behaviors – answering the question of what a healthcare provider actually does – lags behind discussions of definitions and curricula for professionalism. In Wilkinson's blueprint to assess professionalism,[61] nine categories of assessment methods were presented, each of which is applicable to one or more components of professional behavior. At least three fit well under the Miller vernacular of "does" – records of incidents of unprofessional behavior, collated views of coworkers (which could include assessments by supervisors), and opinions of patients. These will be briefly reviewed and one other example will be provided.

Records of incidents of unprofessional behavior

At the broadest level, it is possible to learn which healthcare workers have been disciplined by state licensing boards. There is likely to be little disagreement about the validity of this marker of professionalism, and all of the transgressions would be recognized as "bad" behaviors. The data are available for all states, though one would have to know the states in which a provider was, or had been, licensed in order to use this for a particular purpose. On the other hand, behaviors that warrant this level of intervention are relatively rare and, perhaps more importantly, most definitions of professionalism include behaviors that are unlikely to be flagged at the state licensing board level. Also, these types of data do not exist in a systematic way for professionals in training, thus limiting the options for intervention and remediation.

An alternative to waiting until a transgression has occurred, and one that speaks to the educational enterprise, is to identify behaviors that reliably foreshadow a lack of professionalism. For example, it has been shown that unprofessional behaviors in medical school and low ratings of professionalism in postgraduate training predict later disciplinary actions. In a case control study by Papadakis,[62] 235 graduates of three medical schools who had been disciplined by a state medical board between 1990 and 2003 were matched with controls according to medical school and graduation year. Among multiple predictors was the presence or absence of narratives describing unprofessional behavior during medical school that were included in student records. Strikingly, the odds of disciplinary action by a medical board tripled with prior unprofessional behavior in medical school. The types of unprofessional behavior most strongly linked

with disciplinary action were severe irresponsibility and severely diminished capacity for self-improvement. In a later study, Papadakis et al.[63] found a similar predictive relationship for behaviors identified during postgraduate training. Among 66,171 physicians who entered internal medicine residency training between 1990 and 2000 and subsequently passed the American Board of Internal Medicine certification examination, a low professionalism rating on the annual summary submitted by program directors predicted a record of disciplinary action by a state licensing board. Moreover, as the ratings of professionalism on a nine-point scale increased, there was less risk for subsequent disciplinary actions. These results suggest that records of student behaviors and summary ratings by observers are useful tools for assessment of professionalism.

360° evaluations – collated views of coworkers, peers, supervisors, or patients

As suggested above, another way to assess the "does" aspect of professionalism is to collect views and opinions of coworkers about a colleague's professional behaviors. Peer assessment is thought to be an especially valuable source of information because of frequent interactions among peers, often without a supervisor present. Arnold[64] reviewed some of the psychometric and practical issues with peer ratings, such as moderate inter-rater reliability, high intercorrelations across categories of items, and halo effects. While these are surmountable, implementation issues remain a challenge. Logistics such as how often to assess and who to include as an assessor become quite important. It also takes some effort to make sure that those involved take it seriously and neither "straightline" everyone in a positive or negative manner nor use assessment as an opportunity to hurt a colleague. Best practices would include anonymity, obtaining a wide range of opinions both in numbers (for reliability) and "types" of colleagues (for validity), and making sure the content of the rating form was restricted to observable behaviors. The requirements for high-quality assessment using rating scales are well known, and aggregating multiple data points is central to achieving reproducible scores.[65] In sum, this form of assessment can be very labor intensive, perhaps explaining why it is underutilized.

As a complement to peer assessment, patients' views are sometimes included in 360° evaluations. In fact, in many healthcare systems, patients' opinions are routinely sought and used outside of peer assessments. While the content of the typical survey is often broad and encompasses much more than professionalism (e.g., wait times, ease of getting an appointment, understanding of discharge instructions), most widely used instruments also contain at least a few items related to aspects of the primary provider's professionalism, such as respect and clear communication.[66] The virtues of patient opinions as an assessment tool are debatable. On one hand, there is intuitive appeal in knowing what patients think of their physicians; they are, after all, the most direct consumers of the services. Conversely, many have shown that patient-generated data have relatively weak psychometric characteristics and that a very large number of evaluations would be needed for robust assessment of an individual.[67] Moreover, patients see only a subset of behaviors related to professionalism. Despite these limitations, it is difficult to imagine a complete system of the assessment of professionalism that does not include the experiences and views of patients.

One might also think about including self-assessment as part of a 360° evaluation. The value of self-assessment as a robust form of assessment has been hotly debated for the past decade or so. Despite some rather compelling data that suggest that individuals are not particularly accurate self-assessors, especially when self-assessments are done in the absence of feedback and other data, self-assessment, particularly under the guise of reflection, continues to be an important part of teaching about professionalism and professional identity.[68,28] Closely related to self-assessment is self-reporting of unprofessional behaviors. Self-reporting fits clearly in the "does" category, but it is probably not optimal for many aspects of professionalism, foremost being the reluctance of individuals to disclose their unprofessional behaviors.

Conscientiousness index

This creative tool was developed as a quantitative and objective assessment of some key student behaviors,[70,71] for example, attendance at required sessions, turning in required information (e.g., immunization record) in a timely fashion, completing course evaluation forms, and taking required trainings. Key features were that the tool uses readily available data and the scores correlated with faculty and staff members' independent ratings of professionalism.[70] Similar observations (e.g., completing course evaluations and reporting immunization

compliance) were found to be predictors of professional behavior by Stern et al.[71]

Although this was developed specifically for students, one can imagine how it could be used throughout the continuum of training and practice. Within a clinical setting there is a wealth of information that is reflective of different dimensions of professionalism, for example, attendance at grand rounds, submitting required documentation of licenses, and responding to requests for meetings.

An assessment system for professionalism

Given the multiple purposes for assessing professionalism, the different discourses, the many stakeholders, and the multiple methods of assessment, each with strengths and weaknesses, there is little doubt that a system of assessment is needed by most institutions. Furthermore, capturing and supporting the development of professional identity requires the assessment of values, attitudes, and behaviors as they unfold over time. As a result, there is little likelihood that a single method or system will be acceptable across the spectra of learners and users.

For decades, institutions have employed multiple measures of the same competencies with an emphasis on the quality of each individual instrument. However, systems thinking has risen in prominence over the past few decades and there are now several papers offering advice on creating a program of assessment.[72–74] These differ from reviews of the assessment of professionalism[18,75] in that they are creating the forest and not focusing on the specific trees. Although there are differences, mainly in emphasis, among the various authors, a report of the National Research Council[76] identifies three key characteristics of a balanced assessment system that have direct applicability to health professions education and professionalism: comprehensiveness, coherence, and continuity.

The system must have *comprehensiveness*. It must take a range of approaches to assessing professionalism. As noted earlier, part of the issue is that the construct of professionalism is not black and white; there are multiple varying interpretations and most are very broad and multifaceted.[63] Moreover, there is no clear consensus on either the elements or the specificity of the elements and, in the case of the development of identity, the elements evolve over time. Therefore, rigorous assessment will most certainly require a suite of tools, each better geared toward different aspects of professionalism.[61] No single measure provides sufficient information to assess all aspects of professionalism across all contexts, to provide feedback that promotes learning and reflection, and to make decisions about whether learners are safe and competent.

Of course, decisions about how to create a system of assessment rely on the development of clear learning goals that are broadly communicated. And, the nature of the assessments themselves must produce information that is reliable, valid, and fair in aggregate. That said, methods that address the "knows" level of the pyramid should play a role, with their prominence decreasing as time in training and practice increases. In contrast, methods that address the "does" level of the pyramid should increase in prominence toward the end of training and into practice. Methods in the other two levels of the pyramid have applicability across the continuum but might be emphasized during clinical training when the development of professional identity is occurring most rapidly.

The system must have *coherence*. Assessment must be aligned with both the curriculum objectives and instructional methods. For example, if the summative assessments are composed solely of methods that test knowledge and reasoning, learners will devalue those parts of the curriculum aimed at the acquisition of communication skills. Similarly, if the formative assessment that is delivered in the clinical workplace is at odds with an instructor's unprofessional attitudes and behavior, learners will model those behaviors and render the aim of the assessment ineffective.

A coherent system will play an important role during the development of professional identity. It is especially important to locate the developmental stage of trainees, offer them insight to their values, attitudes, and behavior, and expose them to the types of experiences that support further development. This implies a system that is rich in formative assessment, with summative assessments playing a more prominent role toward the end of training when patient safety and institutional accountability take precedence.

Finally, the system must have *continuity*. It must be ongoing, produce regular feedback, and provide an assessment of progress toward the desired outcomes. Single assessments, or assessments too broadly spaced in time, will limit effectiveness, especially of feedback.

Likewise, failure to integrate assessments across medical school and postgraduate training will produce a disjointed learning experience. This is particularly critical during the periods when the development of professional identity is occurring most rapidly.

Lessons learned and future directions

Reflection on the state of assessment of professionalism leads to a few summary lessons. First, it is simply not realistic to think that stakeholders in the evaluation process will agree to a single definition of professionalism. They come from too many different disciplines steeped in different traditions, values, and vocabularies. That said, there is probably a relatively short list of common knowledge elements, attitudes, skills, and behaviors that cut across the values and definitions of the stakeholders. These should form the core elements of an assessment system.

Second, given the complexity of professionalism and the values that underlie it, there is a need for systems of assessment, and those systems must be comprehensive, coherent, and continuous. In developing such systems, the emphasis needs to shift from summative to formative assessment with a focus on supporting identity formation. Both are essential, but the potential for formative assessment to generate significant educational gains is largely untapped.

Third, to populate the systems there are a few excellent assessment tools, dozens of very good tools, and a few creative but understudied tools. We do not need many more tools. It is time to stop developing additional methods and focus our efforts on refining those we have and tailoring them for different purposes and for use throughout the learning continuum.

Fourth, to be done well, assessment requires considerable resources. With exceptions, as assessment methods move up levels in Miller's pyramid, they become less efficient and thus more expensive. This is not an argument against creating a system that samples from all levels; rather, it is an argument to pool and share resources and increase planned evaluation. Further, it would be helpful if future work focused on the development of item and case pools, rather than individual instruments created by consortia of institutions. This is an efficient way of supporting a broader range of needs.

Fifth, many of the activities needed to support an assessment system rely on the effort, skill, and judgments of faculty. Yet, these efforts are often uncompensated and we spend little if any time training them. Support and faculty development are the keystones of a well-functioning system of assessment.

In terms of the future, several key questions and issues come to mind:

- A truly robust assessment system must have standards, likely multiple standards as befitting levels of learners and multiple types of assessments. Research on standard setting in this context is needed. Particularly when one assesses identity, what methods for standard setting can fairly conclude that one's identity is wrong or insufficient? It is one thing to say that a learner lacks knowledge or exhibits an inappropriate or immature behavior. It is quite another to state that the core of a person, what they are, is subpar.

- Little has been done about combining, aggregating, or weighting the results of multiple assessments. This issue becomes especially complex when the assessments are conducted at multiple points in time, using multiple methods for multiple purposes. Historically, clinical competence committees have been charged with this responsibility and while this is probably the best mechanism, considerably more research is needed.

- Data ownership, data sharing, and data confidentiality are issues. For example, are outcomes observed (or scores obtained or attitudes revealed) when one is a medical student, to be shared with potential postgraduate training programs? Are they shared before or after acceptance into the program? Who gets to decide?

The assessment of professionalism offers the possibility to make a positive difference in the training of physicians, the accountability of the profession, and the quality of patient care. For doctors, it offers a route to the development of professional identity and the identification of strengths and weaknesses. For the profession, it can fulfill an obligation to society. For patients, it provides a safeguard that their doctors will treat them in the way that they deserve. But as Colton warns us, it is important that we use them in a wise way.

Examinations are formidable even to the best prepared, for the greatest fool may ask more than the wisest man can answer.   *Charles Colton*

References

1. Frank, JR, Jabbour, M, Tugwell, P, Boyd, D, Labrosse, J, MacFadyen, J. Skills for the new millennium: report of the societal needs working group, CanMEDS 2000 Project. *Ann R Coll Physicians Surg Can*. 1996; **29**(4):206–16.

2. Medical Council of India. *Salient Features of Regulations on Graduate Medical Education*. New Delhi, IN: Medical Council of India; 2012. [Accessed Jan. 2, 2015.] Available from www.mciindia.org/Rules andRegulations/GraduateMedicalEducationRegulatio ns1997.aspx.

3. General Medical Council. *Good Medical Practice*. London, UK: General Medical Council; 2001.

4. Leach, DC. A model for GME: shifting from process to outcomes. A progress report from the Accreditation Council for Graduate Medical Education. *Med Educ*. 2004; **38**(1):12–14.

5. Tekian, A, Hodges, BD, Roberts, TE, Schuwirth, L, Norcini, J. Assessing competencies using milestones along the way. *Med Teach*. 2015; **37**(4):399–402.

6. Norcini, J, Burch, V. Workplace-based assessment as an educational tool: AMEE Guide No. 31. *Med Teach*. 2007; **29**(9):855–71.

7. Marcia, JE. Development and validation of ego-identity status. *J Pers Soc Psychol*. 1966; **3**(5):551–58.

8. Erikson, EH. *The Life Cycle Completed*. New York, NY: WW Norton; 1982.

9. Bosk, CL. *Forgive and Remember*. Chicago, IL: University of Chicago Press; 1979.

10. Monrouxe, LV. Identity, identification and medical education: why should we care? *Med Educ*. 2010; **44**(1):40–49.

11. Cruess, RL, Cruess, SR, Boudreau, JD, Snell, L, Steinert, Y. Reframing medical education to support professional identity formation. *Acad Med*. 2014; **89**(11):1446–51.

12. Stern, DT. A framework for measuring professionalism. In Stern, DT, ed. *Measuring Medical Professionalism*. New York, NY: Oxford University Press; 2006:3–14.

13. Hodges, BD, Ginsburg, S, Cruess R, Cruess, S, Delport, R, Hafferty, F, Ho, MJ, Holmboe, E, Holtman, M, Ohbu, S, Rees, C, Ten Cate, O, Tsugawa, Y, Van Mook, W, Wass, V, Wilkinson, T, Wade, W. Assessment of professionalism: recommendations from the Ottawa 2010 Conference. *Med Teach*. 2011; **33**(5):354–63.

14. Miller, GE. The assessment of clinical skills/ competence/performance. *Acad Med*. 1990; **65**(9 Suppl):S63–S67.

15. Cruess, RL, Cruess, SR, Steinert, Y. Amending Miller's pyramid to include professional identity formation.

Acad Med. 2015. Sept. 1, 2015. ['Online First': DOI 10.1097/ACM.0000000000000913].

16. Norcini, JJ, Swanson, DB, Grosso, LJ, Shea, JA, Webster, GD. A comparison of knowledge, synthesis, and clinical judgment. Multiple-choice questions in the assessment of physician competence. *Eval Health Prof.* 1984; **7**(4):485–499.

17. Cruess, RL, Cruess, SR. Teaching professionalism: general principles. *Med Teach.* 2006; **28**(3):205–08.

18. Veloski, JJ, Fields, SK, Boex, JR, Blank, LL. Measuring professionalism: a review of studies with instruments reported in the literature between 1982 and 2002. *Acad Med.* 2005; **80**(4):366–70.

19. Kao, A. Ethics, law, and professionalism: what physicians need to know. In Stern, DT, ed. *Measuring Medical Professionalism.* Oxford, UK: Oxford University Press; 2006:39–52.

20. CITI Program. Collaborative Institutional Training at the University of Miami. [Accessed Dec. 26, 2014.] Available from www.citiprogram.org/.

21. Nunnally, JC, Bernstein, IH. *Psychometric Theory.* Third edition. New York, NY: McGraw-Hill; 1994.

22. Streiner, DL, Norman, GR. *Health Measurement Scales: A Practical Guide to their Development and Use.* Fourth edition. Oxford, UK: Oxford University Press; 2008.

23. Barry, D, Cyran, E, Anderson, RJ. Common issues in medical professionalism: room to grow. *Am J Med.* 2000; **108**(2):136–42.

24. Stobo, JD, Blank, LL. ABIM's project professionalism: staying ahead of the wave. *Am J Med.* 1994; **97**:1–3.

25. Kesselheim, JC, McMahon, GT, Joffe, S. Development of a Test of Residents' Ethics Knowledge for Pediatrics (TREK-P). *J Grad Med Educ.* 2012; **4**(2):242–45.

26. Blue, AV, Crandall, S, Nowacek, G, Luecht, R, Chauvin, S, Swick, H. Assessment of matriculating medical students' knowledge and attitudes towards professionalism. *Med Teach.* 2009; **31**(10):928–32.

27. Swick, HM. Toward a normative definition of medical professionalism. *Acad Med.* 2000; **75**(6):612–16.

28. Niemi, PM. Medical students' professional identity: self-reflection during the preclinical years. *Med Educ.* 1997; **31**(6):408–15.

29. Rademacher, R, Simpson, D, Marcdante, K. Critical incidents as a technique for teaching professionalism. *Med Teach.* 2010; **32**(3):244–49.

30. Stark, P, Roberts, C, Newble, D, Bax, N. Discovering professionalism through guided reflection. *Med Teach.* 2006; **28**(1):e25–e31.

31. Jha, V, Bekker, HL, Duffy, SR, Roberts, TE. A systematic review of studies assessing and facilitating attitudes towards professionalism in medicine. *Med Educ.* 2007; **41**(8):822–29.

32. Veloski, J, Hojat, M. Measuring specific elements of professionalism: empathy, teamwork, and lifelong learning. In Stern, DT, ed. *Measuring Medical Professionalism.* Oxford, UK: Oxford University Press; 2006:117–46.

33. Kohlberg, L. *The Meaning and Measurement of Moral Development (Volume 13).* Worcester, MA: Clark University Press; 1981.

34. Gibbs, JC, Arnold, KD, Morgan, RL, Schwartz, ES, Gavaghan, MP, Tappan, MB. Construction and validation of a multiple-choice measure of moral reasoning. *Child Dev.* 1984; **55**(2):527–36.

35. Rest, JR. Longitudinal study of the defining issues test of moral judgment: a strategy for analyzing developmental change. *Dev Psychobiol.* 1975; **11**(6):738–48.

36. Rees, CE, Knight, LV. The trouble with assessing students' professionalism: theoretical insights from sociocognitive psychology. *Acad Med.* 2007; **82**(1):46–50.

37. Hojat, M, Mangione, S, Nasca, TJ, Cohen, MJM, Gonnella, JS, Erdmann, JB, Veloski, J, Magee, M. The Jefferson scale of physician empathy: development and preliminary psychometric data. *Educ Psychol Meas.* 2001; **61**(2):349–65.

38. Hojat, M, Fields, SK, Veloski, JJ, Griffiths, M, Cohen, MJ, Plumb, JD. Psychometric properties of an attitude scale measuring physician-nurse collaboration. *Eval Health Prof.* 1999; **22**(2):208–20.

39. Hojat, M, Veloski, J, Nasca, TJ, Erdmann, JB, Gonnella, JS. Assessing physicians' orientation toward lifelong learning. *J Gen Intern Med.* 2006; **21**(9):931–36.

40. Hojat, M, Gonnella, JS, Nasca, TJ, Fields, SK, Cicchetti, A, Lo Scalzo, A, Taroni, F, Amicosante, AM, Macinati, M, Tangucci, M, Liva, C, Ricciardi, G, Eidelman, S, Admi, H, Geva, H, Mashiach, T, Alroy, G, Alcorta-Gonzalez, A, Ibarra, D, Torres-Ruiz, A. Comparisons of American, Israeli, Italian and Mexican physicians and nurses on the total and factor scores of the Jefferson scale of attitudes toward physician–nurse collaborative relationships. *Int J Nurs Stud.* 2003; **40**(4):427–35.

41. Kohlberg, L. *The Development of Modes of Moral Thinking and Choice in the Years 10 to 16.* Unpublished doctoral dissertation. Chicago, IL: University of Chicago; 1958.

42. Kohlberg, L. Stage and sequence: the cognitive-developmental approach to socialization. In Goslin, DA, ed. *Handbook of Socialization Theory and Research.* Chicago, IL: Rand McNally; 1969:347–480.

43. Kohlberg, L, Candee, D. The relationship of moral judgment to moral action. In Kurtines, WM, Gewirtz, JL, eds. *Morality, Moral Behavior and Moral Development.* New York, NY: Wiley; 1984:52–73.

44. Baldwin, DC Jr, Self, DJ. The assessment of moral reasoning and professionalism in medical education and practice. In Stern, DT, ed. *Measuring Medical Professionalism*. New York, NY: Oxford University Press; 2006:75–93.

45. McDaniel, MA, Hartman, NS, Whetzel, DL, Grubb III, WL. Situational judgment tests, response instructions, and validity: a meta-analysis. *Personnel Psychology*. 2007; **60**(1):63–91.

46. Lievens, F, Buyse, T, Sackett, PR. The operational validity of a video-based situational judgment test for medical college admissions: illustrating the importance of matching predictor and criterion construct domains. *J Appl Psychol*. 2005; **90**(3):442–52.

47. Aukes, LC, Geertsma, J, Cohen-Schotanus, J, Zwierstra, RP, Slaets, JP. The development of a scale to measure personal reflection in medical practice and education. *Med Teach*. 2007; **29**(2–3):177–82.

48. Crossley, J, Vivekananda-Schmidt, P. The development and evaluation of a Professional Self Identity Questionnaire to measure evolving professional self-identity in health and social care students. *Med Teach*. 2009; **31**(12):e603–e607.

49. Norcini, JJ, McKinley, DW. Assessment methods in medical education. *Teaching and Teacher Education*. 2007; **23**(3):239–50.

50. Swanson, DB, Clauser, BE, Case, SM. Clinical skills assessment with standardized patients in high-stakes tests: a framework for thinking about score precision, equating, and security. *Adv Health Sci Educ Theory Pract*. 1999; **4**(1):67–106.

51. Barrows, HS, Abrahamson, S. The programmed patient: a technique for appraising student performance in clinical neurology. *J Med Educ*. 1964; **39**:802–05.

52. Harden, RM, Gleeson, FA. Assessment of clinical competence using an objective structured clinical examination (OSCE). *Med Educ*. 1979; **13**(1):41–54.

53. van Zanten, M, Boulet, JR, Norcini, JJ, McKinley, D. Using a standardised patient assessment to measure professional attributes. *Med Educ*. 2005; **39**(1):20–29.

54. Klamen, D, Williams, R. Using standardized clinical encounters to assess physician communication. In Stern, DT, ed. *Measuring Medical Professionalism*. Oxford, UK: Oxford University Press; 2006:53–74.

55. Norcini, JJ, Blank, LL, Arnold, GK, Kimball, HR. The mini-CEX (clinical evaluation exercise): a preliminary investigation. *Ann Intern Med*. 1995; **123**(10):795–99.

56. Cruess, R, McIlroy, JH, Cruess, S, Ginsburg, S, Steinert, Y. The Professionalism Mini-evaluation Exercise: a preliminary investigation. *Acad Med*. 2006; **81**(10 Suppl):S74–S78.

57. Kogan, JR, Holmboe, ES, Hauer, KE. Tools for direct observation and assessment of clinical skills of medical trainees: a systematic review. *JAMA*. 2009; **302**(12):1316–26.

58. Al Ansari, A, Ali, SK, Donnon, T. The construct and criterion validity of the mini-CEX: a meta-analysis of the published research. *Acad Med*. 2013; **88**(3):413–20.

59. Hawkins, RE, Margolis, MJ, Durning, SJ, Norcini, JJ. Constructing a validity argument for the mini-Clinical Evaluation Exercise: a review of the research. *Acad Med*. 2010; **85**(9):1453–61.

60. Tsugawa, Y, Ohbu, S, Cruess, R, Cruess, S, Okubo, T, Takahashi, O, Tokuda, Y, Heist, BS, Bito, S, Itoh, T, Aoki, A, Chiba, T, Fukui, T. Introducing the Professionalism Mini-Evaluation Exercise (P-MEX) in Japan: results from a multicenter, cross-sectional study. *Acad Med*. 2011; **86**(8):1026–31.

61. Wilkinson, TJ, Wade, WB, Knock, LD. A blueprint to assess professionalism: results of a systematic review. *Acad Med*. 2009; **84**(5):551–58.

62. Papadakis, MA, Teherani, A, Banach, MA, Knettler, TR, Rattner, SL, Stern, DT, Veloski, JJ, Hodgson, CS. Disciplinary action by medical boards and prior behavior in medical school. *N Engl J Med*. 2005; **353**(25):2673–82.

63. Papadakis, MA, Arnold, GK, Blank, LL, Holmboe, ES, Lipner, RS. Performance during internal medicine residency training and subsequent disciplinary action by state licensing boards. *Ann Intern Med*. 2008; **148**(11):869–76.

64. Arnold, L. Assessing professional behavior: yesterday, today, and tomorrow. *Acad Med*. 2002; **77**(6):502–15.

65. Norcini, JJ. Peer assessment of competence. *Med Educ*. 2003; **37**(6):539–43.

66. Consumer Assessment of Healthcare Providers and Systems. *CAHPS Clinician & Group Surveys*. Rockville, MD: Agency for Healthcare Research & Quality; 2011. [Accessed Dec. 30, 2014.] Available from https://cahps.ahrq.gov/surveys-guidance/survey2.0-docs/1355a_Adult_Visit_Eng_20.pdf.

67. Donnon, T, Al Ansari, A, Al Alawi, S, Violato, C. The reliability, validity, and feasibility of multisource feedback physician assessment: a systematic review. *Acad Med*. 2014; **89**(3):511–16.

68. Eva, KW, Regehr, G. Self-assessment in the health professions: a reformulation and research agenda. *Acad Med*. 2005; **80**(10 Suppl):S46–S54.

69. Mann, K, Gordon, J, MacLeod, A. Reflection and reflective practice in health professions education: a systematic review. *Adv Health Sci Educ Theory Pract*. 2009; **14**(4):595–621.

70. McLachlan, JC, Finn, G, Macnaughton, J. The conscientiousness index: a novel tool to explore students' professionalism. *Acad Med*. 2009; **84**(5):559–65.

71. Stern, DT, Frohna, AZ, Gruppen, LD. The prediction of professional behavior. *Med Educ.* 2005; **39**(1):75–82.

72. Shumway, JM, Harden, RM. AMEE Guide No. 25: The assessment of learning outcomes for the competent and reflective physician. *Med Teach.* 2003; **25**(6):569–84.

73. Birenbaum, M, Breuer, K, Cascallar, E, Dochy, F, Dori, Y, Ridgway, J, Wiesemes, R. A learning integrated assessment system. *Educational Research Review.* 2006; **1**(1):61–67.

74. van der Vleuten, CP, Schuwirth, LW, Driessen, EW, Dijkstra, J, Tigelaar, D, Baartman, LK, van Tartwijk, J. A model for programmatic assessment fit for purpose. *Med Teach.* 2012; **34**(3):205–14.

75. Lynch, DC, Surdyk, PM, Eiser, AR. Assessing professionalism: a review of the literature. *Med Teach.* 2004; **26**(4):366–73.

76. Pellegrino, JW, Chudowsky, N, Glaser, R, eds. *Knowing What Students Know: The Science and Design of Educational Assessment.* Committee on the Foundations of Assessment Report: National Research Council. Washington, DC: National Academy Press; 2001.

Remediation of unprofessional behavior

Louise Arnold, Christine Sullivan, and Jennifer Quaintance

Around the time of publication of the book *Teaching Medical Professionalism*,[1] literature on remediation of unprofessional behavior of learners and practitioners in medicine had just begun to emerge in earnest, no doubt reflecting developments in accreditation of graduate medical education programs and health facilities as well as concern for patient safety. The book's chapter on the topic[2] summarized the extant publications, along with the authors' experience in addressing professional lapses of learners in academic medicine. Much of the work covered in the chapter provided prescriptions for how to proceed with the process of remediation: general approaches to remediation, policies to follow, steps to take including the development of a detailed remediation plan, and suggestions for specific remediation techniques. Apparent themes emphasized changing the behavior of the individual learner or practitioner and the crucial role of assessment in identifying and defining a lapse, as well as determining whether remediation had been successful. Factors thought to predict success or failure of the attempt to correct unprofessional behavior were proposed, including the individual's recognition that a problem exists, her subscription to the values of medical professionalism, a genuine desire to change her behavior, acceptance of the responsibility to participate in remediation, and her demonstration of accountability during the process.[2] Program factors predictive of remediation success included early recognition of the problem, creation of a remediation plan with transparent goals, specific remediation activities, and frequent performance feedback under the guidance of a mentor–advisor who models professional behavior, administers the plan consistently, and in fact gives frequent feedback.[2] Despite the existence of this wisdom from experts, there was recognition that remediation of unprofessional behavior was challenging and not always successful, with the likelihood of relapses and outright failures.

In the years since publication of *Teaching Medical Professionalism* to the present, the remediation literature has grown substantially. An emphasis on steps in the remediation process and techniques to address unprofessional behavior remains,[3–21] while recognition of the relationship between professional lapses and patient safety has grown.[9,16,18,22–25] Appreciation of the role of the environment has intensified, and specific recommendations for building environments supportive of effective remediation as well as professionalism have been formulated.[9,15–18,25–28] Attention paid to the interaction between the environment and the individual in causing, addressing, and preventing unprofessional behavior has emerged.[7,19,22,23,28–30] And well-considered advice about conducting remediation of unprofessional behavior has become increasingly elaborated.[9,19,20,31] A summary of the advice available in the extant literature appears at the end of this chapter.

Several articles report that remediation of unprofessional behavior has been effective,[18,32,33] but the recognition continues of how challenging successful remediation can be.[3,33,34] Difficulties previously discussed in the literature endure: a belief that unprofessional behavior is not fixable; reluctance to report professional lapses based on questions about the definition and assessment of professionalism including whether altruism is tenable; concern about the validity of allegations; poor knowledge about procedural matters and remediation techniques; distaste for confrontation; fear of litigation; and indecision about when unprofessional behavior becomes so intolerable that the learner or practitioner has no place in medicine.

Although the literature and experience with remediation of professional lapses have blossomed, a major gap exists: carefully researched evidence on best practices is typically missing.[8,11,35] An exception is the Vanderbilt University Medical Center's considerable work that is a model for studies of the effectiveness of remediation policies and practices, as well as a model for those policies and practices in and of themselves.[18] Still, effective remediation is not ensured.

Perhaps an antidote to limited success with remediation and gathering evidence for effective intervention lies in a new trend in the remediation literature. The trend begins to apply social science theories about social and psychological development in adulthood to conceptualizing and implementing remediation of unprofessional behavior. Theories of self-determination, self-efficacy, constructivism, development of moral reasoning and behavior, and especially formation of professional identity are promising.

Thus, this chapter examines remediation of unprofessional behavior through a theoretical lens, particularly that of professional identity development. It addresses how the theories of professional identity formation could frame general approaches to remediation by:

- Explaining components of the theories relevant to remediation;
- Exploring the implications of these theoretical insights for changing how we think about remediation;
- Describing current practices compatible with identity development and remediation;
- Specifying next steps to advance the application of identity formation theory to remediation policies and practices and potentially enhance the success of remediation efforts and the development of professional identity among learners and practitioners in medicine;
- Suggesting future research studies; and
- Summarizing lessons already learned.

Components of identity formation theories relevant to remediation of unprofessional behavior

The psychological and sociocultural processes underlying professional identity formation and their implications for professionals and professional students have received increased attention over the past few years and have been thoroughly presented elsewhere.[36-39] There are several components of identity formation theories that are especially relevant to remediation of unprofessional behavior. Identification and discussion of these components follow.

Fundamental to remediation of unprofessional behavior is the view that professional identity formation is a life-long process consisting of a near constant negotiation between an individual's own internal values, adopted roles, personality and external influences, including other individuals, communities of practice (workplaces, institutions, professional organizations, medical profession),[40] and explicit and implicit cultural messages from the environment.[37-39] Another basic concept in professional identity formation is that individuals advance and regress along three interdependent levels: the individual, the environment, and the interaction between the individual and the environment.[37-39] These three sets of processes occur simultaneously, but for the sake of providing an organizational structure of this chapter each will be discussed in turn.

The individual

Theories of professional identity formation describe the journey that an individual takes to build her own professional identity. They recognize that learners in medicine do not enter training programs as a blank slate ready to adopt the professional identities endorsed by their eventual communities of practice.[39] Rather, they arrive with a set of ascribed identities, such as "Woman," "Hispanic," and "Heterosexual," that have been cultivated almost from birth. They also bring their own set of achieved identities, such as "Musician," "Athlete," and "Scholar." Everyone has multiple identities, and the ways in which individuals reconcile those identities have implications for professional identity formation. Social identity complexity theory categorizes the ways in which individuals reconcile multiple identities in terms of the extent to which the identities are perceived as overlapping.[41] At the most simplified level, the individual views others who are members of the same set of social identities as in-group members (intersection). For example, a heterosexual, Hispanic medical student will see other heterosexual, Hispanic medical students as part of her in-group; everyone else is part of the out-group. At the most complex level, the individual views others who hold any one social identity in common as in-group members (merger). The heterosexual, Hispanic medical student would see anyone who is heterosexual, or Hispanic, or a medical student as part of her in-group. Individuals with more complex social identity structures tend to be more open to experiences, tolerant of ambiguity, and accepting of differences than individuals with more simple social identity structures. It is important to note that when individuals are experiencing stress, or are engaged in activities that require substantial cognitive effort, they tend to resort to more simplified social identity structures even if their typical social identity structure may be more complex. As explained later, this set of idiosyncratic identities has implications for an individual's ability to construct a professional identity sanctioned by his or her community of practice.[41]

The theories often describe the individual's journey of identity formation as moving from one stage to the next. For example, Kegan's[42] identity development stage theory posits that on their way to developing an internalized, self-authored identity where they are able to successfully negotiate and integrate their multiple identities including the values of the profession (stage 4), individuals first move through a stage focused on achieving external goals to meet their own needs (stage 2) and a stage where they define themselves through the relationships they have (stage 3). Some argue that Kegan's stage 5, where individuals are able to fully contextualize their identity and understand that there are multiple valid ways to act in accordance with one's core beliefs, is very rarely achieved and remains aspirational for most.[36,38] These stage theories, including Kegan's model, provide useful benchmarks that indicate where individuals fall along the continuum of professional identity formation.

Other theories point to mechanisms that can promote movement from one stage to the next. Constructivist learning theory in particular underscores the importance of knowing the stage of individuals' development as a necessary first step in facilitating movement toward an integrated, internalized identity. Given that knowledge, the right amount of challenge can be provided to move individuals into a state of disequilibrium along with the scaffolding necessary to keep individuals in their zone of proximal development.[43] A primary mechanism that guides development is indeed scaffolding, when more experienced members of the social environment provide assistance or model appropriate behavior or thought processes. Additionally, the potential for growth is greatest when the individual is in the zone of proximal development, a state in which the individual can complete a given task with scaffolding. The zone of proximal development lies in the space between where the individual can complete a task

independently and where the individual cannot complete the task even with expert guidance. In short, balancing the levels of challenge and of support is crucial for encouraging growth without overwhelming individuals to such an extent that they are not able to cope.[43]

In addition, other theories posit (and empirical studies suggest) that the flow from one stage to the next is not always seamless.[36,38,44] The learners' road to becoming a physician is perilous, consisting of a series of discontinuities and crises to work through as they internalize what it means to be a student, resident, and physician.[38] Each discontinuity and each crisis present an opportunity for growth and for making mistakes. Likewise, individuals who are dealing with a major stressor may stagnate on their developmental trajectory or even regress to a more familiar way of thinking about and acting in their environment, manifesting in behavior deemed unprofessional by the community of practice.[41] Given the discontinuities and crises encountered during the process of professional identity formation, individuals experience a wide range of emotions, both negative and positive, that medical educators often have not taken into account.[45]

Finally, individual learners and practicing physicians may not be as far along the developmental continuum as might be intuitively expected. Research has shown that many individuals do not reach the higher stages of identity development until they are well into adulthood.[36,46] Because identity development is a process of negotiation involving inputs from the environment that are ever changing, including shifting roles throughout the life cycle and the task of integrating various aspects of the self into a coherent whole, identity development may be most properly conceptualized as not only ongoing but also life-long.

The environment

Professional identity formation theory maintains that the socialization process that takes place when individuals enter into and maintain their membership in a community of practice acts on individuals in a powerful way.[37-39] Foremost are the influences of role models (peers, near peers, practicing physicians) and mentors and participation in apprenticeships offering authentic experiences with ever increasing integration into communities of practice.[47] Environments characterized by positive institutional cultures, clearly articulated policies and practices, and zero tolerance of frank substandard professional behavior are also key.[16] Other recognized environmental factors include opportunities for learners and practitioners to observe behavior, talk about experiences in safe environments, reflect on those experiences under the guidance of seasoned professionals, and self-assess one's own behavior.[47]

Self-determination theory (SDT) offers recommendations to structure our environments in ways that can foster positive growth in professional identity formation.[48,49] Individuals who wish to join or maintain membership in a particular community of practice will work toward engendering a sense of relatedness with the community by internalizing and integrating the community's beliefs, practices, and values. The explicit and implicit socialization processes employed within communities of practice have varying degrees of success in facilitating individuals' internalization and integration of the communities' norms and values. Central to SDT is the role the environment plays in facilitating whether an individual is motivated to act by her own internalized and integrated goals and values (autonomous motivation) or by external pressures such as rewards and punishments (controlled motivation). The behaviors and activities that are driven by autonomous motivation are the ones most likely to contribute to positive identity formation. Environments that foster a sense of competence, autonomy, and relatedness (i.e., when individuals believe that they can be successful in the activities they choose to engage in and feel personally connected to others in their environment) tend to promote autonomous motivation. On the other hand, when individuals feel externally controlled and disconnected from leaders in the community of practice and are required to engage in activities that are either under- or overly challenging, the likelihood that they will internalize the desired behaviors and values is quite low; rather, they tend to exhibit the desired behaviors only when pressured externally.[48,49]

Role modeling and mentoring are potent mechanisms that transmit the characteristics of the environment to individuals. Theory and empirical work show that role models have a substantial impact on learners' and physicians' professional behavior.[47,50–56] Students, residents, and faculty have reported that the primary way they learn professionalism is through role modeling.[50,53–55] See Chapter 6. Further, individuals report the influence on learning professionalism not just from positive role models but also negative role models.[50,52–55] Role modeling often has a powerful and positive influence on individuals' professional behavior; however, role models are not always positive models. Individuals regularly witness faculty members, residents, and students engaging in unprofessional behavior.[54,57–62] The role that negative role models play in influencing professionalism has the potential to be deleterious.[52,57,58,61,62]

The interaction between the individual and the environment

An individual's unique set of ascribed and achieved identities, coupled with his or her current stage of identity formation, interacts with the environment and leads individuals to construct their unique professional identity.[39,63] In some cases, the match between the individual's identity and the community of practice's notions of what it means to be a member are congruent, making it relatively painless to begin to integrate. For others, the match-up is not so straightforward, often leading the individual into a state of identity dissonance, where she struggles to negotiate between maintaining her identity and adopting the professional identity being imposed by the community of practice.[63]

Identity dissonance is a mechanism that causes some individuals to restructure their identity, much like cognitive disequilibrium functions for constructivists. Others who experience identity dissonance may actively reject the professional identity being imposed by the community of practice, frequently leading to alienation and sometimes extreme struggles within their community of practice.[63] Working through a state of identity dissonance can often cause major emotional and cognitive upheaval[63] and may be a ripe time to make professionalism lapses; likewise, others' reactions to a professional lapse may be enough to push an individual into a state of identity dissonance. Individuals who are not able to successfully work through a state of intense identity dissonance to a place of identity congruence are precisely the individuals who need special attention in the form of a remediation plan.

In addition to tensions between already internalized identities and identities that are being prescribed by the environment, there are also tensions between competing messages sent by the environment. There are conflicting discourses within medical schools; one focused on standardization, as exemplified by a competency approach, and the other focused on diversity, as exemplified by admissions committees' beliefs that each student is unique and brings singular gifts to the educational experience that enrich others in the environment.[64] The two discourses are in tension, although both aim at providing the best possible care to patients. The way learners internalize the competing discourses is strongly influenced by the identities and the social identity structures they have already constructed, leading them to embrace one discourse over the other, or meld the two.[64]

Implications of professional identity formation theory for remediation

If identity formation is an ongoing process, then remediation might best be considered as a life-long continuous quality improvement activity for the development of a professional identity, incumbent upon each member of the profession, including the student and the resident through to the most senior of physicians. An unexamined identity would not be acceptable, since such an identity ignores changes during the life cycle of roles.

Remediation of behavior incompatible with identities accepted by communities of practice, including the professional lapse caused by issues with professional identity formation and the lapse due to other factors such as illness of the individual, a toxic environment, or a mismatch between the individual and the environment, becomes a matter of continuous quality improvement. This conceptualization of remediation then transforms the goal of remediation as not only a matter of changing inappropriate behavior, but also of developing a professional identity accepted by the community of practice. In other words, remediation for professional lapses would become a special case of continuous quality improvement, since all members of the profession must participate in ongoing professional identity assessment and development. Given that, remediation of a professional lapse may lose some of its stigma, and the process may proceed more easily.

In the paradigm shift toward looking at professionalism remediation through the lens of professional identity development, another important stigma to overcome is the very common belief that professionalism is an innate quality not amenable to change. Labeling behavior as bad is a social process often coupled with the notion that professionalism is innate and cannot be taught or changed, leading us to label the individual as bad or unprofessional. Using the new framework, we can shift our understanding of unprofessional behavior from innate and immutable to a normal part of an individual's development toward an identity that has more fully internalized and integrated the practices, beliefs, and values of the community of practice. That being said, it is still important for a community of practice to establish its own red line, so individuals understand that some kinds of behavior are unacceptable and will not be tolerated. Each school of medicine and clinical practice needs to have clear codes of conduct for professional behavior and accompanying policies that delineate the consequences for individuals when their behavior crosses the red line. It is up to individual communities of practice to determine under what contexts and with which behaviors it is appropriate to engage continuous professional development or remediation strategies and when the behaviors require disciplinary action.

Viewing professional lapses through the lens of professional identity formation might point to more fundamental issues that are problematic, involving not only the content of a learner's values and attitudes but also the way in which the individual structures those values and attitudes.[42] For example, in an early stage of professional identity development, a medical student subscribes to the pursuit of excellence, an aspirational value of medical professionalism. But in aiming at achieving outstanding performance of valued role behaviors such as high scores on examinations, the medical student does not collaborate on a group project (which contributes little value to a final course grade), but chooses to prepare for an end-of-semester test by herself in order to "ace" it (which is most heavily weighted in the computation of a final grade). Her focus derives from her own need to achieve that external goal of top grade, and it defines who she is. She is not concerned about how her peers regard her: she believes they cannot help her achieve a top score on the test and indeed that working with them on the project could diminish her chances for getting the top grade. The remediation process then might usefully involve discussions about higher levels of professional identity that go beyond a preoccupation with one's own needs and interests, and thus may get at the core of the student's problem rather than just a discussion of meeting expectations for attendance and participation in group projects. As this example illustrates, identity formation theory provides deeper insight into a possible cause of unprofessional behavior: arrested development reflecting achievement of only beginning stages of the journey to a professional identity acceptable to the community of practice.

Theories of identity formation identify yet another potential trigger of unprofessional behavior because this behavior brings to the fore the possibility that the individual has not yet fully achieved a coherent sense of self that resolves potential conflicts between various identities to the point of fully subscribing to aspirational professional values as primary drivers. In particular, as an example, learners' and clinicians' discomfort with or outright rejection of altruism as service to others may be understood as a manifestation of an unsettled clash between the professional identity and family identities such as spouse, parent, or child. This disequilibrium or dissonance brings its own emotional upheaval, but also might be a spur to further development of the professional identity. By viewing the cause of the clash in terms of achieving a coherent sense of self, the magnitude of the task of improving the alignment of aspirations toward professional values as part of the self with other identities is recognized, but is also perhaps a source of resolution, aligning aspirations with professional values. As the example suggests, identity development theory not only identifies a cause of unprofessional behavior but also offers leverage into creation of a more appropriate remediation plan.

In addition, the theory underscores the importance of environmental factors, already recognized as contributing to professional behavior and discussed above. Identity formation theory suggests the need, not widely acknowledged, for educational opportunities to learn about, discuss, and reflect on the process of identity formation itself, its course and characteristics, and ways to fashion a trajectory moving toward the final aspirational stage. Mentors sharing their journeys can be powerful tools in this regard.

The goal in fostering positive professional identity formation is that individuals embody the norms, beliefs, and practices valued by the community of practice and do so of their own volition, and in all of the contexts in which they find themselves. That is, we want individuals to act from a place of autonomous motivation after having fully internalized and integrated the community of practice's highest aspirational professionalism principles.[48,49] However,

environments in medicine and medical education are sometimes criticized for being structured in such a way as to elicit motivation through controlling and coercive methods rather than through methods that SDT labels as autonomy-supportive, leading individuals to act in desirable ways only when externally pressured to do so.[49] The characteristics of an ideal environment for facilitating autonomous motivation and the internalization of practices and values include:

- Taking individuals' perspectives into account;
- Communicating expectations in an empathetic manner;
- Explaining the rationale for implementing new policies and practices;
- Allowing individuals to choose their own activities and behaviors whenever possible; and
- Providing opportunities to participate in reasonably challenging activities with the provision of nonjudgmental feedback.[48,49]

The theory's emphasis on the environment prompts the suggestion that any plan to enable individuals to move to a more advanced stage of development or to remediate unprofessional behavior must be built upon identification of which environmental elements that could promote growth have been missing in the individual's experience. In other words, investigation of which environmental factors mentioned above have been missing or inadequate in the experience of the learner or practicing physician could guide more targeted selection of solutions to the problem and shape a potentially more effective remediation plan.

Current practices compatible with identity development formation theory and remediation

If educators, supervisors, physicians in training, and even practicing physicians embrace the concept of identity formation as a continuous process of growth and development, it follows that this belief can be incorporated into the view of a physician's professionalism as a life-long improvement opportunity. Within this model, even exemplars of professionalism can strive to enhance their skills and work on taking their achievements beyond their own identity and influencing professionalism within systems and organizations. Therefore, within this framework, the process of remediation of individuals who do not meet professionalism standards becomes more readily accepted as a quality improvement activity in which everyone participates – in contrast to a punitive process. However, even in this model, it would be necessary to accept that there are unprofessional behaviors that might not be amenable to remediation.

Practical expressions of the continuous performance improvement model can readily be seen in expectations set for the development of medical students, residents and fellows, practicing physicians, and for the environment itself. Reviewing some current practice examples can frame the concept of professionalism as a continuous improvement opportunity throughout the life of a physician and the organizations and systems in which he or she practices.

The individual

For medical students, the Association of American Medical Colleges has developed core "entrustable professional activities" (EPAs) as a set of requisite skills that students must demonstrate by the time of graduation to help ensure successful transition from the role of student to that of resident.[65] Critical to the development and implementation of all the EPAs is the foundation of student trustworthiness and self-awareness of personal limitations paired with self-directed guidance to improve.[65] As an example, to fulfill the expectations of the EPA "[c]ollaborate as a member of an interprofessional team," students must not only demonstrate their role and acknowledge their limits as a team member, they must also accept that the team supersedes their personal interests and that they have a responsibility to assist team members.[65] While the EPAs describe expected behaviors, the demonstration of those behaviors helps define the identity of a successful student prepared to transition to residency. The Association of Faculties of Medicine of Canada (AFMC) has similarly worked to define requirements during critical transition stages in the life of physician development from student to resident to independent practice.[66]

The Accreditation Council for Graduate Medical Education (ACGME) recognizes that development of skills in residents and fellows is a progression with certain expectations to be mastered by the time of completion of training. As part of the Next Accreditation System, milestone landmarks have been crafted for each specialty, including achievements in professionalism.

Training programs are required to measure the achievement "level" of the milestones for each trainee every six months until she completes the program.[67] The milestones are intended to demonstrate the progression of a resident's individual knowledge, skills, and attitudes as she achieves competence to enter independent practice.[68] For this discussion of professionalism as a continuous improvement process, we reviewed the milestones in professionalism of the core hospital-based, medical, and surgical specialties. The specialties (anesthesiology, diagnostic radiology, emergency medicine, family medicine, internal medicine, pathology, pediatrics, psychiatry, obstetrics and gynecology, ophthalmology, orthopedic surgery, and surgery) differed in the number of milestones devoted to professionalism but shared themes representing highest achievements.[69-80] The aspirational or uppermost accomplishments in professionalism describe individuals taking professionalism beyond actions and behaviors of themselves and relationships with patients to include contributions to and impacts on systems, teams, and organizations.[69-80] Examples include developing policies and procedures regarding professionalism, serving as a resource and mentor for those not meeting standards (such as working with impaired colleagues), fostering collegiality to promote teamwork, and modeling constructive feedback (both providing and receiving criticism).[69-80] Such individuals are viewed as leaders and mentors for professionalism.

By implementing milestone assessment for their learners, residency programs can determine if an individual trainee is progressing, is stagnant, or is regressing in professionalism achievements. In doing so, the milestones can provide guidance to program directors (PDs) regarding the current expression of professionalism in each resident or fellow and serve as a first step to recommending remediation goals for those not meeting standards. The professionalism lapse can then be viewed as an opportunity for growth and development in each learner.

Practicing physicians know that maintenance of certification for both the American Board of Medical Specialties (ABMS) and the Royal College of Physicians and Surgeons of Canada requires the practitioner to participate in performance improvement and life-long learning activities. For physicians certified by the ABMS, the diplomate must demonstrate a commitment to professional responsibilities including adherence to ethical principles and the demonstration of humanism, compassion, and acceptance of diversity to patients, healthcare teams, and physician self-care.[81] The AFMC further mandates physician self-regulation, both individually and collectively, as an obligation to the profession including remediation and discipline of those not meeting predefined standards.[82]

Environment

Institutions are required to implement continuous quality improvement activities related to the environments in which students, residents, fellows, and practicing physicians work and learn. The Liaison Committee for Medical Education (LCME) and ACGME require, as part of the accreditation process, educational programs to conduct self-studies examining the effectiveness of professionalism current practices and identifying opportunities for improvement. The ACGME has implemented the Clinical Learning Environment Review (CLER) process as an assessment of the current system in which residents and fellows learn. This process encourages institutions and hospital systems to work cooperatively in a continuous quality improvement effort to enhance the learning environment for GME.[83] Professionalism is one of the six focus areas examined in the clinical setting. Specifically, the review investigates how residents, fellows, and faculty are educated about professionalism; which attitudes, beliefs, and skills of residents and fellows are related to professionalism; how faculty are engaged in professionalism training; and how the clinical site monitors professionalism.[84] The goal of the CLER is to enhance the integration of residents, fellows, and faculty members in hospital systems to promote the learning environment and patient care.

Perhaps the greatest example of practicing continuous quality improvement of healthcare environments are the changes in the healthcare delivery and monitoring systems that arose from initiatives by The Joint Commission (TJC) and other organizations to improve patient quality care and safety. It has become all too common for healthcare professionals to work in silos disconnected from their colleagues, which undermines their sense of relatedness in the work environment. The recent and welcome focus on interprofessional collaboration and education may be a boon to individuals who feel isolated and disconnected. Working in a team on which all members are valued for their individual contributions could go a long way toward building a sense of relatedness.

Concern for quality care and patient safety has also prompted proposals to construct a culture supportive of professional behavior in educational and clinical settings. One proposal views respect as the essential ingredient in achieving a nurturing environment and stipulates that institutions must develop effective methods for responding to episodes of disrespectful unprofessional behavior while initiating cultural changes necessary to prevent such episodes.[16] An excellent model of a comprehensive approach to this task, including the remediation of unprofessional behavior, entails three programs nested in a center for patient and professional advocacy.[28] The center advances the institution's values for safety, quality, and professionalism; offers continuing medical education courses; and sponsors a faculty physician wellness program, a physician assessment program focusing on fitness for duty, and a committee for awareness intervention. Perhaps at the pinnacle of that institution's approach is a carefully tested mentoring program for physicians who do not meet professionalism standards, which demonstrates how the institution actively implemented an environmental process to promote professionalism among physicians.[18] Physicians who were identified by patients' and families' complaints as not meeting professionalism standards received intervention and intense mentoring by trained peer mentors. The process included sharing of the complaint, physician self-reflection, and on-going advising and feedback regarding patient interactions. The authors concluded that intensive, persistent, and professional sharing with physician outliers acknowledged the fact that they differed from their peers and the prospect that they could improve their performance was necessary to successful remediation. Promoting accountability of every physician for her actions could ultimately enhance the overall environment.

Interaction between the individual and the environment

Another ongoing practice in medicine, root cause analysis (RCA), is relevant to remediation of unprofessional behavior, an idea that our previously published chapter introduced.[2] Healthcare organizations utilize this technique to understand the cause of medical harm and error through identifying primary and contributing factors to that harm. It emphasizes system issues, examines the relationships between individual team members as members of larger systems, and avoids placing blame on individuals. The goal of the process is to prevent future incidents by educating patient providers, implementing changes in the system to promote safe practices, and clearly defining expectations and accountability.[85–88]

With the understanding of RCA as a tool to examine systems and promote quality improvement, its application in the context of remediation framed in terms of professional identity formation deserves special mention. Its use as a device to support remediation prompts an examination of the individual and the environment as well as the interaction between the two when determining factors causing professional lapses. It leads to recommendations, based on the review of the behaviors and processes involved, to improve and further the professionalism of not only the individual but also the environment. The end result is the professionalism development of both the individual and the system with a focus on how they can interact successfully to improve the care of patients.

Next steps

Although current practices just reviewed are compatible with adapting professional identity development theories to remediation of unprofessional behavior, they only facilitate that prospect. What can be done, then, to directly incorporate professional identity formation into the processes of remediating professional lapses? A number of concrete steps are immediately at hand that constitute an approach to remediation with professional identity development as a core element. Table 12.1 presents these steps. They encompass a series of suggested actions to analyze individual, environmental, and interactional factors that contribute to the behavior of learners and seasoned clinicians plus a series of possible responses to the findings that the analyses uncover. The steps can be applied in concert with the hard-won wisdom in the literature.[2–31] The following scenario illustrates the suggested approach:

A PD receives several complaints from nurses that a resident has been rude to patients and healthcare team members. As the PD investigates the complaint, he finds that the resident's unprofessional behavior only occurred during high-volume times in the clinic. During the investigation and formulation of remediation strategies, the PD reviews the complaints with the resident and allows her to respond. When he shares with her the finding that her behavior occurs only when patient volume is high, the opportunity to

discuss emotional triggers for stress with her emerges. That conversation raises questions about her professional identity: how she sees herself as a physician and the conflicts she experiences among her need to excel in patient care while expanding her clinical skills and assuming a leadership role on the team, the team's need to accommodate the patient load, and the patients' need for efficient timely care. Then it expands to her perception of the environmental support she receives: how well it helps her to create a coherent sense of professional self through strengthening her clinical competence, her autonomy, leadership, and connection to the team to ease her stress. Replying to her negative perceptions, the PD first recounts his struggles in his journey to physicianhood and then discusses strategies that she and the residency program can use to prevent future unprofessional behavior and assist her professional identity development. The resident asks for help to better recognize and react to inherent stressors in her work. She also requests clarification of team members' roles and her role of leader. Together they discuss possible referral to counseling for stress management; a small group on team building; and assignment of a mentor who models teamwork, monitors her professional behavior, and explores her progress in developing a coherent professional identity. The resident and the PD agree to her participation in these strategies. In closing, the PD states that the program should recognize when an imbalance arises between furthering the resident's clinical skills and increasing the number of patients she is expected to see in clinic and offer her relief.

Back in his office, the PD examines the work flow processes and resources in the environment and detects room for improvement during times of high patient volume. Because he believes that the professionalism of all team members and the environment could be raised if changes could be made, he meets with the clinic director to explore the issue. Also, due to the resident's questions about team roles, he requests that the director evaluate the roles and responsibilities of the team members. Together they lay plans to involve the team in adapting ways to facilitate patient care during high-volume times. Further, because the PD suspects that the nurses reporting the resident's behavior were under duress themselves and lacked adequate assistance with their identity development, he speaks to their supervisor about more education for the nurses concerning identity formation and professionalism, its assessment, and the role and responsibilities of the resident in the clinic system.

The PD hopes that adaptive work flow processes and professional development education in the clinic

Table 12.1. A proposed approach to professionalism lapses and remediation based on professional identity, self-determination, and constructivist theories

Contributing Factors	Investigate	Respond
The individual	1. Where is the individual in her professional identity development? Is her identity focused only on her own needs, derived from relationships she has with a healthcare team, or fully integrated with the values of the profession across multiple identities? Does she not understand how to view her identity beyond self; does she lack knowledge about her role as a member of a team or community of practice? Is she physically, emotionally, and mentally well? 2. Has the reporter of the professional lapse or supervisor or advisor considered the individual's perspective? Does the individual feel supported by the environment in the development of her identity? Does she feel appropriately challenged to reach autonomy and a self-authored integrated identity or does she feel pressured to work beyond her current capabilities?	1. Consider need for referrals to physician assistance programs or counseling, education regarding expectations, and professional identity growth provided in an empathetic and supportive manner. Normalize the process of remediation as continuous quality improvement in which everyone participates. Encourage sharing of struggles on the journey to physicianhood. 2. Assign to the individual a role model or mentor who can provide nonjudgmental feedback, enhance her understanding of what it means to be part of the larger healthcare system and the profession of medicine, and create a plan for growth that builds on the individual's current identity while providing appropriate challenge and support for development.
The environment	1. Did the current system contribute to or cause the lapse? 2. What is the current state of professionalism in the environment? Are educators, advisors, teams, and systems supportive of professionalism? 3. How amenable are individuals to reframing professionalism remediation as continuous quality improvement? How pervasive is the attitude that an individual who behaved unprofessionally is innately bad? Is there reluctance to report unprofessional behavior and change it? 4. In what ways does the environment advance and inhibit professional identity formation?	1. Take a comprehensive approach to investigating factors, consider root cause analysis. Consider the need to implement changes in policies and systems to promote professionalism, the reporting of professional lapses, and remediation of unprofessional behavior. 2. Administer environmental inventories and use results to implement action plans to improve the environment as indicated. Enhance support systems for individuals working in the environment. Consider creating wellness programs for individuals across the continuum. 3. Improve the institution's education about and faculty development for professionalism and identity formation. Train advisors, supervisors, and team members in identity development and increase their skills in assessment of professionalism and identity formation. Train mentors, advisors, and supervisors in designing remediation that takes into account issues in identity development when indicated. 4. Consider the specific guidelines suggested by self-determination theory, discussed in this chapter. If indicated,

Table 12.1. (cont.)

Contributing Factors	Investigate	Respond
		amend current policies and practices to include growth in professional identity formation of learners and healthcare professionals.
Interaction between the individual and the environment	1. Is there a lack of understanding about how the environment interacts with the individual to trigger unprofessional behavior and to impede professional identity formation? 2. What instances generate stress and compromise professionalism of the individual and the environment? 3. How can the individual and environment together promote professionalism?	1. Educate individuals and team members about their roles and responsibilities as members and leaders of teams to include supporting professionalism. 2. Consider giving additional resources and support to the system during certain instances of stress on the individual or system. Implement team building to promote a sense of belonging to the community of practice by all members of the team or community. Ensure that advisors and mentors have skills to assist an individual to negotiate and form acceptable identities for her environment and for herself. Promote acceptance of the diversity of team members' identities within the limits of core professional standards. 3. Explain the rationale for implementing new policies and practices to the individual and the team.

might improve patient care in the clinic through minimizing stress within the team and reducing future incidents of the resident's unprofessional behavior. But, by using this approach, the PD does learn that the resident has been able to recognize the conflicts in her identity and to see that remediation is an opportunity for growth and development. The resident also told him that through her small group, stress management counseling, support by her mentor, and better workflow processes, she feels she is not labeled as "bad" or "unprofessional" and views the program as facilitating her growth in competence, autonomy, leadership, and relatedness to the group while increasing the professionalism of the team as a whole.

Once concrete steps are underway in applying identity formation theory to remediation and continuous quality improvement for all, local initiatives should be documented and outcomes noted. In that way, an evidence-based foundation can be built to identify which remediation practices work at each institution. However, we await more long-term initiatives to discern the efficacy of incorporating identity formation into remediation on a broader scale.

Future research studies

Theoretical and empirical studies of remediation considered through the lens of professional identity formation are essential to address underlying questions about reframing remediation as a special case of identity development throughout a physician's career. Guidance for future studies is suggested below.

A number of theoretical traditions are apparent in the literature on professional identity development. From these traditions, this chapter has selected those elements that seem relevant to informing remediation practices, without noting similarities and reconciling differences among the theories. However, clarification of these theories of professional identity formation, particularly their differences, could elucidate which of them, or which aspects thereof, would result in the most effective remediation of unprofessional behavior. In particular, dialogue among theorists and educators should strive to achieve lucidity about the concept of professional identity itself – its definition and measurement. This dialogue should pinpoint critical differences in how various theories characterize the processes of professional identity formation; investigate ways in which a unified theory of identity formation could be created; and project the consequences that various versions of a unified theory would hold for undertaking the remediation of unprofessional behavior.

While theories of professional identity formation in remediation are generated, empirical studies based on these perspectives should begin to answer such questions as the following. Are there stages in a physician's journey toward embracing a mature appropriate professional identity? What do they look like? What individual and environmental factors elicit movement from one stage to another, regression, and stagnation? Do individuals with diverse backgrounds and diverse selves have equal chances to form appropriate professional identities in a particular environment? What sorts of environments support diverse individuals' sense of autonomy, sense of competence, and belonging to a community of practice so they can develop and demonstrate identities compatible with their community? What are the relationships, if any, between the various stages of professional identity development and unprofessional behavior? Depending upon context, are some types of professional identities more likely to evoke unprofessional behavior than others? Which remediation is most effective: one that helps an individual to subscribe to a professional identity more appropriate for her environment or one that focuses only on behavioral change of the individual? What intervention techniques are most effective when issues of professional identity are implicated in unprofessional behavior and in what contexts? Answers to these questions are necessary to gauge the utility of looking at remediation through the lens of professional identity formation and to discern how to design and administer remediation plans that take identity development into account.

Research that produces credible answers to these questions is a complex task. The number of individuals who require formal remediation is not large, while the need to tailor remediation to the individual, the unprofessional behavior, and the environment further reduces the number of instances of remediation available for generalizability. Instruments to characterize individuals' professional identities and their behaviors expressing those identities, and tools to describe aspects of the environment that support identity formation, need to be located (several are available[44,89]) or created and tested. Faculty need to be trained to promote professional identity development and incorporate it into the remediation they offer individuals for whom they have responsibility. Collaboration across institutions, together with material support, would enable this research to commence. In the meantime, the advice culled from the literature is available to tide us over until well-tested identity formation theories enlighten the practices of remediation of unprofessional behavior.

Lessons learned

When faced with the special case of an individual who may have acted unprofessionally, the process of remediation needs to be nested in the policies, steps, and practices distilled through experience.[2–31]

Definition of professional lapse

Before a professional lapse can be identified and addressed, it must first be defined. Institutional policy or professional organizations can serve as the framework to derive a definition regarding behaviors that are standard and acceptable, and those that are not, including behaviors beyond the "red line." As an example, unprofessional behavior that interferes with patient care may be defined as critical and emergent to address, whereas untimely record keeping may be deemed less critical and urgent while still being viewed as substandard.

General approach

Unprofessional behavior should be identified and addressed as early as possible lest it become refractory to change. To encourage reporting, the complainant needs a safe environment and should receive acknowledgement that her report is under investigation. To maximize success of the process, the supervisor of the individual identified as unprofessional should express genuine concern in an atmosphere of support, not discipline. Furthermore, the supervisor should encourage the individual to share her perspective and involve her throughout. Adherence to due process and documentation is paramount and will protect all those involved.

Investigation and characterization of the lapse

Before remediation is implemented, the lapse must be fully investigated, characterized, and documented.

Sound professionalism assessment measures and fact finding are important in verifying the unprofessional behavior. Further, consultation to assess the reliability of the report and determine its severity is recommended. To assist in the development of the remediation plan, exploration of the cause(s) of the lapse is critical: are behavioral, interpersonal, and attitudinal issues; stress; impairment resulting from medical, cognitive, psychological, or psychiatric problems or substance abuse; or family concerns involved? Finally, consideration of the role of the environment as a cause or contributing factor should be undertaken.

Remediation process

The remediation begins with the initial meeting to notify the individual of the complaint and to define and characterize the unprofessional behavior. Allow the individual to reflect, respond, and provide her perspective. This meeting should be documented. A graduated approach should be utilized:[90] for less serious first-time lapses, the meeting with the individual may serve as a "wake-up call" providing education, and may in fact be all that is necessary to correct the behavior. However, when there are more serious, frequent, or recurrent lapses, or when informal remediation has been unsuccessful, a more formal remediation must be implemented. In designing a plan, the supervisor should discuss with the individual the plan's rationale and expectations and elicit her suggestions. Subsequently, the plan should be formalized, based on the nature of the lapse, its cause, credible information from multiple sources, and the perspective of the individual.

The supervisor should specify remediation activities that include frequent discussion with an advisor; intensive mentoring; continuous performance feedback, preferably from multiple sources; and self-reflection by the individual. Referrals for educational programs, such as team building or effective communication practices, might be indicated depending on the nature of the lapse. Evaluation or formal counseling using motivational interviewing or cognitive behavioral therapy may be appropriate for certain lapses and their cause(s).

Critical to the remediation plan are clear goals, transparent expectations, and a definite timeframe. Consistency and adherence to the plan by the individual, the person administering the process, and the institution must be understood, accepted by all, and documented. Goals and measures of successful remediation must be formalized. Additionally, consequences for failure to achieve goals and participate in the plan must be clear.

Verify outcomes of remediation

With goals, expectations, and defined timeframe of the process predetermined, monitoring during the remediation by the supervisor is crucial. Feedback and issues discovered during the process may indicate the need for a modification of the plan to meet the remediation needs of the individual. As an example, intensive mentoring may disclose an additional cause of the lapse that may require attention. At the conclusion of the remediation, outcomes should be determined by using reliable assessment methods. Successful remediation and conclusion of the process may still require additional monitoring for relapse and should be discussed with the individual. If the plan is not successful, an extension of the existing plan or modifications to address the lapse may be required. Additionally, if remediation is determined to be unsuccessful or additional lapses or relapse occur, disciplinary action may be initiated.

Conclusion

For now, current wisdom can inform remediation of unprofessional behavior. At the same time, incorporating theories of professional identity formation into remediation may advance our efforts. But, doing so is fraught with immense challenges. It demands a paradigm shift away from remediation as discipline focused only on modification of observable behavior of abnormal individuals to remediation as just a special case of ongoing professional identity development and renewal, viewed as a normal process incumbent upon all members of a community of practice moving toward aspirational values of medical professionalism. Therein, however, lies an exhilarating opportunity. The key to achieving it entails cultural, social, and individual change. That will be accomplished only in the long term. Nevertheless, a sound beginning may be at hand in the appearance of the second edition of *Teaching Medical Professionalism*.

References

1. Cruess, RL, Cruess, SR, Steinert, Y, eds. *Teaching Medical Professionalism*. New York, NY: Cambridge University Press; 2009.

2. Sullivan, C, Arnold, L. Assessment and remediation in programs of teaching professionalism. In Cruess, RL,

Cruess, SR, Steinert, Y, eds. *Teaching Medical Professionalism.* New York, NY: Cambridge University Press; 2009:124–49.

3. Adams, KE, Emmons, S, Romm, J. How resident unprofessional behavior is identified and managed: a program director survey. *AM J Obstet Gynecol.* 2008; **198**(6):692.e1–4;692.e4–5.

4. Belitz, J. How to intervene with unethical and unprofessional colleagues. In Roberts, LW, ed. *The Academic Medicine Handbook: A Guide to Achievement and Fulfillment for Academic Faculty.* New York, NY: Springer; 2013:183–89.

5. Buchanan, AO, Stallworth, J, Christy, C, Garfunkel, LC, Hanson, JL. Professionalism in practice: strategies for assessment, remediation, and promotion. *Pediatrics.* 2012; **129**(3):407–09.

6. Elnicki, DM. *Remediation in Medical Education.* Pittsburgh, PA: Academy of Master Educators, University of Pittsburgh School of Medicine; 2011. [Accessed Feb. 21, 2015.] Available from www.ame.pitt.edu/documents/remediation_elnicki_000.pdf.

7. Guerrasio, J. *Remediation of Poor Professional Behaviors among Practicing Physicians.* Federation of State Physician Health Program Annual Meeting; 2013. [Accessed Feb. 21, 2015.] Available from www.fsphp.org/Guerrasio%20Presentation.pdf.

8. Hauer, KE, Ciccone, A, Henzel, TR, Katsufrakis, P, Miller, SH, Norcross, WA, Papadakis, MA, Irby, DM. Remediation of the deficiencies of physicians across the continuum from medical school to practice: a thematic review of the literature. *Acad Med.* 2009; **84**(12):1822–32.

9. The Joint Commission. *Behaviors that Undermine a Culture of Safety.* Sentinel Event Alert. Issue 40; 2008. [Accessed Feb. 21, 2015.] Available from www.jointcommission.org/assets/1/18/SEA_40.pdf.

10. Katz, ED, Dahms, R, Sadosty, AT, Stahmer, SA, Goyal, D; CORD-EM Remediation Task Force. Guiding principles for resident remediation: recommendations of the CORD remediation task force. *Acad Emerg Med.* 2010; **17** Suppl 2:S95–S103.

11. Kalet, A, Tewksbury, L, Ogilvie, JB, Yingling, S. An example of a remediation program. In Kalet, A, Chou, CL, eds. *Remediation in Medical Education: A Mid-Course Correction.* New York, NY: Springer; 2014:17–37.

12. White, MK, Barnett, P. A five step model of appreciative coaching: a positive process for remediation. In Kalet, A, Chou, CL, eds. *Remediation in Medical Education: A Mid-Course Correction.* New York, NY: Springer; 2014:265–81.

13. Caligor, E, Levin, Z, Deringer, E. Preparing program directors to address unprofessional behavior. In Kalet, A, Chou, CL, eds. *Remediation in Medical Education: A Mid-Course Correction.* New York, NY: Springer; 2014:285–96.

14. Kalet, A, Zabar, S. Preparing to conduct remediation. In Kalet, A, Chou, CL, eds. *Remediation in Medical Education: A Mid-Course Correction.* New York, NY: Springer; 2014:311–22.

15. Guerrasio, J. "The prognosis is poor": when to give up. In Kalet A, Chou CL, eds. *Remediation in Medical Education: A Mid-course Correction.* New York, NY: Springer; 2014:323–38.

16. Leape, LL, Shore, MF, Dienstag, JL, Mayer, RJ, Edgman-Levitan, S, Meyer, GS, Healy, GB. Perspective: a culture of respect, part 2: creating a culture of respect. *Acad Med.* 2012; **87**(7):853–58.

17. Tennessee Medical Foundation. *Model Policy for Distressed Physician Behavior.* Brentwood, TN: Tennessee Medical Foundation. [Accessed Feb. 21, 2015.] Available from www.e-tmf.org/mpdpb.php.

18. Pichert, JW, Moore, IN, Karrass, J, Jay, JS, Westlake, MW, Catron, TF, Hickson, GB. An intervention model that promotes accountability: peer messengers and patient/family complaints. *Jt Comm J Qual Patient Saf.* 2013; **39**(10):435–46.

19. Reynolds, NT. Disruptive physician behavior: use and misuse of the label. *Journal of Medical Regulation.* 2012; **98**(1):8–19.

20. Sagin, T. *Addressing Unprofessional Conduct: A Guide for Physician Leaders.* Salem, WI: HG Healthcare Consultants; 2012. [Accessed Feb. 21, 2015.] Available from www.hughsdigest.com/wp-content/uploads/2012/07/Addressing-Unprofessional-Conduct.pdf.

21. Sanfey, H, Darosa, DA, Hickson, GB, Williams, B, Sudan, R, Boehler, ML, Klingensmith, ME, Klamen, D, Mellinger, JD, Hebert, JC, Richard, KM, Roberts, NK, Schwind, CJ, Williams, RG, Sachdeva, AK, Dunnington, GL. Pursuing professional accountability: an evidence-based approach to addressing residents with behavioral problems. *Arch Surg.* 2012; **147**(7):642–47.

22. Gallagher, TM, Levinson, W. Physicians with multiple patient complaints: ending our silence. *BMJ Qual Saf.* 2013; **22**(7):521–24.

23. Leape, LL, Shore, MF, Dienstag, JL, Mayer, RJ, Edgman-Levitan, S, Meyer, GS, Healy, GB. Perspective: a culture of respect, part 1: the nature and causes of disrespectful behavior by physicians. *Acad Med.* 2012; **87**(7):845–52.

24. Shojania, KG, Dixon-Woods, M. 'Bad apples': time to redefine as a type of systems problem? *BMJ Qual Saf.* 2013; **22**(7):528–31.

25. Speck, RM, Foster, JJ, Mulhern, VA, Burke, SV, Sullivan, PG, Fleisher, LA. Development of a professionalism committee approach to address unprofessional medical staff behavior at an academic

medical center. *Jt Comm J Qual Patient Saf.* 2014; **40**(4):161–67.

26. Nothnagel, M, Reis, S, Goldman, RE, Anandarajah, G. Fostering professional formation in residency: development and evaluation of the "forum" seminar series. *Teach Learn Med.* 2014; **26**(3):230–38.

27. Shapiro, J, Whittemore, A, Tsen, LC. Instituting a culture of professionalism: the establishment of a center for professionalism and peer support. *Jt Comm J Qual Patient Saf.* 2014; **40**(4):168–77.

28. Swiggart, WH, Dewey, CM, Hickson, GB, Finlayson, AJ, Spickard, WA Jr. A plan for identification, treatment, and remediation of disruptive behaviors in physicians. *Front Health Serv Manage.* 2009; **25**(4):3–11.

29. Kalet, A, Chou, CL. Preface. In Kalet, A, Chou, CL, eds. *Remediation in Medical Education: A Mid-Course Correction.* New York, NY: Springer; 2014:xiii.

30. Samenow, CP, Worley, LL, Neufeld, R, Fishel, T, Swiggart, WH. Transformative learning in a professional development course aimed at addressing disruptive physician behavior: a composite case study. *Acad Med.* 2013; **88**(1):117–23.

31. Kalet, A, Chou, CL, eds. *Remediation in Medical Education: A Mid-Course Correction.* New York, NY: Springer; 2014.

32. Guerrasio, J, Garrity, MJ, Aagaard, EM. Learner deficits and academic outcomes of medical students, residents, fellows, and attending physicians referred to a remediation program, 2006–2012. *Acad Med.* 2014; **89**(2):352–58.

33. Zbieranowski, I, Takahashi, SG, Verma, S, Spadafora, SM. Remediation of residents in difficulty: a retrospective 10-year review of the experience of a postgraduate board of examiners. *Acad Med.* 2013; **88**(1):111–16.

34. Sullivan, C, Murano, T, Comes, J, Smith, JL, Katz, ED. Emergency medicine directors' perceptions on professionalism: a Council of Emergency Medicine Residency Directors survey. *Acad Emerg Med.* 2011; **18** Suppl 2:S97–S103.

35. Papadakis, MA, Paauw, DS, Hafferty, FW, Shapiro, J, Byyny, RL; Alpha Omega Alpha Honor Medical Society Think Tank. Perspective: the education community must develop best practices informed by evidence-based research to remediate lapses of professionalism. *Acad Med.* 2012; **87**(12):1694–98.

36. Forsythe, GB. Identity development in professional education. *Acad Med.* 2005; **80**(10 Suppl):S112–S117.

37. Goldie, J. The formation of professional identity in medical students: considerations for educators. *Med Teach.* 2012; **34**(9):e641–e648.

38. Jarvis-Selinger, S, Pratt, DD, Regehr, G. Competency is not enough: integrating identity formation into the medical education discourse. *Acad Med.* 2012; **87**(9):1185–90.

39. Monrouxe, LV. Identity, identification and medical education: why should we care? *Med Educ.* 2010; **44**(1):40–49.

40. Wenger, E. *Communities of Practice: Learning, Meaning, and Identity.* Cambridge, UK: Cambridge University Press; 1998.

41. Roccas, S, Brewer, MB. Social identity complexity. *Pers Soc Psychol Rev.* 2002; **6**(2):88–106.

42. Kegan, R. *The Evolving Self: Problem and Process in Human Development.* Cambridge, MA: Harvard University Press; 1982.

43. Vygotsky, LS. *Mind in Society: The Development of Higher Psychological Processes.* Cambridge, MA: Harvard University Press; 1978.

44. Bebeau, MJ, Faber-Langendoen, K. Remediating lapses in professionalism. In Kalet, A, Chou, CL, eds. *Remediation in Medical Education: A Mid-Course Correction.* New York, NY: Springer; 2014:103–27.

45. Helmich, E, Bolhuis, S, Dornan, T, Laan, R, Koopmans, R. Entering medical practice for the very first time: emotional talk, meaning and identity development. *Med Educ.* 2012; **46**(11):1074–86.

46. Baxter Magolda, MB. *Making Their Own Way: Narratives for Transforming Higher Education to Promote Self-Development.* Sterling, VA: Stylus; 2001.

47. Kenny, NP, Mann, KV, MacLeod, H. Role modeling in physicians' professional formation: reconsidering an essential but untapped educational strategy. *Acad Med.* 2003; **78**(12):1203–10.

48. Ryan, RM, Deci, EL. On assimilating identities to the self: a self-determination theory perspective on internalization and integrity within cultures. In Leary, MR, Tangney, JP, eds. *Handbook on Self and Identity.* New York, NY: Guildford Press; 2003:253–74.

49. Williams, GC, Saizow, RB, Ryan, RM. The importance of self-determination theory for medical education. *Acad Med.* 1999; **74**(9):992–95.

50. Baernstein, A, Oelschlager, AM, Chang, TA, Wenrich, MD. Learning professionalism: perspectives of preclinical medical students. *Acad Med.* 2009; **84**(5):574–81.

51. Cruess, RL, Cruess, SR. Teaching professionalism: general principles. *Med Teach.* 2006; **28**(3):205–08.

52. Hojat, M, Vergare, MJ, Maxwell, K, Brainard, G, Herrine, SK, Isenberg, GA, Veloski, J, Gonnella, JS. The devil is in the third year: a longitudinal study of erosion of empathy in medical school. *Acad Med.* 2009; **84**(9):1182–91.

53. Moyer, CA, Arnold, L, Quaintance, J, Braddock, C, Spickard, A 3rd, Wilson, D, Rominski, S, Stern, DT. What factors create a humanistic doctor? A nationwide

survey of fourth-year medical students. *Acad Med.* 2010; **85**(11):1800–07.

54. Murinson, BB, Klick, B, Haythornthwaite, JA, Shochet, R, Levine, RB, Wright, SM. Formative experiences of emerging physicians: gauging the impact of events that occur during medical school. *Acad Med.* 2010; **85**(8):1331–37.

55. Park, J, Woodrow, SI, Reznick, RK, Beales, J, MacRae, HM. Observation, reflection, and reinforcement: surgery faculty members' and residents' perceptions of how they learned professionalism. *Acad Med.* 2010; **85**(1):134–39.

56. Weissmann, PF, Branch, WT, Gracey, CF, Haidet, P, Frankel, RM. Role modeling humanistic behavior: learning bedside manner from the experts. *Acad Med.* 2006; **81**(7):661–67.

57. Brainard, AH, Brislen, HC. Viewpoint: learning professionalism: a view from the trenches. *Acad Med.* 2007; **82**(11):1010–14.

58. Feudtner, C, Christakis, DA, Christakis, NA. Do clinical clerks suffer ethical erosion? Students' perceptions of their ethical environment and personal development. *Acad Med.* 1994; **69**(8):670–79.

59. Ginsburg, S, Kachan, N, Lingard, L. Before the white coat: perceptions of professional lapses in the pre-clerkship. *Med Educ.* 2005; **39**(1):12–19.

60. Ginsburg, S, Regehr, G, Stern, D, Lingard, L. The anatomy of the professional lapse: bridging the gap between traditional frameworks and students' perceptions. *Acad Med.* 2002; **77**(6):516–22.

61. Satterwhite, RC, Satterwhite, WM 3rd, Enarson, C. An ethical paradox: the effect of unethical conduct on medical students' values. *J Med Ethics.* 2000; **26**(6):462–65.

62. Satterwhite, WM 3rd, Satterwhite, MA, Enarson, CE. Medical students' perceptions of unethical conduct at one medical school. *Acad Med.* 1998; **73**(5):529–31.

63. Costello, CY. *Professional Identity Crisis: Race, Class, Gender, and Success at Professional Schools.* Nashville, TN: Vanderbilt University Press; 2005.

64. Frost, HD, Regehr, G. "I am a doctor": negotiating the discourses of standardization and diversity in professional identity construction. *Acad Med.* 2013; **88**(10):1570–77.

65. Association of American Medical Colleges. *Core Entrustable Professional Activities for Entering Residency: Faculty and Learners' Guide.* Washington, DC: AAMC; 2014. [Accessed Aug. 10, 2014.] Available from https://members.aamc.org/eweb/upload/Core%20EPA%20Faculty%20and%20Learner%20Guide.pdf.

66. The Association of Faculties of Medicine of Canada. *The Future of Medical Education in Canada (FMEC): A Collective Vision for MD Education.* Ottawa, ON: AFMC; 2012. [Accessed Jan. 19, 2015.] Available from www.afmc.ca/future-of-medical-education-in-canada/medical-doctor-project/pdf/collective_vision.pdf.

67. Nasca, TJ, Philibert, I, Brigham, T, Flynn, TC. The next GME accreditation system–rationale and benefits. *N Engl J Med.* 2012; **366**(11):1051–56.

68. Sullivan, G, Simpson, D, Cooney, T, Beresin, E. A milestone in the milestones movement: the JGME milestones supplement. *J Grad Med Educ.* 2013; **5**(1 Suppl 1):1–4.

69. The anesthesiology milestone project. *J Grad Med Educ.* 2014; **6**(1 Suppl 1):15–28.

70. Vydareny, KH, Amis, ES Jr, Becker, GJ, Borgstede, JP, Bulas, DI, Collins, J, Davis, LP, Gould, JE, Itri, J, LaBerge, JM, Meyer, L, Mezwa, DG, Morin, RL, Nestler, SP, Zimmerman, R. Diagnostic radiology milestones. *J Grad Med Educ.* 2013; **5**(1 Suppl 1):74–78.

71. Beeson, MS, Carter, WA, Christopher, TA, Heidt, JW, Jones, JH, Meyer, LE, Promes, SB, Rodgers, KG, Shayne, PH, Wagner, MJ, Swing, SR. Emergency medicine milestones. *J Grad Med Educ.* 2013; **5**(1 Suppl 1):5–13.

72. The family medicine milestone project. *J Grad Med Educ.* 2014; **6**(1 Suppl 1):74–86.

73. Iobst, W, Aagaard, E, Bazari, H, Brigham, T, Bush, RW, Caverzagie, K, Chick, D, Green, M, Hinchey, K, Holmboe, E, Hood, S, Kane, G, Kirk, L, Meade, L, Smith, C, Swing, S. Internal medicine milestones. *J Grad Med Educ.* 2013; **5**(1 Suppl 1):14–23.

74. The pathology milestone project. *J Grad Med Educ.* 2014; **6**(1 Suppl 1):182–203.

75. Carraccio, C, Benson, B, Burke, A, Englander, R, Guralnick, S, Hicks, P, Ludwig, S, Schumacher, D, Vasilias, J. Pediatrics milestones. *J Grad Med Educ.* 2013; **5**(1 Suppl 1):59–73.

76. The psychiatry milestone project. *J Grad Med Educ.* 2014; **6**(1 Suppl 1):284–304.

77. The obstetrics and gynecology milestone project. *J Grad Med Educ.* 2014; **6**(1 Suppl 1):129–43.

78. The ophthalmology milestone project. *J Grad Med Educ.* 2014; **6**(1 Suppl 1):146–61.

79. Stern, PJ, Albanese, S, Bostrom, M, Day, CS, Frick, SL, Hopkinson, W, Hurwitz, S, Kenter, K, Kirkpatrick, JS, Marsh, JL, Murthi, AM, Taitsman, LA, Toolan, BC, Weber, K, Wright, RW, Derstine, PL, Edgar, L. Orthopaedic surgery milestones. *J Grad Med Educ.* 2013; **5**(1 Suppl 1):36–58.

80. The general surgery milestone project. *J Grad Med Educ.* 2014; **6**(1 Suppl 1):320–28.

81. American Board of Medical Specialties. *Standards for the ABMS Program for Maintenance of Certification (MOC).* Chicago, IL: ABMS; 2014. [Accessed Dec. 15, 2014.] Available from www.abms.org/media/1109/standards-for-the-abms-program-for-moc-final.pdf.

82. ABIM Foundation, American Board of Internal Medicine; ACP-ASIM Foundation, American College of Physicians-American Society of Internal Medicine; European Federation of Internal Medicine. Medical professionalism in the new millennium: a physician charter. *Ann Intern Med.* 2002; **136**(3):243–46.

83. Weiss, KB, Wagner, R, Bagian, JP, Newton, RC, Patow, CA, Nasca, TJ. Advances in the ACGME Clinical Learning Environment Review (CLER) program. *J Grad Med Educ.* 2013; **5**(4):718–21.

84. Accreditation Council for Graduate Medical Education. *Clinical Learning Environment Review (CLER).* Chicago, IL: ACGME; 2014. [Accessed Dec. 15, 2014.] Available from www .acgme.org/acgmeweb/Portals/0/PDFs/CLER/CLER_ Brochure.pdf.

85. Longo, DR, Hewett, JE, Ge, B, Schubert, S. The long road to patient safety: a status report on patient safety systems. *JAMA.* 2005; **294**(22):2858–65.

86. Yates, GR, Bernd, DL, Sayles, SM, Stockmeirer, CA, Burke, G, Merti, GE. Building and sustaining a systemwide culture of safety. *Jt Comm J Qual Patient Saf.* 2005; **31**(12):684–89.

87. Lee, A, Mills, PD, Neily, J, Hemphill, RR. Root cause analysis of serious adverse events among older patients in the Veterans Health Administration. *Jt Comm J Qual Patient Saf.* 2014; **40**(6):253–62.

88. Grissinger, M. Building patient-safety skills: avoiding pitfalls in conducting a root cause analysis. *P T.* 2013; **38**(12):728–29.

89. Pitkala, KH, Mantyranta, T. Professional socialization revised: medical students' own conceptions related to adoption of the future physician's role – a qualitative study. *Med Teach.* 2003; **25**(2):155–60.

90. Hickson, GB, Pichert, JW, Webb, LE, Gabbe, SG. A complementary approach to promoting professionalism: identifying, measuring, and addressing unprofessional behaviors. *Acad Med.* 2007; **82**(11):1040–48.

Professional identity formation, the practicing physician, and continuing professional development

Jocelyn Lockyer, Janet de Groot, and Ivan Silver

Mary is a fifty-year-old family physician who has worked for nearly two decades in a large suburban multidisciplinary family medicine clinic with eight other family physicians as well as nurses, pharmacists, and a dietician. Many of her patients and their families have been with her for several years. To better enjoy and support her children and aging parents, she has recently left the clinic to join a group of medical and radiation oncologists in a breast cancer clinic where she will be the only family physician providing primary care and counseling to their patients who don't have a family physician. She wonders how she will adapt to this work environment in which other family physicians are not available on location to discuss cases with and calibrate her work. She is feeling anxious about working exclusively with cancer physicians, given how specialized their work is, and she does not know any other family physicians who have assumed this type of a role in a specialty clinic.

John is a forty-six-year-old MD-PhD working in a medical school. He has just been promoted to professor in his medical school based on the quality of his work as judged by peers within the medical school and internationally. However, he struggles to combine clinical work, teaching, research, and committee work. He frequently works twelve to fourteen-hour days to fulfill the responsibilities of his various roles and succeeds partly by compartmentalizing his work. When he is on clinical service, he tries to focus on being a physician and clinician educator to the medical students and residents on his service. When he is in the lab, he tries to focus on his research, getting grants, running the lab and ensuring graduate students are making progress. As a professor, he is now expected to bring in larger, more complex grants from international agencies and to support postdoctoral

fellows as well as graduate students. Many days are difficult as he finds himself pulled with questions from his lab or from the clinic when he is not there. Hospital meetings occur regularly and he is expected to actively participate in quality assurance committee work. Dealing with the new expectations associated with the promotion has been difficult; he feels pulled in too many directions and is not staying on top of his work.

Introduction

A physician's identity is a representation of self, achieved in stages over time during which the characteristics, values, and norms of the medical profession are internalized, resulting in an individual thinking, acting, and feeling like a physician.[1]

Physicians who have completed postgraduate medical education (residency) training and attained certification or independent practice continue to develop their professional identity throughout the rest of their careers and into retirement. While the formation of professional identity may be considered a phenomenon that occurs primarily during formal periods of learning, people do change over a career. It is critical to recognize the concept of professional identity as a process that continues throughout a physician's life.

Professional identity is shaped by many forces. As Jarvis-Selinger et al.[2] note, professional identity occurs at two levels: the individual level, which involves the psychological development of the person; and the collective level, which involves a socialization of the person into appropriate roles and forms of participation in the community's work. Similarly, Sabel et al.[3] note that it is helpful to think of identity within the context of social identity theory to bring

---

Teaching Medical Professionalism, 2nd Edition, ed. Richard L. Cruess, Sylvia R. Cruess and Yvonne Steinert.
Published by Cambridge University Press. © Cambridge University Press 2016.

together the self, internalized identity, and the identity that is co-constructed through social interactions. People work to integrate their roles (e.g., cardiologist, retired physician, "new" family physician) and status, along with their diverse experiences, into a coherent image of themselves, thus achieving their professional identity that continues to evolve.

Physician identity is achieved in stages and parallels adult psychological development. While the formative years for psychological development are during childhood, the potential for further development and change continues throughout adult life. In this regard, the formation of a physician's identity begins in early adult life, within the context of prior psychosocial development, and is influenced by the individual's specific generational and sociocultural environments.[2,4] A consideration of theories of adult development that emphasize different aspects of psychological growth, and may influence how physicians engage with their role in society, helps to further understand facets of professional identity formation.

For example, Erikson's[5] widely known and influential theory of healthy adult male psychological development described step-wise resolution of task-related conflicts beginning in early childhood and extending throughout adult life. The stages relevant to professional identity begin in late adolescence with identity versus role confusion, followed by adult developmental stages of intimacy versus isolation (ages eighteen–forty), generativity versus stagnation (ages forty–sixty-five), and integrity versus despair (over sixty-five). Failure to successfully complete a stage can result in a reduced ability to complete further stages. Emphasizing the fluidity of identity formation, these stages, however, can be resolved successfully at a later time in the life cycle. Vaillant's[6] longitudinal study of healthy adult male development notes the importance of work and love over seven decades. Building on Erikson's theoretical framework, Vaillant[7] added two developmental tasks: career consolidation and keeper of meaning. Following mastery of intimacy, wherein the capacity for interdependence, reciprocity, and commitment in romantic relationships and friendship is matured, career consolidation is characterized by commitment, competence, contentment, and compensation, and the career contributes to the same enjoyment as did play in childhood.[7] Subsequent to the stage of generativity, characterized by serving as a mentor or consultant, Vaillant's[7] description of the keeper of meaning task

emphasizes the preservation of culture through tradition and history. This stage may be more evident in retirement.

Levinson[8] developed a highly influential, although controversial, theory of life structure, with sequential life stages for both men and women.[8,9] Early, mid, and late adult life are three eras lasting about twenty-five years each, and requiring several years to complete the transition. Mid-life, which at the time of his research was not well understood, was of great interest to Levinson and his research team. The theme of tension between individuation and attachment is present in all eras, but particularly important in the middle period. Individuation refers to being separate from the world and its attachments, and to being self-generating. It also gives one the confidence and understanding to have more intense attachments in the world and to those one interacts with, to feel more fully a part of society, and, in turn, to help to further shape one's identity. He also discussed vitalizing "dreams" that developed in the early to mid-twenties among men and developed creativity and life satisfaction. However, a careful review suggested that the "dream" among women was less vitalizing and thought to be subverted to an early sense of expectations of family responsibilities.[10]

Kohlberg's[11] theory of moral development is also useful to consider, given the importance of values and norms to physician identity. In Kohlberg's model of justice-based morality, the highest level of moral development requires the use of principles to resolve ethical conflicts. Gilligan,[12] who studied with both Kohlberg[11] and Erikson,[5] wrote the highly influential book *In a Different Voice*, which described a more relational approach to resolving moral dilemmas through an ethic of care. Her research and its interpretation have been soundly critiqued, and yet have stimulated further research that shows that women's and men's moral development is less polarized, and that ethical dilemmas may require evaluation of both care and justice. In this regard, Held[12] beautifully articulates how moral reasoning best includes both care that considers the context of human dependence and value of emotions, and justice that upholds rational, abstract principles. To achieve a more nuanced physician identity, grappling with these considerations of morality is important.

As the preceding discussion indicates, adult psychological development influences personal identity. The potential gender differences described are more likely based on socialization interacting with biology.[14] In this regard, socialization is also very important to professional identity, and how socialization interacts with the unique variation between individual physicians is important to consider. In fact, a gender-similarities hypothesis that finds that men and women are more similar than different has been upheld with recent meta-synthesis research[15] on more than 100 meta-analyses. The remaining psychological differences included women's greater interest in peer attachment and people than things, and among men, greater aggression and confidence in physical abilities.

With respect to socialization and female adult development, the typical role of women in relation to family has significant implications. That is, women's roles in society and the role of female physicians have evolved greatly to accommodate white middle-class females[16] as they have cracked the "glass ceiling" or navigated the labyrinth of leadership.[18] This has required negotiating societal views about the role of professional women[17] as well as a mothering ideology.[19] Feminist research indicates that perspectives on "mothering" over the past seventy years have been strongly informed by the 1950s post-war stereotype of a white suburban family.[19,20] From this perspective, mothering is viewed as highly child centered and best provided by a mother (Hays, 1996). Further, a mother's identity is intertwined with balancing paid work and childcare.[20]

In this chapter, we begin by positioning professional identity within what is known about the topic, recognizing that it is situated within a broader context of adult development. We move next to considering the transitions within a physician's career because they provide a useful way of thinking about professional identity. Transitions represent periods of change in which physicians must make sense of their new settings and experiences in order to re-form their identity. We will discuss some of the other phenomena that influence physicians' identity, including personal, specialty, and work-setting characteristics that may influence professional identity given the interplay between the individual and the collective setting. We will then discuss the role that continuing professional development (CPD) appears to play in forming professional identity. We conclude with lessons learned and future directions.

Transitions

Transitions are common in medicine. They are a dynamic process[21] representing a period of change or movement between one state of work and another[22] or one set of circumstances and another.[21] Common transitions include changing one's work or specialty or geographical location.[22] Generally, transitions are "critically intense learning periods"[22] associated with a limited time in which a major change occurs and that change results in a transformation. During transitions, people re-form their way-of-being and their identity in fundamental ways. Thus, transitions represent a process which involves a fundamental reexamination of one's self, even if the processing occurs at a largely unconscious level.[23] In transition periods, people enter into new groups or "communities of practice."[24] This involves adopting shared, tacit understandings; developing competence in the skilled pursuits of the practice; and assuming a common outlook on the nature of the work and its context.[24] It is in this new site, or community of practice, that identities evolve.[24]

While transitions can be highly stressful and involve negative emotions, they also provide individuals with opportunities for rapid personal development and new behavioral responses to cope with the discontinuity in one's life space.[21] In a medical career, three critical transitions have been identified: the periods of "getting in," "fitting in," and "getting out."[25] However, while "getting in" and "getting out" may be more clearly marked periods, there are many transitions that physicians make during the course of practice that require attention and contribute to professional identity.

Entry to independent practice

Entry to independent practice is a particularly challenging phase. It is as difficult as the transitions that took physicians into and through medical school and residency.[23,25–28] During this period, physicians must come to terms with their identity in a new role as an independent licensed physician with new expectations for patient care and workplace relationships.[23,26,28] Many will feel confident about their clinical tasks.[21,29] Others will struggle to feel as competent in the nonclinical tasks of their work that include teaching, management, and finance. These skills are often not taught or poorly taught in residency but are needed to assume new roles and expectations. Some physicians will enter into arrangements in which they need to hire or supervise staff. Others working with medical students and residents will assume responsibility as the senior physician for care in a teaching unit.[21,29,30]

Westerman's[26] description of the transition from resident to attending physician identifies three themes that interacted during the longitudinal process as the new identity was assumed. First, there were the disruptive elements of the new environment, which included both nonclinical tasks not previously learned as well as supervisory roles in which the physician carried the final medical responsibility for care. There was perception and coping, which included being medically well prepared but not well prepared for nonclinical tasks and having to reduce stress and feelings of incompetence. Last, there was personal development and outcome, in which the feelings of incompetence diminished and task mastery developed over time. As the physicians clarified their roles over time, they developed task mastery adjusted to the culture of the institution and its expectations. Nonetheless, more stress was experienced by those for whom the discrepancy between the tasks of residency and practice were the greatest.

Transitions in practice

The transitions that physicians experience during the course of a career occur in many ways. For example, they can occur in response to a community or personal need in which the physician narrows a clinical practice to a focused area (e.g., general obstetrics to infertility). Scientific advances may require additional training and supervision by those who need to maintain currency in the discipline. Physicians can assume new roles as researchers, administrators, or educators. Some physicians will move to a new community or country. Others will reenter practice following a leave or the identification of a need for remedial training.[31] Further, as the healthcare system and expectations change, physicians must adapt to workplace changes, which are likely to include working more closely with other medical and health disciplines. While the transitions may be planned for some, for others they may be incremental, unplanned, and opportunistic.[32]

Several studies describe transitions into different "communities of practice" or work settings and how the physicians adapt and, in so doing, assume new identities. For example, Loh's[32] examination of transitions into management roles describes how physicians often take on these roles in incremental ways in order to have an impact on a larger population than would be possible if they continued as a clinician seeing individual patients. He noted that physicians can have an identity problem as their clinical colleagues do not see medical management as a real medical specialty, creating a dissonance for the transitioning physician who may have few role models and mentors. Research involving physicians who immigrate describes the hurdles the physicians must overcome to master the practice of medicine in a new country.[33] This study showed that the immigrant physician may lack the tacit knowledge that their Canadian trained colleagues had learned through common experiences in medical school, residency, and professional networking. As the immigrant physician enters the new culture and setting, tacit knowledge has to be gained by trial and error based on feedback from colleagues, other healthcare professionals, and patients. Initially, this leaves the physician frustrated because it is difficult to calibrate his or her work to meet expectations. Things become easier over time as the physicians assume the work expected and gain confidence, seeing themselves in new ways. McLean's[34] study of physicians from other nations who became medical educators in the Middle East describes the development of identity as a cyclical process in which, through experiences and reflection, individual world views and perspectives are continually modified and developed. Transitioning geographically within a country can also be challenging. One study of physicians moving within Canada suggested that some physicians, particularly those who were pragmatic about the move, had moved previously, had supportive spouses, or had previously lived in the city appeared to be less challenged personally by the move and more able to integrate and assume new working roles quickly. Conversely, those physicians who did not come to a job, did not have a previously established network, or moved due to a spousal move took longer to establish themselves because they had to manage both personal and professional integration.[35]

It is common in medicine to assume more than one role; physicians often perform work as clinicians while maintaining roles as researchers, educators, and administrators. A recent study examined the experiences of physician and basic science educators who conducted faculty development workshops. They found that these individuals had faculty educator identities as well as their (clinician) professional identity. Their faculty educator identity evolved over time and tended to merge with their professional identity.[36] However, there were variations. Some physicians had a compartmentalized identity: at times one was a physician and at other times an educator. Some adopted a hierarchical identity, which placed being a physician–scientist above being a physician–educator or vice-versa. For others, there were parallel identities that existed simultaneously but without conscious overlap, and merged identities in which both roles were integrated and coexisted simultaneously.[36] In another study of early career medical educators, the authors observed that this group understood their medical-educator role to be secondary to their roles as a scientist or clinician and had not developed an emotional attachment to the field, maintaining their relationship at an operational one revolving around roles and responsibilities.[3]

Transitions out of practice

Leaving practice or retiring from practice is another period of transition in which professional identity is also challenged. Many fear the potential loss of the identity they have assumed over many years. Some find it difficult to change roles, give up roles, bring others along, or negotiate new roles.[37] Further, the decision to retire or reduce work leading to retirement is likely to be accompanied by significant decision-making that can be accompanied by recognized declines in cognitive function,[38,39] financial concerns,[40] succession planning,[37] and continuing to work as workload expectations change.[40] For example, there may be changes in cognitive function as cognitive performance may decline with age.[38,39] Older age can be accompanied by a loss of skill and confidence. A large ten-year UK study of cardiac surgery identified an increased risk of mortality in patients operated on by longer serving surgeons.[41] Similarly, a study of anesthesiologists found a higher frequency of litigation and a greater severity of injury in patients treated by anesthesiologists in the age sixty-five or older group.[42] It can be stressful to remain in positions as the organization's needs change or to redirect one's work given previous decisions the physician may have made to reduce or focus the scope of work.[43] Physicians may also find it difficult to manage heavy patient loads and night work.[40] For physicians who are employed or dependent on group earnings, there may be pressure to leave, particularly if the physician is not able to meet workload expectations or obtain research grants.[43] Physicians whose professional identity is tightly linked to their professional roles often find it difficult to "let go."[37] Retirement is not always accompanied by a sense of loss or fear. For some, retirement offers an opportunity to grow in different ways using medical expertise to volunteer or do part-time teaching. For many, it is a time of reinvention, choice, and opportunity to explore new, otherwise dormant, or previously restricted activities.[44]

Transitions are periods when physicians have a chance to reflect and determine how they will move ahead and into new roles and responsibilities. Along the way, physicians will work toward a new sense of who they are.

Personal identity and life stages

As discussed in relation to adult development, personal identity (e.g., gender, ethnic background, religious orientation, sexual preference) and life stages intersect and interact with and influence ongoing socialization in relation to physician identity.

Being a woman and a physician can influence career consolidation and professional identity as a physician. For example, while the last fifty years have witnessed a tremendous increase in the proportion of women in full-time work, and men are more involved in raising children, including as single parents,[45] female physicians with children are less likely to work full time than their male counterparts with children.[46] Similarly, with respect to adult female development, another significant mid- to late-life role common to women is that of providing or managing care for elderly parents or disabled spouses.[47]

There is some adverse socialization through discrimination that women may experience from patients and healthcare workers. For example, among Canadian general internists, women physicians are more likely than men physicians to report gender discrimination that is not influenced by the woman's age, community size, or academic affiliation.[48] Fortunately, there may be a generational shift in the healthcare context[16] in that physician daughters of mothers who are physicians report lower rates of gender, racial, and ethnic discrimination than did their mothers. Despite this improvement, they reported similar rates of sexual harassment and overall, gender discrimination rates remained high. These adverse experiences within the healthcare system associated with lower career satisfaction may interfere with consolidation of physician identity. Female physicians find opportunities to reflect on the intersection of their personal and professional identities through online discussion boards (e.g., American College of Surgeons – Women Surgeons), blogs, and professional development programming developed specifically for women physicians.[52]

There are other examples of how personal identity intersects with physician identity. A moving and reflective account by a transcultural psychiatrist[49] conveys how her ethnicity and early experiences with bullying and an outsider identity led to working in her chosen field. In this account, Madelyn Hicks, a part-Chinese, part-Caucasian American academic psychiatrist and mother working in London, chooses to call her field cross-cultural to convey what she describes as intentional interaction with difference, including within personal and professional identities. Her experience as an outsider and with racism promoted her capacity to care for the vulnerable and to uphold ethics. Hicks' experience evokes Symonds'[50] description of a "divided or uncertain sense of identity" as she maintains her academic career through part-time work, job-sharing, and taking a break from clinical work to maintain her research and writing. Her narrative role models the value of reflecting, connecting with mentors and peers, and engaging with relevant literature to process challenging and complex experiences.

The intersection of the healthcare environment with personal identity may interfere with physician identity. Medical students and residents who are lesbian, gay, bisexual, transgender, or queer (LGBTQ) describe the healthcare environment as frequently homophobic. They face rarely discussed challenges throughout their career, including remaining closeted to avoid expulsion, being denied supportive recommendations from advisors, and being exposed to blatant prejudices from colleagues that affect patient care.[51] Identity concealment is particularly problematic as it has been shown to have significant negative effects on physical and mental well-being.[51] Homophobic remarks by patients or other members of the healthcare team were reported by forty percent of internists.[48] For some gay medical students and residents, their experiences as "outsiders" in a conservative environment had the potential to enhance their capacity for identifying patients' inner conflicts, recognizing bias against minorities, and making a choice to use inclusive language as part of their professional identity.[52] Established practitioners who are open about their LGBTQ identity may find greater integration between the elements of their personal and physician identities.

Other phenomena that influence identity

Physicians are also shaped by the teams within which they work, the context of their work, and their specialization.

Teams

As healthcare evolves, there is a great emphasis on working in interdisciplinary teams. Work in multispecialty clinics has been shown to affect specialists' perceptions of identity with some specialties affected more than others.[53]

As Molleman et al.[53,54] note, specialists with a strong professional identity derive part of their self-view from belonging to their specialty as they see their specialty in a positive light. This can affect their team functioning and identity differentially. Some will adopt common expertise norms and behaviors within the team more easily. Others will want to demonstrate the importance of their work for patient care, and this can be challenged by other members of the team. Molleman et al. note that identity threat is more likely to occur when different specialties have competing opinions about treatment in complex healthcare situations, when new specialties enter the domain of existing specialties, and when technological developments shift the boundaries between specialties.[3]

Working in and collaborating in interdisciplinary teams requires team skills (e.g., attitudes and behaviors focused on collaboration and communication for effective team care). These latter attitudes and behaviors may be different than those expected in other settings, where the physician may be more autonomous. This may require a shift in how physicians see themselves. For example, Wright et al.[55] found that family physicians working on geriatric teams struggled with but held a continuum of beliefs about the role they should play on teams, including whether the family physician should be autonomous or a collaborative decision-maker, work inside or outside the team, and be leaders or members of the team. In another setting where physicians were given explicit training to enhance team skills, it was clear that physicians changed their perceptions of themselves and of the team over the training period. They identified personal and professional growth as outcomes of the program. Some assumed new roles as developers of team skills within the medical school curriculum and members of group research grant teams.[56]

Certainly contemporary management of chronic diseases is challenging traditional perceptions of identity, as physicians recognize that identity centered on autonomy, authority, and the ability to "heal" may be counterproductive in chronic disease care, which demands interdependency between physicians, their patients, and teams of multidisciplinary healthcare providers.[57]

Context

The context of physician practice has been shown to affect identity in a number of settings. For example, in settings in which physicians provide care to indigenous populations, physician effectiveness appears to depend on developing a more "fluid" identity so that the physician's cultural and professional beliefs and practices can intersect with the expectations of culturally safe practice shaped by the indigenous context. In these settings, identity is negotiated through differences in language, role expectation, practice, status, and identification. In another example, physicians trained in a modality of complementary and alternative medicine integrate complementary and alternative medicine and biomedical medicine to develop a hybrid professional identity that comprises two sets of healthcare values.[58] An exploration of how physicians experience and cope with vulnerability facing the life and death aspects of their clinical work, and how such experiences affect their professional identities, showed that they could deal with death and mostly keep it at a distance. In these settings, vulnerability was closely linked to professional responsibility and identity, perceived as a burden to be handled.[59] However, physicians who direct their focus to the humanistic aspects of care in the physician-patient relationship, and physicians who administer needed interventions to reduce pain and suffering at the end of life, have the privilege of experiencing particularly poignant moments with patients nearing death.[60] In this regard, competence in psychosocial aspects of care and acceptance that dying is a part of life may enhance the humanistic aspect of physician identity.

Specialization

The type of physician one is and becomes is also linked to professional identity. In moving from medical school through residency, physicians begin to adopt the identity of their teachers along with the appropriate knowledge and behaviors. In doing so, they differentiate themselves from other disciplines in this community of practice.[61] It is not always an easy transition. For example, neonatal residents described the conflicts experienced in becoming neonatologists as they learned to care for very sick and dying babies. In this study, they identified multiple conflicts of identity as members of the neonatology team, as members of the medical profession, as members of their own families, and as members of society. These conflicts often led them to question their own morals and their role in the medical profession.[62] The transformation into a specialty can also be detrimental, as Jin et al.[63] point out in their examination of surgeons' professional identity, which they note is constructed and negotiated within a surgical culture. The hidden curriculum, which calls for displaying confidence and certainty, gives rise to "appropriate" surgical behavior, which can impact surgical judgment and decision-making. Identity formation takes time, often extending beyond residency. Gendron et al.[64] found that professional identity as a gerontologist took time, and that success could be predicted by length of time in the field, age, satisfaction with coworkers, and satisfaction with opportunities for advancement.

Physicians will also construct their identity within their specialty in response to changes made by the speciality. Specialties change boundaries. As noted in a retrospective analysis of the disciplines of medical oncology and hematology, the work and the professional identities of physicians in both disciplines changed when medical oncologists, in pursuit of specialty status, claimed wide-ranging expertise over the treatment of all patients suffering from malignant disease.[65] Currently family medicine is struggling for a clear identity between generalist and specialist roles. On the one hand are physicians who would preserve all the professions' traditional functions while adapting to changing contexts. Other physicians would like to concentrate on areas of expertise and moving toward creating "specialist" general practitioners, in response to a rapidly expanding scope of practice and to the high value attributed to specialization by society and the professional system.[66]

Summary

Many factors affect how physicians see and identify themselves within the profession of medicine. Identity formation is influenced by the transitions that occur through work and a physician's personal life. It is affected by gender, age, and family. The type and setting of practice as well as specialty also have an influence. In the next section, we will explore how the requirement that physicians keep up their learning through continuing professional development activities can and should enhance identity.

Continuing professional development and professional identity

Physicians have a responsibility to develop their competence through focused learning activities throughout their careers. As noted in Chapter 14, this obligation is mandated through maintenance of competence, certification, and relicensure programs established by professional organizations and by regulatory bodies who require varying forms of evidence. Two cases were described at the beginning of the chapter – Mary and John. Both are within transition periods. Both need to reflect on the changes in their lives and focus their learning activities to meet the new demands. Mary is trying to enhance how she integrates her home and professional life through changing her clinical work context. While each person in transition needs to find the best approach to ease the transition, Mary might find it helpful to shadow surgeons, medical and radiation oncologists, and other members of the healthcare team with whom she is now working, to learn about their work in order to fit into the team more comfortably. National or regional oncology meetings may be useful in identifying family physicians in comparable positions as potential mentors, as well as in helping her gain knowledge of breast cancer and oncology. Given that she is providing primary care services within the clinic, she will need to maintain her own competence as a family physician, albeit while working in a nontraditional context. She may enjoy meeting with peers in a study group, to help her manage the emotions evoked in her new work context. John's situation is different as he struggles to achieve a better balance among his commitments and to feel comfortable in the role of "Professor" with its emerging demands. Mentorship from other faculty members who have successfully made the transition and appear to be able to juggle various commitments may be helpful. They may also help him understand the complexity and feasibility of writing grant applications for international funding. Discussions with his department head may be necessary to determine workload, gain a commitment for

protected time, and establish realistic expectations. Education related to time and personnel management may prove helpful. In both cases, the physician's identity – as a family physician with expertise in breast cancer and as an MD-PhD academic – is evolving to meet the new work challenges.

Along with literature concerning the identification of transitions and the difficulties that physicians face as they work through transitions, there is a literature about the types of things that help physicians at both the individual and the group level. Regardless of the type of transition, several themes recur. Ensuring clinical competence is important. This may require additional intensive formal training, which improves confidence,[67] or training that might occur longitudinally through workshops, discussions, and reading. For physicians who are moving into a very different clinical system or setting (e.g., country to country, small to large clinic), formal orientation and mentorship programs are warranted.[33,68] Most physicians benefit from the support of friends and colleagues.[28,67] While physicians who join functioning units appear to have fewer problems, it appears that physicians who appear to have more difficulty with transitional periods often are those who join dysfunctional groups, those without clearly defined roles, those without professional networks in the city, and those entering community rather than an institutional practice.[35] Collegial, continuing professional development, and institutional and systems support can clearly benefit physicians as they make sense of their emerging professional identity.

Continuing professional development (CPD) or continuing medical education consists of educational activities that serve to maintain, develop, or increase the knowledge, skills, and professional performance and relationships that a physician uses to provide services for patients, the public, or the profession.[69] As examples, CPD activities include conferences, courses, rounds, traineeships, mentoring relationships, online learning, self-assessment programs, reading, and discussions with colleagues. In the same way that physicians are shaped by periods of transition, the natural progressions of adulthood, and other phenomena that define their lives and work, the CPD the physician undertakes can also shape professional identity. CPD can influence professional identity at the individual level by maintaining the physician's competence through activities they determine will enhance the quality of their work as well as through activities in which the physician is a member of a group and is learning from others within that group. Skilled CPD designers need to recognize that both individual and group learning activities are critically important facets of development and need to be built into educational programming. Similarly, physicians need help learning how they will benefit from both individual and group activities in which they strive to develop the skills they need for competent practice as individuals as well as from being part of a learning community of physicians and other health-care team members.

Individual CPD

Research on self-assessment reveals that adults have difficulty accurately self-assessing in domains of knowledge and skills in which they are less competent.[70,71] Physicians with competency gaps are those most in need of CPD but are less likely to seek it out because they do not or cannot acknowledge gaps in their knowledge and skills. To address this, physicians require benchmarks of competent practice, including feedback about their knowledge, skills, performance, and behaviors. Self-assessment quizzes and certifying-body testing can help physicians identify and address knowledge gaps. Simulation labs with task trainers and high-performance simulators can provide feedback on skills. Physicians' own practice performance data allows physicians to more clearly see how their practice outcomes compare to others.[72] Clinical audit data helps physicians enhance clinical expertise. Multisource feedback data provides information about professionalism, communication skills, collaboration, and team effectiveness. Data from these and other sources can be a powerful motivator for physicians to address gaps in their practices and therefore fulfill their professional responsibilities to remain competent. Increasingly, assessment data is being adopted as a requirement in relicensure and maintenance of competence.[73,74]

As physicians grow in awareness of their learning needs, educational programs may be helpful to maintain and improve their clinical competence. In addition, some will benefit from formalized mentorship programs, particularly as they enter independent practice, are gaining new skills, or are remediating.[75–78] As Harrison et al.[76] note, mentorship may prevent or reduce active failures, be used to identify patient safety threats in the local working environment, and encourage a healthier safety culture.

Similarly, coaching has been advocated as another way physicians can improve their work and identity as physicians.[79–81] Helping physicians to identify and seek out role models is also important. By seeking out role models and observing them, the cognitive and behavioral processes associated with successfully internalizing roles (e.g., the good doctor–medical educator) begin to be embodied[82] and become part of professional identity.

Group CPD

Drawing on educational theory, particularly theories that suggest new approaches to support physicians in their alignment with the values of the profession can be helpful in conceptualizing how collective activities can support the development of professional identity. In this, we draw on three related theories and conceptual frameworks that seem particularly relevant: social constructivism, communities of practice, and transformational learning. Collectively, these theories provide support for continuous group learning. Social constructivism theory implies that groups construct knowledge for one another; individuals in a group work collaboratively to create common understanding and shared meanings. This theory predicts that (simply) providing opportunities for physicians to congregate to share their practice experiences can be a significant learning opportunity.[83] As noted earlier, communities of practice are groups of people who share a concern or a passion for something they do and learn how to do it better as they interact regularly, and they are a robust method of constructing and further developing personal identity in the context of a community.[84] Last, transformative learning theory emphasizes individual meaning making, in which practitioners become aware through life challenges of the need to question themselves and their common assumptions. Adults move in and out of their social practices as they grow older and as their professional identity grows. There are natural tensions and conflicts that develop in the process of meaning making that can be mitigated by joining a longitudinal practice-based group.

Several approaches seem particularly useful in supporting the continuous development of identity. For example, the Balint group model within Family Medicine is an excellent example of the application to practice of all three of these frameworks for learning.[85] More than fifty years old, it has adherents in many European countries and in North America.

Balint groups meet regularly (often monthly) and sometimes over a physician's entire career. Case presentations, drawn by group members from their practices and supplemented by group discussion, focus on enabling physicians to be more psychologically aware of the emotional content of the doctor-patient relationship. The longitudinal nature of the group meetings enables the professional identity of these physicians to be continually reviewed and incrementally adjusted over time. Similarly, practice-based small group (PBSG) learning, popularized by the College of Family Physicians of Canada but adopted internationally, offers another example whereby small groups of family physicians meet on a monthly basis. In PBSG groups, the physicians begin with a discussion of challenging clinical cases, supported by evidence-based clinical modules and guided by trained peer facilitators.[86] Other examples of communities of practice in CPD include study groups within specific medical disciplines that emerge either formally connected with a medical school or form spontaneously for continuous learning in community and rural practices.[87] Through regular meetings, the physicians form a professional identity within the "community" along with shared approaches to clinical practice.

While groups often meet face to face, medical communities of practice can also function online, where the learning experience can occur widely across disciplines and include every aspect of medical practice and are longitudinal and available 24/7. Ongoing social professional networks develop that can take advantage of many aspects of learning that an online environment can uniquely deliver interprofessionally. Longitudinal online environments can enrich communities of practice because they transcend the "learn first/transfer later" binary that is embedded in face-to-face CPD.[88]

The role that group teaching and traditional CPD plays in professional identity is less clear. Traditional conferences, courses, and other large-group events have come under scrutiny and their effectiveness has been questioned.[89,90] While large-group events may change knowledge and validate current practices, the impact on practice and clinical skills is often limited.[89,90] As CPD becomes increasingly evidence based, there is a recognition that CPD that is interactive, practice based, and longitudinal will pay greater dividends.[89,90] Hand in hand with changes in format, there has been an increased recognition that education funded through pharmaceutical company sponsorship, with its inherent potential for bias, presents a professionalism challenge for CPD providers, sets up conflicts of interest within and between physicians, and erodes public trust in physicians.[91,92]

To overcome the challenges inherent in large-group learning and the need to develop educational programs based around clinical need that provide physicians with quality data, several approaches have been taken to improve the uptake and potential of these programs to help physicians practice safely and appropriately within the contexts of their specialty. It is becoming more common for CPD providers to partner with patient safety or quality assurance groups to provide effective CPD. For example, in North America, the AAMCs Ae4Q, Aligning and Educating for Quality Initiative program, supports the alignment of data sources (financial, quality, referral, utilization, patient-centered-outcomes research, and other data) with educational programming to improve the quality of patient care.[93] Similarly, CPD providers are increasingly incorporating quality improvement methodology into traditional CPD activities.[94] This serves to both improve the quality of educational offerings and ensure that those reached by the programs are encouraged to identify with and adopt practices and behaviors consistent with contemporary medical practice. Large national meetings provide networking breakfasts and lunches, "hot" topics, and workshop and practical sessions as ways to make programming more relevant at an individual level as well as conveying appropriate approaches. Enabling physicians to connect to national meetings via synchronous and asynchronous Internet also helps physicians recognize the changes occurring in practice and may stimulate physicians' needs for further inquiry and study to ensure that their work is aligned with professional expectations.

Closer to the physician's practice base, rounds are a proven way for groups of physicians working within an institution or group of institutions to get together on a weekly basis. Morbidity and mortality rounds are common in the surgical and medical specialties and provide a model and framework for a limited group of professionals to systematically review challenging, complex patients and, at times, their unexpected outcomes. Medical-error rounds provide a similar opportunity for review and reflection on medical practice with resultant prescription for changes in everyday processes and procedures. General "weekly" or "monthly" rounds are increasingly being enhanced by clinical audit data or by evidence-based data such as Clinical Care Pathways that provide a framework for evidence-based interprofesional practice. Clinical Care Pathways have been found to reduce the rate of in-hospital complications, improve documentation, and maintain hospital efficiencies.[95] By getting together regularly, physicians can calibrate their own practices, have their values and beliefs challenged, and reaffirm their alignment with the profession and its expectations.

Certainly CPD providers must continue to examine their development work and see how they can draw on innovations in the field to improve care and ensure that physician performance is optimal. Recently, the American Board of Internal Medicine's *Choosing Wisely* program, which focuses on educating patients about unnecessary tests, treatments, and procedures, cosponsored a *Teaching Value and Choosing Wisely Competition* and elicited 70 "best ideas" for reducing healthcare costs and inefficiencies from front-line physicians.[96] CPD planners have a role in partnering with this type of campaign to support the content delivery, advise about the best methods to deliver the patient education, and cosponsor healthcare resource competitions in order to provide physicians with incentives and reinforce the fact that they are working within a community of practice that includes themselves, the patients, other healthcare professionals, and systems.

Lessons learned

The body of literature reviewed and analyzed for this chapter identified a number of aspects of physician professional identity, which occurs at two levels: the individual level, which involves the psychological and professional development of the person, and the collective level, which involves a socialization of the person into appropriate roles and forms of participation within the community and its work. It is clear that physicians grow in conjunction with career transitions, new career opportunities, and other phenomena related to geography and specialty. These changes are affected by and interact with the changes and identity formation that occurs in conjunction with the adult life cycle and other phenomena (e.g., gender). Through this, professional identity is shaped.

Physicians will describe their identity in many ways. For some, it will be related to their specialty (e.g., cardiologist), concurrent roles (e,g., physician researcher or medical scientist), geographic location (e.g., rural family physician), family roles (e.g., physician and mother), and current and past roles (e.g., president of medical staff, retired physician). In some cases, the roles are well integrated and fluid. In other cases, there is a hierarchy of roles or a compartmentalization of roles.

Identity within the profession is critical because it helps ensure and maintain alignment with the professional values, beliefs, and practices inherent in being a physician. It can be relatively easy for some physicians entering groups that are well established and inclusive. Others will be challenged by poorly developed and nonsupportive institutional structures. CPD can play a role; however, one must recognize that CPD is a broad term that encompasses any and all activities that physicians use to validate performance, to improve, and to change. Further, CPD operates at both the individual level and the group level. At the individual level, it provides feedback about performance, helps the physician get the necessary knowledge and skill, and guides the physician through mentorship and role modeling. At the group level, CPD enables the physicians to have formal and informal opportunities to gain skills in social settings, verify practices, and regularly and frequently interact with a group of physicians.

Effective CPD must recognize that programming and activities need to be provided both to support the individual's specific learning needs and to ensure that physicians have a "home" or "community of practice" in which they can safely learn, exchange ideas, receive feedback, and develop their identities as competent and safe practitioners. Individuals and their professional and regulatory organizations must all assume responsibility for physician learning and change to support patient care.

Future directions

There has been relatively little attention paid to how physicians maintain and change their professional identity over the course of a career. Work in the area of transitions through medical careers helps delineate some of the challenges physicians face as they assume new roles. Further, the general literature on the psychology of adulthood also illuminates the natural trajectory of life. There appear to be other important factors, such as specialty, geography, clinical setting, gender, and family, that interact with and affect professional identity. It will be important to encourage research that specifically asks physicians about their perceptions of professional identity, how it is sustained, and how it changes over the course of a career.

While it appears that colleagues, friends, mentors, and the organization itself influence professional identity, the current investment in CPD by individuals, industry, physician employers, and professional societies make it imperative to discern the roles that CPD can play. It is recognized that CPD plays many roles in physician competence and also that it can be variable in its effectiveness. A clearer understanding of how CPD influences professional identity over the span of a physician's career would be useful in enhancing educational programs and facilitating informal and formal communities of practice.

Conclusion

This chapter began by presenting two physicians, Mary and John. Mary had recently left a well-established family medicine practice and joined a subspecialty group, to gain more control over her clinical work and thus free up time to meet family obligations. John was feeling the pressure that his newly gained professorial rank had given him while trying to balance clinical, research, and service obligations. The two cases set the stage for exploring the literature on professional identity, recognizing that considerations of professional identity formation are situated within a broader context of adult development and related phenomena including gender, specialty, and geography, and operate at both the individual and the collective level. Transitions provide a useful way to examine professional identity because they describe periods of intense learning resulting in a transformation of identity. Continuing professional development in its broadest sense can help physicians form, maintain, and make changes in their identity, but attention needs to be paid to the quality of these activities to ensure they are embracing physicians in safe and competent practice within the healthcare system.

References

1. Cruess, RL, Cruess, SR, Boudreau, JD, Snell, L, Steinert, Y. Reframing medical education to support professional identity formation. *Acad Med.* 2014; **89**(11):1446–51.

2. Jarvis-Selinger, S, Pratt, DD, Regehr, G. Competency is not enough: integrating identity formation into the medical education discourse. *Acad Med.* 2012; **87**(9):1185–90.

3. Sabel, E, Archer, J; Early Careers Working Group at the Academy of Medical Educators. "Medical education is the ugly duckling of the medical world" and other challenges to medical educators' identity construction: a qualitative study. *Acad Med.* 2014; **89**(11):1471–80.

4. Frost, HD, Regehr, G. "I am a doctor": negotiating the discourses of standardization and diversity in professional identity construction. *Acad Med.* 2013; **88**(10):1570–77.

5. Erikson, EH. *The Life Cycle Completed.* New York, NY: WW Norton; 1997.

6. Vaillant, GE. *Triumphs of Experience: The Men of the Harvard Grant Study.* Cambridge, MA: Harvard University Press; 2012.

7. Vaillant, GE. Mental health. *Am J Psychiatry.* 2003; **160**(8):1373–84.

8. Levinson, DJ, Darrow, CN, Klein, EV, Levinson, MH, McKee, B. *The Seasons of a Man's Life.* New York, NY: Knopf; 1978.

9. Levinson, DJ, Levinson, JD. *The Seasons of a Woman's Life.* New York, NY: Knopf; 1996.

10. Kittrell, D. A comparison of the evolution of men's and women's dreams in Daniel Levinson's theory of adult development. *J Adult Dev.* 1998; **5**(2):105–15.

11. Kohlberg, L. *The Psychology of Moral Development: The Nature and Validity of Moral Stages (Essays on Moral Development, Volume 2).* San Francisco, CA: Harper and Row; 1984.

12. Gilligan, C. *In a Different Voice: Psychological Theory and Women's Development.* Cambridge, MA: Harvard University Press; 1982.

13. Held, V. *The Ethics of Care: Personal, Political, and Global.* Oxford, UK: Oxford University Press; 2006.

14. Eagly, AH, Wood, W. The nature-nurture debates: 25 years of challenges in understanding the psychology of gender. *Perspect Psychol Sci.* 2013; **8**(3):340–57.

15. Zell, E, Krizan, Z, Teeter, SR. Evaluating gender similarities and differences using metasynthesis. *Am Psychol.* 2015; **70**(1):10–20.

16. Shrier, DK, Zucker, AN, Mercurio, AE, Landry, LJ, Rich, M, Shrier, LA. Generation to generation: discrimination and harassment experiences of physician mothers and their physician daughters. *J Womens Health (Larchmt).* 2007; **16**(6):883–94.

17. Eagly, AH, Carli, LL. *Through the Labyrinth: The Truth About How Women Become Leaders.* Boston, MA: Harvard Business Review Press; 2007.

18. Eagly, AH, Carli, LL. Women and the labyrinth of leadership. *Harv Bus Rev.* 2007; **85**(9):62–71.

19. Hays, S. *The Cultural Contradictions of Motherhood.* New Haven, CT: Yale University Press; 1996.

20. Dillaway, H, Paré, E. Locating mothers: how cultural debates about stay-at-home versus working mothers define women and home. *J Fam Issues.* 2008; **29**(4):437–64.

21. Teunissen, PW, Westerman, M. Opportunity or threat: the ambiguity of the consequences of transitions in medical education. *Med Educ.* 2011; **45**(1):51–59.

22. Kilminster, S, Zukas, M, Quinton, N, Roberts, T. Learning practice? Exploring the links between transitions and medical practice. *J Health Organ Manag.* 2010; **24**(6):556–70.

23. Wilkie, G, Raffaelli, D. In at the deep end: making the transition from SpR to consultant. *Adv Psychiatr Treat.* 2005; **11**:107–14.

24. Lave, J, Wenger, E. *Situated Learning: Legitimate Peripheral Participation.* Cambridge, UK: Cambridge University Press; 1991.

25. Bennett, NL, Hotvedt, MO. Stage of career. In Fox, RD, Mazmanian, PE, Putnam, RW, eds. *Changing and Learning in the Lives of Physicians.* New York, NY: Praeger; 1989:65–77.

26. Westerman, M, Teunissen, PW, van der Vleuten, CP, Scherpbier, AJ, Siegert, CE, van der Lee, N, Scheele, F. Understanding the transition from resident to attending physician: a transdisciplinary, qualitative study. *Acad Med.* 2010; **85**(12):1914–19.

27. McKinstry, B, Macnicol, M, Elliot, K, Macpherson, S. The transition from learner to provider/teacher: the learning needs of new orthopaedic consultants. *BMC Med Educ.* 2005; **5**(1):17.

28. Brown, JM, Ryland, I, Shaw, NJ, Graham, DR. Working as a newly appointed consultant: a study into the transition from specialist registrar. *Br J Hosp Med (Lond).* 2009; **70**(7):410–14.

29. Beckett, M, Hulbert, D, Brown, R. The new consultant survey 2005. *Emerg Med J.* 2006; **23**(6):461–63.

30. Higgins, R, Gallen, D, Whiteman, S. Meeting the non-clinical education and training needs of new consultants. *Postgrad Med J.* 2005; **81**:519–23.

31. Lockyer, J, Silver, I, Oswald, A, Bullock, G, Campbell, C, Frank, JR, Taber, S, Wilson, J, Harris, KA. The continuum of medical education. In Harris, KA, Frank, JR, eds. *Competence by Design: Reshaping Canadian Medical Education.* Ottawa, ON: Royal College of Physicians and Surgeons of Canada; 2014:135–37. [Accessed March 5, 2015.] Available from www.royalcollege.ca/portal/page/portal/rc/advocacy/educational_initiatives/competence_by_design.

32. Loh, E. How and why doctors transition from clinical practice to senior hospital management: a case research study from Victoria, Australia. *The International Journal of Clinical Leadership.* 2013; **17**(4):235–44.

33. Lockyer, J, Hofmeister, M, Crutcher, R, Klein, D, Fidler, H. International medical graduates: learning for practice in Alberta, Canada. *J Contin Educ Health Prof.* 2007; **27**(3):157–63.

34. McLean, M, McKimm, J, Major, S. Medical educators working abroad: a pilot study of educators' experiences in the Middle East. *Med Teach.* 2014; **36**(9):757–64.

35. Lockyer, J, Wycliffe-Jones, K, Raman, M, Sandhu, A, Fidler, H. Moving into medical practice in a new community: the transition experience. *J Contin Educ Health Prof.* 2011; **31**(3):151–56.

36. O'Sullivan, PS, Irby, DM. Identity formation of occasional faculty developers in medical education: a qualitative study. *Acad Med.* 2014; **89**(11):1467–73.

37. Frugé, E, Margolin, J, Horton, T, Venkateswaran, L, Lee, D, Yee, DL, Mahoney, D. Defining and managing career challenges for mid-career and senior stage pediatric hematologist/oncologists. *Pediatr Blood Cancer.* 2010; **55**(6):1180–84.

38. Choudhry, NK, Fletcher, RH, Soumerai, SB. Systematic review: the relationship between clinical experience and quality of health care. *Ann Intern Med.* 2005; **142**(4):260–73.

39. Durning, SJ, Artino, AR, Holmboe, E, Beckman, TJ, van der Vleuten, C, Schuwirth, L. Aging and cognitive performance: challenges and implications for physicians practicing in the 21st century. *J Contin Educ Health Prof.* 2010; **30**(3):153–60.

40. Goldberg, R, Thomas, H, Penner, L. Issues of concern to emergency physicians in pre-retirement years: a survey. *J Emerg Med.* 2011; **40**(6):706–13.

41. Hickey, GL, Grant, SW, Freemantle, N, Cunningham, D, Munsch, CM, Livesey, SA, Roxburgh, J, Buchan, I, Bridgewater, B. Surgeon length of service and risk-adjusted outcomes: linked observational analysis of the UK National Adult Cardiac Surgery Audit Registry and General Medical Council Register. *J R Soc Med.* 2014; **107**(9):355–64.

42. Tessler, MJ, Shrier, I, Steele, RJ. Association between anesthesiologist age and litigation. *Anesthesiology.* 2012; **116**(3):574–79.

43. Moss, AJ, Greenberg, H, Dwyer, EM, Klein, H, Ryan, D, Francis, C, Marcus, F, Eberly, S, Benhorin, J, Bodenheimer, M, Brown, M, Case, R, Gillespie, J, Goldstein, R, Haigney, M, Krone, R, Lichstein, E, Locati, E, Oakes, D, Thomsen, PE, Zareba, W. Senior academic physicians and retirement considerations. *Prog Cardiovasc Dis.* 2013; **55**(6):611–15.

44. Byles, J, Tavener, M, Robinson, I, Parkinson, L, Smith, PW, Stevenson, D, Leigh, L, Curryer, C. Transforming retirement: new definitions of life after work. *J Women Aging.* 2013; **25**(1):24–44.

45. Barnett, RC, Hyde, JS. Women, men, work, and family. An expansionist theory. *Am Psychol.* 2001; **56**(10):781–96.

46. Buddeberg-Fischer, B, Stamm, M, Buddeberg, C, Bauer, G, Hämmig, O, Knecht, M, Klaghofer, R. The impact of gender and parenthood on physicians'

careers – professional and personal situation seven years after graduation. *BMC Health Serv Res.* 2010; **10**:40.

47. Cassel, CK, Neugarten, BL. A forecast of women's health and longevity. Implications for an aging America. *West J Med.* 1988; **149**(6):712–17.

48. Cook, DJ, Griffith, LE, Cohen, M, Guyatt, GH, O'Brien, B. Discrimination and abuse experienced by general internists in Canada. *J Gen Intern Med.* 1995; **10**(10):565–72.

49. Hicks, MH. "What are you?" A recurring question in a cross-cultural psychiatrist's life and career. *Transcult Psychiatry.* 2011; **48**(1–2):37–52.

50. Symonds, A. Emotional conflicts of the career woman: women in medicine. *Am J Psychoanal.* 1983; **43**(1):21–37.

51. Mansh, M, Garcia, G, Lunn, MR. From patients to providers: changing the culture in medicine toward sexual and gender minorities. *Acad Med.* 2015; **90**(5):574–80.

52. Risdon, C, Cook, D, Willms, D. Gay and lesbian physicians in training: a qualitative study. *CMAJ.* 2000; **162**(3):331–34.

53. Molleman, E, Broekhuis, M, Stoffels, R, Jaspers, F. Consequences of participating in multidisciplinary medical team meetings for surgical, nonsurgical, and supporting specialties. *Med Care Res Rev.* 2010; **67**(2):173–93.

54. Molleman, E, Rink, F. Professional identity formation amongst medical specialists. *Med Teach.* 2013; **35**(10):875–76.

55. Wright, B, Lockyer, J, Fidler, H, Hofmeister, M. Roles and responsibilities of family physicians on geriatric health care teams: health care team members' perspectives. *Can Fam Physician.* 2007; **53**(11):1954–55.

56. Magrane, D, Khan, O, Pigeon, Y, Leadley, J, Grigsby, RK. Learning about teams by participating in teams. *Acad Med.* 2010; **85**(8):1303–11.

57. Bogetz, AL, Bogetz, JF. An evolving identity: how chronic care is transforming what it means to be a physician. *Acad Psychiatry.* May 9, 2014. ['Online First': DOI 10.1007/s40596-014-0141-8]

58. Keshet, Y. Dual embedded agency: physicians implement integrative medicine in health-care organizations. *Health (London).* 2013; **17**(6):605–21.

59. Aase, M, Nordrehaug, JE, Malterud, K. "If you cannot tolerate that risk, you should never become a physician": a qualitative study about existential experiences among physicians. *J Med Ethics.* 2008; **34**(11):767–71.

60. Khan, L, Wong, R, Li, M, Zimmermann, C, Lo, C, Gagliese, L, Rodin, G. Maintaining the will to live of patients with advanced cancer. *Cancer J.* 2010; **16**(5):524–31.

61. Lingard, L, Reznick, R, DeVito, I, Espin, S. Forming professional identities on the health care team: discursive constructions of the "other" in the operating room. *Med Educ.* 2002; **36**(8):728–34.

62. Boss, RD, Geller, G, Donohue, PK. Conflicts in learning to care for critically ill newborns: "it makes me question my own morals." *J Bioeth Inq.* 2015; **12**(3):437–48.

63. Jin, CJ, Martimianakis, MA, Kitto, S, Moulton, CA. Pressures to "measure up" in surgery: managing your image and managing your patient. *Ann Surg.* 2012; **256**(6):989–93.

64. Gendron, TL, Myers, BJ, Pelco, LE, Welleford, EA. Promoting the development of professional identity of gerontologists: an academic/experiential learning model. *Gerontol Geriatr Educ.* 2013; **34**(2):176–96.

65. Krueger, G, Canellos, G. Where does hematology end and oncology begin? Questions of professional boundaries and medical authority. *J Clin Oncol.* 2006; **24**(16):2583–88.

66. Beaulieu, MD, Rioux, M, Rocher, G, Samson, L, Boucher, L. Family practice: professional identity in transition. A case study of family medicine in Canada. *Soc Sci Med.* 2008; **67**(7):1153–63.

67. McKinstry, B, Macnicol, M, Elliott, K, Macpherson, S. The transition from learner to provider/teacher: the learning needs of new orthopaedic consultants. *BMC Med Educ.* 2005; **5**(1):17.

68. Curran, V, Hollett, A, Hann, S, Bradbury, C. A qualitative study of the international medical graduate and the orientation process. *Can J Rural Med.* 2008; **13**(4):163–69.

69. American Medical Association. H-300.988 – *Restoring Integrity to Continuing Medical Education.* [Accessed March 2, 2015.] Available from www.ama-assn.org/ssl3/ecomm/PolicyFinderForm.pl?site=www.ama-assn.org&uri=/resources/html/PolicyFinder/policyfiles/HnE/H-300.988.HTM.

70. Eva, KW, Regehr, G. "I'll never play professional football" and other fallacies of self-assessment. *J Contin Educ Health Prof.* 2008; **28**(1):14–19.

71. Eva, KW, Regehr, G. Effective feedback for maintenance of competence: from data delivery to trusting dialogues. *CMAJ.* 2013; **185**(6):463–64.

72. Silver, I, Campbell, C, Marlow, B, Sargeant, J. Self-assessment and continuing professional development: the Canadian perspective. *J Contin Educ Health Prof.* 2008; **28**(1):25–31.

73. Campbell, CM, Parboosingh, J. The Royal College experience and plans for the maintenance of certification program. *J Contin Educ Health Prof.* 2013; **33** Suppl 1:S36–S47.

74. Holmboe, ES. Maintenance of certification, revalidation, and professional self-regulation. *J Contin Educ Health Prof.* 2013; 33 Suppl 1:S63–S66.

75. Shollen, SL, Bland, CJ, Center, BA, Finstad, DA, Taylor, AL. Relating mentor type and mentoring behaviors to academic medicine faculty satisfaction and productivity at one medical school. *Acad Med.* 2014; **89**(9):1267–75.

76. Harrison, R, Anderson, J, Laloë, PA, Santillo, M, Lawton, R, Wright, J. Mentorship for newly appointed consultants: what makes it work? *Postgrad Med J.* 2014; **90**(1066):439–45.

77. Harrison, R, McClean, S, Lawton, R, Wright, J, Kay, C. Mentorship for newly appointed physicians: a strategy for enhancing patient safety? *J Patient Saf.* 2014; **10**(3):159–67.

78. Ontario College of Family Physicians. *The Centre of Excellence and Innovations in Mentoring and Coaching: The OCFP's Collaborative Care CME/CPD Networks.* Toronto, ON: OCFP. [Accessed Jan. 31, 2015.] Available from http://ocfp.on.ca/docs/publications/the-centre-of-excellence-and-innovation-in-mentoring-and-coach ing--the-ocfps-collaborative-care-cme-cpd-networks .pdf?sfvrsn=2.

79. Gazelle, G, Liebschutz, JM, Riess, H. Physician burnout: coaching a way out. *J Gen Intern Med.* 2015; **30**(4):508–13.

80. Slegers, AS, Gültuna, I, Aukes, JA, van Gorp, EJ, Blommers, FM, Niehof, SP, Bosman, J. Coaching reduced the radiation dose of pain physicians by half during interventional procedures. *Pain Pract.* 2015; **15**(5):400–06.

81. Chase, SM, Crabtree, BF, Stewart, EE, Nutting, PA, Miller, WL, Stange, KC, Jaén, CR. Coaching strategies for enhancing practice transformation. *Fam Pract.* 2015; **32**(1):75–81.

82. Kenny, NP, Mann, KV, MacLeod, H. Role modeling in physicians' professional formation: reconsidering an essential but untapped educational strategy. *Acad Med.* 2003; **78**(12):1203–10.

83. D'Eon, M, Overgaard, V, Harding, SR. Teaching as a social practice: implications for faculty development. *Adv Health Sci Educ Theory Pract.* 2000; **5**(2):151–62.

84. Wenger, E. *Communities of Practice: Learning, Meaning, and Identity.* Cambridge, UK: Cambridge University Press; 1998.

85. Roberts, M. Balint groups: a tool for personal and professional resilience. *Can Fam Physician.* 2012; **58**(3):245.

86. Armson, H, Wakefield, J. Expanding the horizons of practice-based small-group learning: what are we learning? *Educ Prim Care.* 2013; **24**(3):153–55.

87. Parboosingh, JT. Physician communities of practice: where learning and practice are inseparable. *J Contin Educ Health Prof.* 2002; **22**(4):230–36.

88. Singh, G, McPherson, M, Sandars, J. Continuing professional development through reflexive networks: disrupting online communities of practice. Paper presented at ProPEL International Conference: University of Stirling, UK; 2012.

89. Marinopoulos, SS, Dorman, T, Ratanawongsa, N, Wilson, LM, Ashar, BH, Magaziner, JL, Miller, RG, Thomas, PA, Prokopowicz, GP, Qayyum, R, Bass, EB. *Effectiveness of Continuing Medical Education. Evidence Report No. 149.* Agency for Healthcare Research and Quality: Rockville, MD; 2007. [Accessed March 5, 2015.] Available from www.ahrq.gov/clinic/ tp/cmetp.htm.

90. Forsetlund, L, Bjørndal, A, Rashidian, A, Jamtvedt, G, O'Brien, MA, Wolf, F, Davis, D, Odgaard-Jensen, J, Oxman, AD. Continuing education meetings and workshops: effects on professional practice and health care outcomes. *Cochrane Database Syst Rev.* 2009;(2): CD003030.

91. Steinman, MA, Landefeld, CS, Baron, RB. Industry support of CME–are we at the tipping point? *N Engl J Med.* 2012; **366**(12):1069–71.

92. Lo, B, Field, MJ, eds; Institute of Medicine (US) Committee on Conflict of Interest in Medical Research, Education, and Practice. *Conflict of Interest in Medical Research, Education, and Practice.* Washington, DC: National Academies Press; 2009.

93. Davis, NL, Davis, DA, Johnson, NM, Grichnik, KL, Headrick, LA, Pingleton, SK, Bower, E, Gibbs, R. Aligning academic continuing medical education with quality improvement: a model for the 21st century. *Acad Med.* 2013; **88**(10):1437–41.

94. Shojania, KG, Silver, I, Levinson, W. Continuing medical education and quality improvement: a match made in heaven? *Ann Intern Med.* 2012; **156**(4):305–08.

95. Rotter, T, Kinsman, L, James, E, Machotta, A, Gothe, H, Willis, J, Snow, P, Kugler, J. Clinical pathways: effects on professional practice, patient outcomes, length of stay and hospital costs. *Cochrane Database Syst Rev.* 2010;(3):CD006632.

96. Wolfson, D, Tucker, L. *Foundations Supporting Stewardship of Health Care Resources Through Medical Education and Training.* Bethesda, MD: Health Affairs Blog; 2014. [Accessed March 5, 2015.] Available from http://healthaffairs.org/blog/2014/01/22/foundations-supporting-stewardship-of-health-care-resources-through-medical-education-and-training/? cat=grantwatch.

Professionalism, professional identity, and licensing and accrediting bodies

Sir Donald Irvine

Introduction

Because self-regulation or physician-led regulation is a fundamental aspect of being a professional, it is important that those entering the medical profession understand the nature of this regulation, the organizations within medicine mandated to carry out these functions, and how regulation of the profession relates to them as individuals. For these reasons, material relating to the regulatory processes must be included as a part of educational programs designed to support the development of the identities of future physicians so that they may better understand their roles in the profession and in society. While this chapter emphasizes the current state of regulation in the English-speaking world, the trends outlined are found in most developed countries.

Every patient wants to be sure that they have a "good" doctor. No right-thinking person would knowingly choose a bad doctor or even one who they think is barely adequate. The public expects regulators, educators, and employers to provide them with good doctors, to make sure their doctors stay that way, and to act promptly to protect them when they do not. Professor Ron Paterson, former New Zealand Health and Disability Commissioner, said, "It is generally accepted that the vast majority of doctors are well-intentioned and practice safely. But good intentions and generally adequate care are not enough. As a member of the public, and as a potential patient, I want to know that I can rely on the public medical register as assurance that any listed doctor is competent."[1]

Medical regulation in its various forms – licensure, certification, and accreditation in particular – is the means through which the state is expected to make sure that the public is indeed served by doctors who are ethical and competent.[2] In some countries, the United States and British Commonwealth for example, the state has delegated part of its responsibility to

some medical organizations through self-regulation. Self-regulation is thus a privilege, granted by the state, that has to be earned and constantly justified. It is not the right that some doctors think it is.[3,4]

Medical professionalism has been defined as a set of values, behaviors, and relationships that underpin the public's trust in doctors.[5] It is the basis for the profession's "social contract" with the public.[6] Medical education is the principal (but not the only) means whereby professional values and standards are taught, learned, digested, internalized, and continuously refreshed throughout a doctor's career.[7] This is why the relationship among doctors' practice, their medical education, the way they are regulated, and their sense of professional identity is so fundamental.

The basic instrument of professional regulation is licensure. Licensing authorities are statutory bodies that exist to ensure that only people they consider to be properly qualified are allowed to practice medicine. Licenses are granted to new entrants who reach the standard required by the authority and may be restricted or withdrawn from those who do not subsequently maintain the standard. So a license to practice is restrictive – one cannot practice without it.

Certification marks the satisfactory completion of specialist training. Specialty-specific professional bodies such as specialty boards, medical royal colleges, and some professional societies decide the standards needed for entry to practice in their respective fields and the training necessary to achieve those standards. These specialty-specific standards complement the generic standards needed for licensure. Historically, certification has been indicative, that is to say highly desirable but – unlike licensure – not absolutely essential. Employers, insurers, and others may link certification to financial incentives and eligibility for institutional practicing privileges, but there is no automatic bar to practice without it. However,

Teaching Medical Professionalism, 2nd Edition, ed. Richard L. Cruess, Sylvia R. Cruess and Yvonne Steinert.
Published by Cambridge University Press. © Cambridge University Press 2016.

there is a tendency toward making certification more restrictive by linking it to licensure – as has happened already in the United Kingdom through revalidation.

Accreditation is the process whereby designated authorities approve the educational experience and standards of training offered by educational institutions.[8] The U.S. Accreditation Council for Graduate Medical Education (ACGME), which accredits postgraduate training, and the General Medical Council (GMC), which accredits basic medical education and specialist training in the United Kingdom, are examples.

Policy on professional regulation is broadly informed by the public's expectations and experiences of doctors. Describing the relationship between public policy and professional regulation, Klein said, "The aim of public policy is to make the medical profession collectively more accountable for its performance. The aim of professional self-regulation is to make individual practitioners more accountable to their peers. Control over the medical profession collectively is a complement to – not a substitute for – control by the medical profession of its members. The precise balance between the two will depend on the extent to which the medical profession demonstrates that it can be trusted to deliver its part of the bargain."[9]

In Western societies today, the historical notion of passive patient trust in doctors is giving way to the concept of active patient autonomy, empowered and driven as never before by the burgeoning revolution in information technology. With patient autonomy, the argument goes, it is the patient who has the illness and so it is the patient who is – or should be – the final arbiter of what is right for them. It is their body, their mind, their illness, and their life. People who think this way want to be sure that the doctors they consult today are indeed good doctors, fully up to date and fit to practice in their chosen field. Furthermore, some patients, if they choose to, may want to see the evidence confirming their doctor's status for themselves.[10,11] A more robust form of accountability to patients, as well as to peers and employers, enhanced by transparency, is therefore coming to medical practice.

Changing public expectations have potentially far-reaching consequences for professional practice, regulation, and education, and indeed for what it means to be a doctor in the early twenty-first century. The public's and patients' unquestioning trust can no longer be assumed; rather, in the future such trust will have to be continuously earned and justified, by every doctor, as an essential element of everyday medical practice.

Consequently, evolving a new order of professionalism to match this expectation will be critical, both to satisfy patients and to sustain high professional morale, because trust cannot be secured by regulation alone. The big question is whether the profession can summon the collective will to make this cultural change happen or whether, through indifference or outright resistance, it will find itself driven defensively and unhappily by outside forces.

The debate is now engaged and is at the heart of what one might call the politics of the new professionalism. This chapter, which draws particularly on experience in the United Kingdom and North America, considers developments that could lead to a good outcome for both patients and their doctors.

Through patients' eyes: the public expectations of a good doctor

For patients and their relatives, a good doctor is one whom they feel they can trust without having to think about it.[12] They equate "goodness" with clinical and ethical integrity, safety, up-to-date medical knowledge and diagnostic skill, sound judgment, and an ability to form a good relationship with them. For patients, good doctors are clinically expert yet know their limitations. They are honest, interested in their patients, listen to them, will put themselves out for them, and are kind, courteous, considerate, empathetic, respectful, and caring. They are good team players when teamwork is needed. All these attributes matter because patients know their doctors' advice and decisions can affect the outcome of their illness – even make the difference between life and death or between enjoying a speedy recovery and suffering serious disability.

There is ample evidence from patient surveys and focus groups to show that this picture is essentially accurate (e.g., Gerteis et al.,[13] Chisholm et al.,[14] and Coulter[15]). In 2006, the Picker Institute[16] reported the results of surveys across eight European countries to find which qualities patients and relatives looked for in intensive-care doctors. What mattered most to them were medical skill and experience, particularly clinical knowledge, decisiveness in decision-making, and the ability to act calmly in a crisis. Almost equally important were the abilities to exchange information, to communicate effectively, and to deal sensitively with anxious patients and relatives.

Similarly, a systematic review of nineteen studies on patients' priorities in general practice ranked "humaneness" in eighty-six percent of studies, "competence/accuracy" in sixty-four percent, "patient involvement in decisions" in sixty-three percent, and "time for care" in sixty percent.[17] In another study of patients attending the Mayo Clinic, researchers identified seven ideal physician behaviors: according to these patients, good physicians are confident, empathetic, humane, personal, forthright, respectful, and thorough.[18] And patients today want doctors to involve them, to the extent that patients themselves decide appropriate, in decisions about their care.[19,20]

Patients' experiences of doctors

It seems that, generally, patients' experience of their doctors matches their expectations, which is why in so many countries most patients trust their doctors.[21] That is good news. However, the medical profession's historical tolerance of poor practice is fast becoming unacceptable to the public. Professional institutions are trusted less because the public has become more aware of wide variations in doctors' performance, including the profession's toleration of obvious underperformance, which seems difficult and sometimes impossible to justify.

This variation in tolerance is well illustrated in the cluster of behaviors that fall loosely under the headings of communication and professionalism. In a recent study, the Commonwealth Fund has compared patient experience in five countries: the United Kingdom, Australia, Canada, New Zealand, and the United States.[22] The study was based on five examples – doctor-patient communication, involving patients in treatment decisions, giving clear goals and a treatment plan, explaining medication side effects, and giving patients access to their records. Most patients had a positive experience. However, a sizable minority of patients – significant in terms of the millions of people in a population who may be affected – did not experience such care.

Public expectations of professional regulation

In 2005, the UK government commissioned a major study of attitudes to medical regulation among the general public and doctors,[21] in particular the proposal to assess doctors' continuing fitness to practice through the proposed process of revalidation. Three-fifths of people surveyed knew nothing about the assessment of doctors. For them, the inner workings

of licensure and certification were taken on blind trust. Nevertheless, respondents had clear ideas about what aspects of a doctor's practice are important to them and which therefore should be assessed throughout a doctor's career. Nine in ten UK residents want their doctors to show that they have good clinical knowledge and technical skills and, equally, competence in the interpersonal aspects of care. About half wanted these checks done annually.

In Ontario, Canada, a 2006 survey of members of the public and doctors showed that ninety-three percent of public members and fifty-two percent of doctors said there must be regular clinical competence checks to maintain licensure.[23] Similarly, eighty-five percent of public members and forty-four percent of doctors thought that doctors must receive formal feedback from patients about their communication skills. The situation in the United States is similar, with a strong public (but far less certain medical) preference for mandatory knowledge-testing as part of the maintenance of certification.[24]

It is important to listen to what the public is saying. Despite the high levels of overall trust in the profession, patients today want to be sure that their doctors know what they are doing in a consultation. It is that certainty about current competence that is the foundation of a trusting relationship. The clear implication is that doctors who do not measure up must quickly remedy their deficiencies or stop practicing.

Doctors are deeply divided about these matters. Some are in tune with public thinking, but others are hostile, seeing the new forms of accountability as unnecessary, professionally demeaning, and, indeed, as an affront to their sense of identity as doctors.[25] These conflicting views are a huge challenge for professional leaders.

Evolving ideas about professionalism, professional identity, and professional regulation

Most people tend to use the generic word "professional" to describe a combination of strongly positive qualities and attributes including high technical performance, integrity, conscientiousness, commitment, dependability, altruism, and general excellence. In medicine, the earliest interpretations of professionalism were based on the possession of an exclusive body of knowledge held and accessed only by doctors, on doctors' autonomy, and on implicit values and standards of practice and education that were determined almost exclusively by doctors themselves.[3,4]

Abraham Flexner captured the internal ironies and tensions around medicine's unfolding status and self-image as a profession, which have influenced its behavior ever since.[26] He described how medicine simply assumed itself to be a profession. Practitioners who had undergone the necessary training, possessed a basic qualification in medicine, and secured licensure were therefore presumed to be professionals by both the medical community and the public. From that point on in doctors' careers, the particulars of their future practicing styles, their competence, their attitude to patients and colleagues, and their altruism and service ethic were deemed to be largely a matter for individual doctors to decide – after all, they were professionals.

Doctors liked this notion of professional autonomy because it carried with it connotations of trustworthiness, high public esteem, self-worth, self-determination, and self-respect, with no downside. They felt occupationally very secure. Doctors' commitment to near absolute autonomy goes far to explain why poor clinical practice was widely tolerated.

This doctor-centric view of professional identity was taken for granted by both doctors and the public until very recently.[27] It has been the received wisdom among the leaders of the medical schools, postgraduate organizations, colleges, professional associations, and regulatory bodies and has been in the profession's DNA that is passed on to new generations of doctors. The public were willing supporters, not least because they could see the benefits that were flowing from the wonderful new medical science and technology. The medical profession, it seemed, could be trusted to make sure that the public was always served by good doctors who put patients' interests first. The public's relatively uninformed and therefore uncritical endorsement of self-regulation prevailed despite some dissenting voices.[4,25]

Within the last twenty-five years, however, this traditional view of medical professionalism has attracted criticism from within and outside the profession. For example, it became clear that the energetic pursuit of scientific knowledge and skills, especially in academia, had diverted attention from the ethical and human dimensions of medical practice with detrimental effects on the quality of patients' experience.[3,11,21] More generally, as indicated earlier,

patients were more likely to want to take charge of their own lives, as evidenced, for example, by the rapidly evolving consumer's, women's, and civil rights movements in the Western world. These movements spearheaded societal change that emphasized the rights and entitlements of the individual and thus eschewed medical paternalism and patients' passive tolerance of indifferent practice.

In this climate, well-publicized medical disasters in the United Kingdom raised new questions about patient safety. There were questions about whether the profession had the stomach to deal effectively with poorly performing doctors or whether it would continue to give doctors rather than patients the benefit of the doubt.[12,28,29] Patients' trust in individual doctors remained strong in situations in which their personal experience was good. However, their hitherto unquestioning trust of the medical profession to regulate itself effectively began to be replaced by several demands: better protection from poorly performing doctors, more public involvement in regulation, more accountability, more transparency, concrete evidence of consistency of doctors' lifetime competence and performance, and less self-interested protectiveness.[12,29] In the future, trust in the collective profession would have to be evidence based whenever possible and founded on a "patient-centered" culture of medical practice, professional regulation, and medical education.

Doctors have a clear choice. They can accept the validity of the public's criticisms of their professionalism with good grace, adapt their ideas of professional identity and professionalism to meet society's evolving expectations, and so rebuild and reinforce the relationship of trust which both parties want. Or they can reject or ignore the criticisms, or give a grudging, minimalist response, in which event the inevitable consequence will be continuing loss of status and perceived trustworthiness as their wide discretionary clinical and professional privileges are further eroded by managerial control.

Thus far the profession has inclined to favor the former approach and so in several countries is going through the challenging process of moving from a doctor-centered to a patient-centered culture of professionalism, the so-called new professionalism.[30] The change is happening largely because of informal alliances between reforming doctors and progressive patient advocates and patients' organizations that together have sought to push things forward. The change is proving difficult, slow, and emotionally charged. Old habits die hard, not least because medicine is socially still an inward-looking, conservative profession. The present generation of medical students and new doctors, who are the future, will need to promote necessary change because it is the right thing to do. It is in their interests to help create a relationship with the public founded on a new order of trust.

New professionalism, new professional regulation

So what does the profession have to do to rebuild trust? To answer this, it is essential to go back to the public's starting point. As we have seen, when people become ill they expect their doctor to be up to date and to exhibit excellent professional behavior, however long he or she has been qualified. They will assume that the regulatory and medical educational organizations, along with employers, are geared to make sure this happens.

These assumptions, however, are not borne out by the facts. Historically, the mindset and organization of medical education have focused primarily on the selection and preparation of new entrants – making students into doctors and then doctors into specialists. The profession has taken this important phase of preparation very seriously, which is why by and large it has been thorough, rigorous, and effective. This high order of educational professionalism contrasts sharply with the permissive, arbitrary, "do-as-you-please" individualism and, dare one say, amateurism that have characterized the collective approach to the continuing professional development and maintenance of professional standards among career doctors.

Until very recently, the profession has been content to rely on doctors' personal conscience as the main guarantor of their continuing professionalism rather than to take the effective collective responsibility for individual physician performance that Klein[9] wrote about. Sir Robert Francis, in his report on the scandalous events at the United Kingdom's Stafford hospital, said in his opening remarks that the poor medical and nursing care he described would not have happened if doctors and nurses had observed their professional codes of practice conscientiously.[29] His conclusion has general relevance. The price of public trust in the future will be that all members of health professions take this responsibility seriously.

And indeed this is beginning to happen, as the professionalism of the career doctor moves toward the center of the frame, and regulators and employers adjust their sights accordingly. The change in focus sounds simple. In fact, as doctors are now discovering, it is having profound consequences for doctors' sense of professional identity, the governance of the profession particularly at the workplace, the practicing and learning environment, and the design of regulatory and educational processes.

Modernized medical regulation is one result of this change of focus. The new model seeks to be positively patient-centered. It is founded on values, standards, and competencies that should form the basis for doctors' continuing fitness to practice.[2,29,30] Regulation and education assume a new significance because together they become the primary instruments for defining, internalizing, and embedding standards into the professional culture, into the minds and actions of individual doctors, and into the design and operation of effective clinical governance at the workplace. The model embodies the principles of responsibility, accountability, transparency, and partnership with the public, as well as the traditional elements of medical knowledge and skill, ethical values, and service. It is proactive rather than reactive, designed to give continuous attention to professional development and quality improvement through the assessment of performance and, when possible, clinical and patient outcomes, as well as of competence. In this model, medical licensure and certification become more closely aligned to the wider framework of clinical governance, based on continuous quality improvement and quality assurance, at doctors' places of work.

Achieving clarity on professional responsibilities and standards: codes of professional practice

The Hippocratic Oath, formulated in the fourth century BC, is the best-known example in the public mind of a medical code. Amazingly, however, it was only in the last twenty years or so that the medical profession really began to focus on defining the essential principles of medical practice in a way that everyone – doctors and the public alike – could access, understand, and relate to, and to work out how these principles could be implemented wherever doctors practice.

The main driving force was the realization by some leaders of the profession that relying on an implicit understanding among doctors of what a good doctor is was no longer sufficient as the basis for professional practice. Indeed, doctors had difficulty in securing agreement among themselves about some pretty fundamental aspects of their work and so could not always explain themselves to the outside world. Communication, attitudes to relationships with patients, engaging patients in decisions about their care, attitudes to team working, standards of clinical competence and performance, medical audit, transparency, and whistleblowing are all examples of hot topics in regard to which consensus could not be assumed. There was a real crisis of identity. A mechanism for setting out common ground had to be found.

The function of a modern professional code is to describe the standards of knowledge, competence, skills, and conduct expected of those doctors who are licensed to practice.[2] Good codes are critical statements about professional identity – they tell everyone what the profession stands for. Deferring to professional autonomy, early versions of codes were commonly described as "advice" or "guidance," suggesting that they were discretionary rather than a set of rules, a kind of à la carte menu from which doctors could pick and choose – or indeed ignore – according to their personal preferences. However, the profession's regulators in the United Kingdom, the United States, and Canada decided that such a degree of permissiveness was no longer compatible with their objective of bringing a greater measure of consistency to the quality of personal medical practice.

In keeping with this understanding, in 2006 Sir Liam Donaldson, then Chief Medical Officer for England, described the characteristics of a modern professional code of practice for doctors as "a set of clear, unambiguous, and, where possible, assessable set of standards that relate closely to the work of a doctor which at the same time leaves scope for the appropriate exercise of clinical judgment."[31] It should be the vehicle for making sure that doctors know what is and is not expected of them. It should be a benchmark by which patients can test their expectations and judge their experiences and should ensure that all those who contract with doctors have a clear understanding of what they can expect. A code must be capable of being implemented if it was to be of any practical use.[2]

In 2006, the Picker Institute Europe reviewed the qualities of professional codes and standards for doctors used in licensure and certification.[32] Picker found that, although they have different emphases, each of these codes is underpinned by several common principles. These include providing technically good care and keeping up to date, involving patients in their care, and respecting patient autonomy, confidentiality, and consent. The position in the three countries is summarized below.

United Kingdom

Good Medical Practice (GMP) was launched in 1995. With it the GMC signaled that it wanted to replace the traditional doctor-centric culture with a more patient-centered culture of professionalism. Regarded by the GMC as describing "professionalism in action," the code was called "Good" because the GMC wanted everyone to know that it was looking toward optimal generic standards. It was written in plain English, in the second person, so that every licensed doctor would know that it was addressed to him or her personally.

The latest (fifth) edition of Good Medical Practice[33] is grounded on the original set of fundamental principles, Duties of a Doctor, which on one page tells every doctor licensed by the GMC how they are to conduct themselves (see Figure 14.1).

Accompanying this are some sixty generic standards, complemented in separate booklets by more detailed guidance on particular aspects of practice, for example, confidentiality. Good Medical Practice is underpinned by careful research on patients' expectations of doctors. It is the template for the specialty-specific versions now published by most of the UK medical royal colleges.

Good Medical Practice was designed to guide doctors in their everyday practice. It was first used by the GMC as the benchmark against which UK doctors' fitness to practice should be assessed when complaints are made against them. Today, it underpins licensure, certification, and revalidation. It is the foundation of all medical curricula in the United Kingdom.

Every year, on convocation day, the new doctors who have just graduated from Cambridge University stand to commit themselves publically to uphold Duties of a Doctor throughout their practicing lives. The students initiated this moving ceremony fifteen years ago. It would be good if other universities in the United Kingdom followed their example.

Patients must be able to trust doctors with their lives and health. To justify that trust, you must show respect for human life and make sure your practice meets the standards expected of you in four domains.

Knowledge, skills and performance
- Make the care of your patient your first concern.
- Provide a good standard of practice and care.
  - Keep your professional knowledge and skills up to date.
  - Recognise and work within the limits of your competence.

Safety and quality
- Take prompt action if you think that patient safety, dignity or comfort is being compromised.
- Protect and promote the health of patients and the public.

Communication, partnership and teamwork
- Treat patients as individuals and respect their dignity.
  - Treat patients politely and considerately.
  - Respect patients' right to confidentiality.
- Work in partnership with patients.
  - Listen to, and respond to, their concerns and preferences.
  - Give patients the information they want or need in a way they can understand.
  - Respect patients' right to reach decisions with you about their treatment and care.
  - Support patients in caring for themselves to improve and maintain their health.
- Work with colleagues in the ways that best serve patients' interests.

Maintaining trust
- Be honest and open and act with integrity.
- Never discriminate unfairly against patients or colleagues.
- Never abuse your patients' trust in you or the public's trust in the profession.

You are personally accountable for your professional practice and must always be prepared to justify your decisions and actions.

Figure 14.1. The duties of a doctor registered with the General Medical Council[33]

The licensing authorities in Australia[34] and New Zealand[35] have introduced their own versions of Good Medical Practice.

United States

In 2002, distinguished physicians, under the auspices of the ABIM Foundation, the American College of Physicians, and the European Federation of Internal Medicine, published the statement Medical Professionalism in the New Millennium: A Physician's Charter.[36] The Charter explains the underlying rationale, against the background of their heartfelt concern that the principles of medical professionalism were being eroded or even lost in today's managerially driven healthcare.

The authors described three core principles of professionalism, namely, the primacy of patient welfare, patient autonomy, and social justice. They then listed ten commitments that doctors have, including, for example, commitments to professional competence, honesty with patients, patient confidentiality, and maintaining appropriate relations with patients. The Physician's Charter has been seen as a very valuable reminder to doctors of the essentials of contemporary medical professionalism and their central relevance to modern medical practice, and in that sense has been widely appreciated. However, the Charter is a statement of a set of principles; unlike Good Medical Practice, it was not designed to be an operational code.

Perhaps recognizing this, in 2005, the U.S. Federation of State Medical Boards (FSMB) started informal consultations with other interested organizations to promote effective medical regulation. One result was the creation of the National Alliance for Physician Competence, charged with producing a U.S. version of Good Medical Practice. The various bodies responsible for educating, licensing, certifying, and credentialing U.S. doctors all recognized that they had no common language or framework for fulfilling their responsibilities in a consistent way, and that they needed one. GMP-USA was intended to present an agreed statement of professional responsibilities for both U.S. and Canadian doctors, for use in everyday practice. It was published online in 2009[37] but was not adopted by the constituting bodies because of unresolved differences among them about content and purpose. As an exercise in collective self-regulation, the attempt failed – a bridge too far. It seems that unresolved issues about professional identity and responsibility were the problem.

Meanwhile, in 1999, the U.S. Accreditation Council for Graduate Medical Education (ACGME) and the American Board of Medical Specialties (ABMS) together began the Outcome Project to define competencies that would be used in accrediting graduate medical programs.[38] This project identified six general competencies that are widely and successfully used in the United States and elsewhere today. The competencies are the following: professionalism; patient care and procedural skills; medical knowledge; practice-based learning and improvement; interpersonal and communication skills; and systems-based practice. The competencies have provided a durable framework for assessing practice at all levels.

Canada

In 2005, the Royal College of Physicians and Surgeons of Canada created their CanMEDS document around the competencies for training in patient-centered practice.[39] Although not a code of practice, it has nevertheless provided the basis for guiding and tracking doctors' participation in continuing medical education (CME) and in their professional development and is the basis for maintenance of certification by the College – Canadian MOC. A version of the CanMEDS framework is used by the College of Family Physicians of Canada, bringing consistency of purpose across all of Canadian medicine. Interestingly, the CanMEDS and ACGME competencies complement each other.

Holding doctors to account: maintenance of licensure and certification

Having a code of practice is the beginning. Making sure that all doctors observe it conscientiously throughout their active practicing lives is the critical next step. In many countries, professional bodies and employers encourage and support CME and continuing professional development (CPD). However, as with any voluntary undertakings, the uptake over the years has been patchy. For example, a study of twenty-four countries in the Western world has shown that at present, none have completely satisfactory arrangements for ensuring ongoing competence.[40] To try to achieve better results, regulators have therefore started to link the codes directly with evidence-based maintenance of licensure and certification. The three countries that led these developments offer somewhat different approaches.

United Kingdom: maintenance of licensure through revalidation

Revalidation was initially a professional initiative that acquired the backing of Parliament and the National Health Service (NHS). Support for it was strengthened by the recommendations of the three public inquiries mentioned earlier.[12,28,29] The law now requires all British doctors regularly to demonstrate to the GMC that they are currently up to date and fit to practice in their chosen field and are able to provide a good standard of patient care. The license to practice has therefore ceased to be limited to the recognition of a doctor's qualifications on graduation and the attainment of specialist certification at early moments in a doctor's career. Instead, it defines the current status of doctors' practice.[41,42]

Revalidation is the process supporting maintenance of licensure. Through revalidation, doctors must demonstrate their continuing compliance with the standards of Good Medical Practice. It is based on a portfolio of evidence covering CPD, quality improvement activity, significant events, feedback from colleagues and patients, and a summary of complaints and compliments. The updated portfolio is reviewed in an annual workplace appraisal. At the end of the five-year revalidation cycle, a legally designated Responsible Officer at the doctor's workplace submits a recommendation based on the summated results of both the evidence and appraisals. The Responsible Officer decides whether there is sufficient evidence to recommend revalidation. In situations in which there are concerns about a doctor's practice, the GMC will investigate and ultimately decide what to do through its established fitness to practice procedures.

Revalidation is still new. Three big questions remain unanswered. First, will the GMC settle eventually for an optimal standard of practice or accept something less? Second, will the evidence of performance offered by doctors be sufficiently robust to demonstrate compliance convincingly? And third, will the processes for assessing and judging the evidence be equally robust in demonstrating continuing compliance? The answers to these questions should become clearer from the evaluation of the first revalidation cycle.

Incidentally, following the recommendation of the most recent public inquiry,[29] the UK Nursing and Midwifery Council (NMC) is piloting a revalidation scheme for nurses in 2015.[43]

United States: maintenance of certification – MOC

The American Board of Medical Specialties uses a common framework for professional development and assessment based on the ACGME competencies. Following a rigorous review of the existing program, new standards for ABMS Programs for MOC will be implemented in 2015.[44] Each of the twenty-four ABMS specialty boards has adopted the framework. There are four parts:

Part 1. Professionalism and professional standing – the doctor should hold a valid, unrestricted license to practice in a state in the United States, or in Canada. MOC Programs must incorporate professionalism learning and assessment activities.

Part 2. Life-long learning and self-assessment – the doctor should take part in educational and self-assessment programs that meet specialty-specific standards set by the Member Board;

Part 3. Assessment of knowledge, judgment, and skills – showing by the results of examination that the doctor has the necessary knowledge to provide quality care in his or her specialty.

Part 4. Improvement in medical practice – requiring physicians to engage in performance-in-practice assessment (at the individual or system level) with ongoing improvement activities.

To give some idea of performance in MOC, it is helpful to look at the American Board of Internal Medicine (ABIM) MOC requirements as an example. ABIM says that, as of October 2014, of more than 200,000 ABIM professionally active Board-Certified physicians, more than 150,000 are currently enrolled in MOC.[45] The minimum passing score set by ABIM is an absolute standard based on the examination content. Physician subject-matter experts determine how much of that content an examinee must get right to be deemed certified. On average, a physician must answer approximately sixty-five percent of items correctly to achieve a passing score. The Internal Medicine MOC first-taker pass rate in 2013 was seventy-eight percent.[46]

Diplomats in any specialty under the auspices of ABIM who do not pass the exam within the required period are not allowed to describe themselves as "Board Certified" in that discipline.

Maintenance of licensure

The Federation of State Medical Boards (FSMB) has adopted the principle of the maintenance of licensure (MOL) as a condition for license renewal.[47] Physicians will be expected to demonstrate their commitment to lifelong learning that is relevant to their area of practice and contributes to improved healthcare. In 2010, the FSMB's House of Delegates adopted a framework for putting MOL into action, but implementation is estimated to be still several years away. Meanwhile, there is an expectation that participation in MOC will be accepted as representing substantial compliance with MOL, while not a requirement for MOL.

Canada

The Royal College of Physicians and Surgeons of Canada has adopted MOC for Canadian specialists and the Canadian College of Family Medicine has done the same for family physicians. A new version of MOC, CanMEDS 2015 is about to come into use following a meticulous process of development and consultation.[48]

Completion of an RCPSC Fellowship, the mark of certification as a specialist, is dependent upon a physician's commitment to take part in MOC regularly. Fellows who choose not to honor this commitment lose their entitlement to the use of letters FRCP(C), on the grounds that they can no longer demonstrate that they are up to date and fit to practice. A form of collegial fellowship exists for those who are retired from practice but wish to retain their affiliation with the College and the ethical principles it stands for.

In 2006, the Federation of Medical Regulatory Authorities brought the thirteen Canadian jurisdictions together to agree to a set of principles for a Canadian revalidation process.[23] The authorities agreed that "all licensed physicians in Canada must participate in a recognized revalidation process in which they demonstrate their commitment to continued competent performance in a framework that is fair, relevant, inclusive, transferable and formative." Since then, participation in CPD has been adopted as a condition of continued licensure by most jurisdictions. Progress other than this has been slow.

The battle for hearts and minds

Securing agreement to some form of time-limited licensure and certification has been opposed on both sides of the Atlantic, especially when the question of mandated accountability for standards of practice was introduced. The UK and U.S. experiences illustrate the point.

The revalidation decision in 1998 divided the British medical profession. Much has been written about the frantic process of achieving implementation between 1998 and 2012. It is important to understand the nature of the resistance if progress is to be made. Readers wanting to better understand the arguments, and the passion behind them, will find two publications helpful. Sir Donald Irvine, GMC President when revalidation was first proposed, recorded the early argument in detail, and submitted this in 2003 as part of his witness statement to the public inquiry into the practice of a murderous family doctor, Harold Shipman.[49] The other is the report itself, written by a High Court Judge, Dame Janet Smith.[12]

Essentially, the loose coalition of reformers held together by the GMC was the key driver. The profession split between reformers – the GMC, medical royal colleges, and patients' organizations, who wanted a robust, evidence-based, national process with public participation and external scrutiny; and the conservative doctors, led by the British Medical Association (BMA), who wanted to do as little as possible. In particular, the conservatives objected to the linkage of individual performance review with licensure because of the implications for the continuing right to practice of doctors whose performance was an issue. As the battle swayed this way and that,

there was a dramatic intervention in 2004 when Dame Janet said in no uncertain terms that the adoption of watered-down assessments by doctors opposed to revalidation would not comply with the evaluation of practice required by the recently amended Medical Act governing medical practice, which the profession itself had asked for. It was largely as a result of her intervention that the form of revalidation in use today does comply with the law – just barely.

There are parallels in the U.S. experience. The implementation of MOC seemed to have been somewhat uncontentious, while it remained a strictly voluntary undertaking. However, some U.S. physicians are now expressing similar anxieties to their conservative British colleagues, primarily regarding any possible linkage between MOC and MOL, the very idea of MOL itself and in the potential use of MOC by employers, insurers, and other agencies as a lever to influence physicians' behavior and employment conditions. There are other concerns too, particularly, for example, about cost to the physician, the time taken from patients, and the relevance of some of the knowledge testing. Some U.S. physicians are just angry at now being held to account for their current practice. The strength of feeling may be gauged in the views expressed by the Association of American Physicians and Surgeons,[50] the recently formed pressure group Change Board Recertification,[51] and the debate at the time of writing provoked by two papers in the New England Journal of Medicine,[52,53] setting out both sides of the argument.

Lessons for the future

Across the Western world, the balance of power between the medical profession and the public is becoming more equal, more just, more right. We have learned that the change is unstoppable. Patient autonomy and all that it entails is here to stay. Achieving an optimal standard of practice and care from any doctor is the public's defining expectation.

In these circumstances, the medical profession has a choice. It can get a grip, be positive, take the opportunity to redefine its social contract with the public,[6] and paint a positive picture of how doctors see themselves and want to be seen by others, in the early twenty-first century. Or it can sulk, procrastinate, and do as little as possible in order to accommodate its weakest members, and watch the world outside make changes anyway.

In reality, the profession cannot go forward until it is prepared to acknowledge, confront, and deal with the elephant in the room, namely, the deep-seated belief among some doctors that they are entitled, by virtue of who and what they are, to near-total professional autonomy. They will resist any threat to such autonomy. Yet, we have also learned that such autonomy is not compatible with the delivery of optimal medical care for all patients. Moreover, other doctors positively welcome a new relationship with the public and patients and are determined to see this extend to the whole profession. The medical profession is thus divided; it has a crisis of identity.

We have learned that steps must be taken to seek resolution. The most important are described below.

On being a doctor: identity and codes of practice

We have learned from the experience with the ABIM Charter and Good Medical Practice that statements like these are essential for describing and communicating our core values, standards, and responsibilities. They are the outward visible expression of our identity, our professionalism. However, we have also learned that fine words are pointless unless we intend to put principles into practice. Indeed, without such intent, and the means to act on such intent, they could be interpreted at best as wishful thinking, at worst as almost a fraud on the public by promising what cannot be delivered across the practicing profession.

Good Medical Practice is evolving as the main code of professional practice in the English-speaking world. For the public everywhere, the case for a single code is compelling – call it International Good Medical Practice.

Honoring the promise: MOC, MOL, and clinical governance

We have learned that the reactive, complaints-driven approach to licensure and certification is being replaced by a quality-assuring model able to tell the public that all licensed and certificated doctors are currently good doctors, because doctors who have fallen short will have forfeited their practicing license or specialist certification. This new order of rigor, enhanced by a new order of transparency, is what the public is coming to expect from competent medical regulators.

As regulators learn from each other, we should expect more convergence on the kind of evidence and assessment methods to be used.[54] For example, MOC is strong on the assessment of knowledge, whereas revalidation is not. Since knowledge is so important, the GMC needs to close this gap. On the other hand, revalidation is strong on the principle of workplace assessment, whereas MOC is just beginning to lean more in that direction, as evidenced, for example, by the discussions held recently at the Mayo Clinic by a group of high-performing, patient-centered U.S. hospitals.

As workplace clinical governance in health services everywhere becomes more patient centered and more sophisticated, and hospital boards insist on and support high performance from all their clinical staff, we should see both MOC and revalidation require rigorous formative and summative appraisal informed by high-quality data on doctors' competence and personal performance. We should anticipate that much of the ongoing assessment process should merge with everyday practice as data generated through the electronic patient record becomes the norm.

Against this background, it is possible to envisage the kind of evidence that might go into a doctor's MOC and revalidation portfolio in the future. For example, there would be evidence of clinical- and patient-reported outcomes, an assessment of knowledge relevant to the doctor's current practice, multisource feedback from colleagues illuminating clinical judgment and the ability to work in a team effectively, evidence of attitudes to patients and the ability to communicate well drawn from patient-experience data, and evidence of honesty and general trustworthiness.

And so we can foresee a time when a common code of practice informs a common approach to the assessment of continuing fitness to practice. For the citizens of those countries involved, accustomed as they are to moving freely from one country to another, having that kind of guarantee about the quality of their doctors, wherever the patient happens to be, would be a huge step forward.

Specialty standards: leadership by professional societies

Klein[9] reminded us that external control of the profession is a complement to, not a substitute for, control by the profession of its own members. The precise balance between the two will be determined by how successful the profession is at keeping its side of the bargain. This takes us directly to the role of medical colleges and societies. They are, or should be, the natural place to set expert clinical standards in their particular field of practice because it is within their membership that the necessary expertise lies. If not they, who else? The statutory generic regulators do not have the specialized knowledge to do so.

However, colleges and societies are membership organizations, with all that entails in terms of securing agreements based on the best evidence available. Robust leadership can be weakened or overturned. On the other hand, a leaderless group invites outside agencies to step in. The dual function illustrates the inherent tension between setting standards primarily in the public interest and being a quasi-trade union that puts members' interests first.

But it is possible. A good example can be seen in the Society for Cardiothoracic Surgery for Great Britain and Ireland (SCTS). This small society has become a model of how to set optimal standards of practice in cardiac surgery, by publishing the surgeon-specific mortality achieved by every British cardiac surgeon,[55,56] yet at the same time to manage controversial issues openly within the membership and to try and achieve consensus on some current clinical controversies.[57,58] Interestingly, the reaction of the British government and those managing the NHS has been one of immense relief, because the surgeons with the expertise have accepted responsibility for the clinical standards. The significance of this kind of development is that professional societies that fulfill this role successfully become the embodiment of collective professionalism at its best, in a way in which statutory regulators and managers never can.

Leading by example

Educating for the new professionalism is critical. There is one fundamental point at which leadership from the medical schools and postgraduate organizations could be transformative.

In the future, it will be essential that medical faculty members lead by example on professional values and standards. How powerful it would be if every clinical teacher shared their portfolio of evidence and the results of their MOC and revalidation appraisals with their students and junior faculty. What better way to be open about their own practice, and to let the learners see how they manage opportunities and difficulties when they arise?

We wait for the first medical school, with its teaching hospitals and primary care practices, to take such a lead.

Telling the public: engagement through transparency

Lastly, there is the matter of transparency, of letting the light shine on practice. Sir Bruce Keogh, a former British heart surgeon who is now medical director for NHS England, said this recently on launching an NHS website containing data on outcomes from 5,000 NHS surgeons (My NHS, part of NHS Choices): "Anyone who does an intervention on somebody else has a professional and moral responsibility to be able to describe what they do and defend how well they do it. That is the essence of professionalism."[59]

Transparency enables a new order of accountability.[60,61] There is a strong case for making both transparency and accountability explicit duties of a doctor in professional codes of practice.

Transparency is of the modern age. Imagine a world in which patients and employers could look up doctors' names on the regulator's register and on the website of the local hospital or doctors' office. They would learn about doctors' personal practice, what clinical results they achieve, what their patients and colleagues think about their experience with them, and other activities and achievements that seem to make them special. It does not matter whether all patients use the facility. The fact that the information exists, in a highly accessible form, could of itself transform doctors' ideas about personal accountability to patients and fellow clinical team members. Professor Ben Bridgewater, a British heart surgeon, gives a fine personal example.[62] Asked why he does this, he says: "I know everything of relevance about the patient sitting in front of me. Why shouldn't he (or she) know all about me?"

This order of transparency would enhance the quality of the doctor-patient relationship. It would help doctors compete on a reputation for quality of care and make patients' choice of doctor more meaningful.

Conclusion

The new professionalism, grounded firmly on the public's expectations of doctors, is fundamental to the safety and health of patients and the well-being of the medical profession. It is about striving always to do the right thing really well, because that is the right thing to do. Such professionalism offers doctors their best chance of maintaining high public trust in the future. Everybody wins. After all, everyone does want to be sure that they have a good doctor.

References

1. Paterson, R. Regulating doctors: finding the optimal balance between professionalism and self-regulation. In *Revalidation: The Way Ahead*. Publication of proceedings. International Revalidation Symposium: Contributing to the Evidence Base. London, UK: General Medical Council; 2010:3–7. [Accessed Dec. 29, 2014.] Available from www.gmc-uk.org/International_ Revalidation_Symposium_Publication_of_ proceedings.pdf_44014486.pdf.

2. Irvine, D. *Patients, their Doctors and the Politics of Medical Professionalism*. 29th John P. McGovern Award lecture. Oxford, UK: American Osler Society; 2014. [Accessed Dec. 29, 2014.] Available from http:// aosler.org/wp-content/uploads/2014/05/2014-McGov ern-Lecture-Booklet.pdf.

3. Irvine, D. The performance of doctors. I: professionalism and self regulation in a changing world. *BMJ*. 1997:314(7093):1540–42.

4. Freidson, E. *Professionalism Reborn: Theory, Prophecy and Policy*. Cambridge, UK: Polity Press; 1994.

5. Working Party of the Royal College of Physicians. Doctors in society. Medical professionalism in a changing world. *Clin Med*. 2005; 5(6 Suppl 1):S5–S40.

6. Cruess, SR. Professionalism and medicine's social contract with society. *Clin Orthop Relat Res*. 2006:449:170–76.

7. Cruess, RL, Cruess, SR, Johnston, SE. Professionalism: an ideal to be sustained. *Lancet*. 2000:356(9224): 156–59.

8. Lynch, DC, Leach, DC, Surdyk, PM. Assessing professionalism for accreditation. In Stern, DT, ed. *Measuring Medical Professionalism*. New York, NY: Oxford University Press; 2006:265–80.

9. Klein, R. *Regulating the Medical Profession: Doctors and the Public Interest. Healthcare 1997/1998*. London, UK: Kings Fund; 1998.

10. Williamson, C. *Towards the Emancipation of Patients; Patients' Experiences and the Patient Movement*. Bristol, UK: Policy Press; 2010.

11. Robinson, J. The price of deceit: the reflections of an advocate. In Rosenthal, MM, Mulcahy, L, Lloyd-Bostock, S, eds. *Medical Mishaps: Pieces of the Puzzle*. Buckingham, UK: Open University Press; 1999:246–56.

12. The Shipman Inquiry. Fifth report. *Safeguarding Patients: Lessons from the Past, Proposals for the Future*. Chairman Dame Janet Smith. London, UK: Stationery Office; 2004.

13. Gerteis, M, Edgman-Levitan, S, Daley, J, Delbanco, TL, eds. *Through the Patient's Eyes: Understanding and Promoting Patient-Centered Care*. San Francisco, CA: Jossey-Bass; 1993.

14. Chisholm, A, Cairncross, L, Askham, J. *Setting Standards: The Views of Members of the Public and Doctors on the Standards of Care and Practice They Expect of Doctors*. Oxford, UK: Picker Institute Europe; 2006. [Accessed Feb. 2, 2015.] Available from www .gmc-uk.org/Setting_Standards_Exec_Summary_Mar ch06.pdf_25416640.pdf.

15. Coulter, A. What do patients and the public want from primary care? *BMJ*. 2005; 331(7526):1199–1201.

16. Hasman, A, Graham, C, Reeves, R, Askham, J. *What Do Patients and Relatives See as Key Competencies for Intensive Care Doctors?* Oxford, UK: Picker Institute Europe; 2006. [Accessed Feb. 2, 2015.] Available from www.pickereurope.org/wp-content/uploads/2014/10/ What-do-patients-...-see-as-key-competencies....pdf.

17. Wensing, M, Jung, HP, Mainz, J, Olesen, F, Grol, R. A systematic review of the literature on patient priorities for general practice care. Part 1: description of the research domain. *Soc Sci Med*. 1998:47(10);1573–88.

18. Bendapudi, NM, Berry, LL, Frey, KA, Parish, JT, Rayburn, WL. Patients' perspectives on ideal physician behaviors. *Mayo Clin Proc*. 2006; 81(3):338–44.

19. Ellins, J, Coulter, A. *How Engaged Are People in Their Health Care? Findings of a National Telephone Survey*. Oxford, UK: Picker Institute Europe; 2005. [Accessed Feb. 2, 2015.] Available from www.pickereurope.org/ wp-content/uploads/2014/10/How-engaged-are-people-in-their-health-care-....pdf.

20. Coulter, A, Ellins, J. *Patient-Focused Interventions: A Review of the Evidence*. Oxford, UK: Picker Institute Europe; 2006. [Accessed Feb. 2, 2015.] Available from www.health.org.uk/sites/default/files/PatientFocused Interventions_ReviewOfTheEvidence.pdf.

21. IPSOS-MORI. *Attitudes to Medical Regulation and Revalidation of Doctors: Research among Doctors and the General Public*. London, UK: Department of Health; 2005. [Accessed Dec. 1, 2014]. Available from www.ipsos-mori.com/Assets/Docs/Archive/ Polls/doh.pdf.

22. Coulter, A. *Engaging Patients in Their Healthcare: How Is the UK Doing Relative to Other Countries?* Oxford, UK: Picker Institute Europe; 2006. [Accessed Dec. 29, 2014]. Available from www.pickereurope.org/wp-content/uploads/2014/10/Engaging-patients-in-their-healthcare-how-is-the-UK-doing....pdf.

23. College of Physicians and Surgeons of Ontario. *Revalidation Consultation Summary* 2006. Toronto, ON: CPSO; 2006. [Accessed Feb. 2, 2015.] Available

from www.cpso.on.ca/uploadedFiles/downloads/cpso documents/policies/RevalidationConsultSummary Apr06.pdf.

24. The Gallup Organization for the American Board of Internal Medicine. *Awareness of and Attitudes Toward Board-Certification of Physicians.* Princeton, NJ: The Gallup Organization; 2003.

25. Irvine, D. A short history of the General Medical Council. *Med Educ.* 2006; **40**(3):202–11.

26. Flexner, A. *Medical Education in the United States and Canada: A Report to the Carnegie Foundation for the Advancement of Teaching. Bulletin No. 4.* New York, NY: Carnegie Foundation; 1910.

27. Irvine, D, Hafferty, FW. Every patient should have a good doctor. In The Society for Cardiothoracic Surgery in Great Britain & Ireland; Dendrite Clinical Systems Ltd. *Maintaining Patients' Trust: Modern Medical Professionalism 2011.* Henley-on-Thames, UK: Dendrite Clinical Systems Ltd; 2011:64–73. [Accessed Dec. 29, 2014.] Available from www.scts.org/_user files/resources/634420268996790965_SCTS_Professio nalism_FINAL.pdf.

28. Bristol Royal Infirmary Inquiry. *Learning from Bristol: The Report of the Public Inquiry into Children's Heart Surgery at the Bristol Royal Infirmary 1984–1995.* London, UK: Stationery Office; 2001.

29. The Mid Staffordshire NHS Foundation Trust. *Report of the Mid Staffordshire NHS Foundation Trust Public Inquiry. Executive Summary & Volume 3: Present and Future Annexes.* Chaired by Sir Robert Francis. London, UK: Stationery Office; 2013. [Accessed Feb. 2, 2015.] Available from http://midstaffspublicinquiry.com.

30. Stacey, M. *Regulating British Medicine: The General Medical Council.* Chichester, UK: Wiley; 1992.

31. Donaldson, L. *Good Doctors, Safer Patients.* London, UK: Department of Health; 2006.

32. Chisholm, A, Askham, J. *A Review of Professional Codes and Standards for Doctors in the UK, USA and Canada.* Oxford, UK: Picker Institute Europe; 2006. [Accessed Feb. 2, 2015.] Available from www.picker europe.org/wp-content/uploads/2014/10/A-review-of-professional-codes-...-UK-USA-and-Canada.pdf.

33. General Medical Council. *Good Medical Practice.* Fifth edition. London, UK: GMC; 2013.

34. Australian Medical Council. *Good Medical Practice Australia – A Code of Conduct for Doctors in Australia.* Canberra, AU: Australian Medical Council; 2010. [Accessed Jan. 23, 2014.] Available from www.amc.org.au/about/good-medical-practice.

35. Medical Council of New Zealand. *Good Medical Practice New Zealand.* Wellington, NZ: MCNZ; 2013. [Accessed Jan. 23, 2014.] Available from www.mcnz.org.nz/assets/News-and-Publications/good-medical-practice.pdf.

36. ABIM Foundation, American Board of Internal Medicine; ACP-ASIM Foundation, American College of Physicians–American Society of Internal Medicine; European Federation of Internal Medicine. Medical professionalism in the new millennium: a physician charter. *Ann Intern Med.* 2002; **136**(3):243–46.

37. National Alliance for Physician Competence. *Guide to Good Medical Practice – USA.* Dallas, TX: National Alliance for Physician Competence; 2009. [Accessed Dec. 11, 2014.] Available from http://gmpusa.org.

38. Swing, SR. The ACGME outcome project: retrospective and prospective. *Med Teach.* 2007; **29**(7):648–54.

39. Frank, JR, ed. *The CanMEDS 2005 Physician Competency Framework. Better Standards. Better Physicians. Better Care.* Ottawa, ON: Royal College of Physicians and Surgeons of Canada; 2005. [Accessed Feb. 2, 2015.] Available from www.royalcollege.ca/portal/page/portal/rc/common/documents/canmeds/resources/publications/framework_full_e.pdf.

40. Allsop, J, Jones, K. *Quality Assurance in Medical Regulation in an International Context: Report for the Department of Health England.* London, UK: University of Lincoln; 2006.

41. General Medical Council. *The Good Medical Practice Framework for Appraisal and Revalidation.* London, UK: GMC; 2013. [Accessed Feb. 2, 2015.] Available from www.gmc-uk.org/The_Good_medical_practice_framewo rk_for_appraisal_and_revalidation___DC5707.pdf_56235089.pdf.

42. General Medical Council. *Revalidation: What You Need to Do.* London, UK: GMC; 2013. [Accessed Feb. 2, 2015.] Available from www.gmc-uk.org/Revalidation___What_you_need_to_do.pdf_54286567.pdf.

43. Nursing and Midwifery Council. *Revalidation Evidence Report.* London, UK: Nursing and Midwifery Council; 2014. [Accessed Feb. 2, 2015.] Available from www.nmc-uk.org/Documents/Consultations/2014/Revalidation-evidence-report.pdf.

44. American Board of Medical Specialties. *Standards for the ABMS Program for Maintenance of Certification (MOC).* Chicago, IL: American Board of Medical Specialties; 2014. [Accessed Feb. 2, 2015.] Available from www.abms.org/media/1109/standards-for-the-abms-program-for-moc-final.pdf.

45. Baron, RJ, Krumholz, HM, Jessup, M, Brosseau, JL. Board certification in internal medicine and cardiology: historical success and future challenges. *Trends Cardiovasc Med.* 2015; **25**(4):305–11.

46. Yurkiewicz, S. *MOC Watch: Debunking ABIM Pass Rate Myths.* New York, NY: MedPage Today; 2014. [Accessed Jan. 21, 2015.] Available from www.medpa getoday.com/PublicHealthPolicy/MedicalEducation/47601.

47. Chaudhry, HJ, Rhyne J, Cain, FE, Young, A, Crane, M, Bush, F. Maintenance of licensure: protecting the public, promoting quality health care. In *Revalidation: The Way Ahead*. Publication of proceedings: International Revalidation Symposium. London, UK: GMC; 2010:17–24. [Accessed Feb. 2, 2015.] Available from www.gmc-uk.org/International_Revalidation_Symposium_Publication_of_proceedings.pdf_44014486.pdf.

48. Royal College of Physicians and Surgeons of Canada. *CanMEDS 2015*. Ottawa, ON: RCPSC; 2015. [Accessed Jan. 21, 2015.] Available from www.royalcollege.ca/canmeds2015.

49. Irvine, D. *The Doctors' Tale: Professionalism and Public Trust*. Oxon, UK: Radcliffe Medical Press; 2003:139–96.

50. Association of American Physicians and Surgeons. *AAPS Takes MOC to Court*. Tucson, AZ: AAPS; 2015. [Accessed Jan. 23, 2015.] Available from www.aapsonline.org/index.php/article/aaps_takes_moc_to_court/.

51. Change Board Recertification. [Accessed Jan. 23, 2015.] Available from www.changeboardrecert.com/index.php.

52. Irons, MB, Nora, LM. Maintenance of certification 2.0–strong start, continued evolution. *N Engl J Med*. 2015; 372(2):104–06.

53. Teirstein, PS. Boarded to death–why maintenance of certification is bad for doctors and patients. *N Engl J Med*. 2015; 372(2):106–08.

54. Lee, TH. Certifying the good physician: a work in progress. *JAMA*. 2014; 312(22):2340–42.

55. Society for Cardiothoracic Surgery in Great Britain & Ireland; Dendrite Clinical Systems. *Maintaining Patients' Trust: Modern Medical Professionalism 2011*. Henley-on-Thames, UK: Dendrite Clinical Systems Ltd; 2011. [Accessed Dec. 29, 2014.] Available from www.scts.org/_userfiles/resources/634420268996790965_SCTS_Professionalism_FINAL.pdf.

56. Cosgriff, R, Hickey, G, Grant, S, Bridgewater, B, on behalf of the Society for Cardiothoracic Surgery in Great Britain and Ireland. *UK Heart Surgery: What Patients Can Expect from Their Surgeons*. London, UK: Society for Cardiothoracic Surgery in Great Britain and Ireland; 2011. [Accessed Feb. 2, 2015.] Available from www.ucl.ac.uk/nicor/audits/adultcardiac/documents/reports/bluebookforpatients.

57. Westaby S, Baig K, Pepper J. Publishing SSMD: the risks outweigh the benefits. *Bulletin of the Royal College of Surgeons of England*. 2015; 97(4):155–59.

58. Bridgewater, B. Patient-facing data is essential in the digital era. *Bulletin of the Royal College of Surgeons of England*. 2015; 97(4):160–63.

59. Boseley, S. *NHS Chief: Surgeons Have "Moral Responsibility" to Publish Death Rates*. (Interview with Sir Bruce Keogh.) London, UK: The Guardian; 2014. [Accessed Feb. 2, 2015.] Available from www.theguardian.com/society/2014/nov/19/nhs-chief-surgeons-moral-responsibility-publish-death-rates.

60. Tavare, A. Performance data: ready for the public? *BMJ*. 2012; 345(7864):21.

61. Bridgewater, B, Irvine, D, Keogh, B. NHS transparency: not yet perfect, but a huge step forward. *BMJ*. 2013; 347:f4402.

62. Bridgewater, B. Personal communication. Feb. 2, 2015.

The evolution of an undergraduate medical program on professionalism and identity formation

J. Donald Boudreau

Sow an act, and you reap a habit. Sow a habit and you reap a character. Sow a character, and you reap a destiny.

Charles Reade

Introduction

"How can I do that and still be *me*?" Reflections of this nature by medical students are often found in the literature.[1] The belief that medical education has the potential to form, transform, and perhaps even deform a person's core values or sense of self is commonly assumed by learners and teachers alike. The process has been explicated using various concepts, most notably medical character,[2] ethical comportment,[3] moral epistemology,[4] humanism in medicine,[5] and professionalism.[6] More recently, particularly in North America, discussions on the topic have taken a turn toward the conceptual framework of identity.[7]

The concepts of identity and "self-hood" are not new to many academic disciplines, including philosophy, psychology, and anthropology. Identity also has an honorable tradition in medical education. For example, in a research program that culminated in the influential 1957 publication, *The Student Physician*, sociologist Robert Merton and coauthors incorporated psychological perspectives on identity.[8] Of late, however, identity seems to have acquired a privileged status as an analytical tool in understanding the phenomenon of "becoming a doctor." A series of critical inquiries into professional education, funded by the Carnegie Foundation for the Advancement of Teaching, has recently been completed. It has identified the signature pedagogies of various professions and has suggested a clear direction for the teaching of professionalism in the twenty-first century. One of its primary conclusions is that students undergo personal transformations during their educational experiences. The study on educating the clergy focused on "pedagogies of formation."[9] The one that examined nursing practices referred to the teaching of "being, knowing, and doing."[10] The authors of the book on medical education discussed "identity formation," by which was meant the transmission of professional values and commitments.[11] That series has reinforced the conviction of many that medical education should be reframed so that it actively supports professional identity formation.[12,13]

This chapter is focused on the Physicianship Program at McGill University's Faculty of Medicine. It describes the teaching of professionalism from a perspective that is tightly coupled to the development of attributes considered necessary for the good doctor. It will outline key elements of that program, present preliminary findings from evaluation studies, share lessons learned from its implementation, and propose future directions for education and research. In essence, this experience, unfolding over a sixteen-year period, constitutes a case study. The hope is that a retrospective examination of the program's structure and function will illustrate how notions of identity formation can be incorporated into undergraduate medical education. The goal of the chapter is to assist others in developing, redirecting, or enhancing their own efforts with respect to this increasingly salient feature of medical pedagogy.

Before delving into the details of the program, it is important to make known to readers my understanding of "identity." It may appear to be a straightforward concept. In a manuscript previously cited, it was encapsulated using a pithy, common-sense definition derived from the Oxford English Dictionary: "a set of

Teaching Medical Professionalism, 2nd Edition, ed. Richard L. Cruess, Sylvia R. Cruess and Yvonne Steinert.
Published by Cambridge University Press. © Cambridge University Press 2016.

characteristics or a description that distinguishes a person or thing from others."[13] This definition is attractive in its simplicity and suggests an ease of application. However, it is multifaceted. Identity can be understood from two overarching perspectives: (1) theories of psychological, ego, and personality development; or (2) theories of socialization, categorization, and sociocultural development. It can also be considered from a variety of intellectual traditions, including behaviorism, evolutionary biological determinism, psychodynamics, narratology, and moral philosophy (e.g., axiology). It can be viewed as a process or a condition; something that resides internally (inside a person's psyche) or that is primarily outward-directed (meaningful only in interpersonal exchanges); individual, collective, or relational; single or multiple; constructed or discovered. The concept is slippery and some commentators have questioned its utility as an analytical construct, particularly when soft predicates, such as contingency, instability, multiplicity, and fluidity, are emphasized.[14] The operative definition that informed the Physicianship Program is that identity involves a process of identification (with individuals or groups), a conception of self, and a set of self-representations (e.g., the roles that are ascribed or accepted). These all have cognitive and emotional connotations.

Background

McGill introduced a module on medical professionalism in 1998. The catalyst for the curricular innovation was the work of Richard Cruess and Sylvia Cruess, influential advocates for the teaching of professionalism.[15] At the outset, the modules were lecture based, offered to first-year students, and focused on objectives in the cognitive domain. However, the scope expanded very rapidly. Its attention shifted to the promotion of professional behaviors and the support of students in the enculturation process. It relied increasingly on interactive educational strategies such as small-group discussions. By 2002, a module on professionalism, as core curricular content, was present in all four years of McGill's undergraduate program.

The innovations with respect to the teaching of professionalism were complemented by the work of local experts on whole-person care. Under the direction of Balfour Mount, an internationally renowned pioneer in palliative care, a working group was convened. It led efforts aimed at incorporating the concept of healing in the undergraduate program. Lectures and small groups on healing in medicine, including a White Coat Ceremony, were introduced during the 2001–02 academic year. The Physicianship Program itself was introduced in 2005. Some of the key events in the development and deployment of the program, from its precursors to its current form, are identified on a sixteen-year timeline presented in Figure 15.1.

The Faculty adopted the term "physicianship" in order to represent the synthesis of healing with professionalism. The construct of physicianship, as understood at McGill University, refers to the roles of the medical practitioner: the physician as a healer and professional. The healer is considered the primary role whereas professional status is conceived of as the way in which the medical profession has organized its structures and activities to deliver healing services. It is assumed that the two roles are enacted simultaneously; they can, nonetheless, be understood, analyzed, and taught separately.

The Physicianship Program has been described in considerable detail in the academic literature. A philosophical pedigree has been proposed.[16] The process of curricular renewal and the role of faculty development in institutional change have been explored.[17] Patient perspectives on a curriculum grounded in the concepts of the physician as healer and professional were examined and their contributions to program development were reported.[18] The educational blueprint, including its impact on the admissions process, has been outlined.[19] Strategies relating specifically to teaching whole-person care and healing have also been elaborated.[20] The teaching of the healer role, particularly in relation to reflective and mindful practice, is a focus of Chapter 7.

Physicianship also involved changes to certain specific educational practices, for example, in relation to the skills of the clinical method. It led to new approaches to teaching observation skills,[21] attentive listening,[22] and clinical thinking.[23] The program also served as an incentive for the development of novel tools useful in the assessment of professional behaviors, both among students (with the Professionalism Mini-Evaluation Exercise – the PMEX)[24] and teachers (with the Professionalism Assessment of Clinical Teachers – the PACT).[25] In addition, the program delved into attitudinal domains, areas that in pedagogical terms are ill defined. Most notably, it promoted a

Content focus	Professionalism	Professionalism	Professionalism and healing in medicine	Physicianship	Physicianship, identity formation
Teaching strategies	Lecture	Lectures and small groups	Lectures and small groups	Lectures, small groups, apprenticeship groups	Lectures, small groups, apprenticeship groups
Year of the MD program	Med 1	Med 1 and 4	Med 1, 2, 3, 4		
Events occurring in parallel to the MD program	Faculty development workshops on teaching and evaluating professionalism		Working group on "Healing and Healthcare"	Task force on teaching the professional and healer roles	Faculty development workshop on professional identity formation
Academic year(s)	1998	1999–2001	2002–2005	2005–2009	2014

Figure 15.1. Key stages in the development of the Physicianship Program. This timeline identifies key events during the sixteen-year period in which McGill's Physicianship Program was developed. It demonstrates how the focus of the program evolved: from professionalism to physicianship, and, most recently, toward the incorporation of identity formation. It shows how the scope of the program expanded progressively (initially confined to the first-year class and eventually including all four years of the MD program), and how the teaching strategies became more complex. It also notes some of the important developments occurring in parallel to those taking place within the undergraduate medical program. It is important to point out that this schema does not include all relevant developments; for example, the introduction of the White Coat Ceremony (in 2001), the Physicianship Portfolio (in 2005), and modules in interprofessionalism (in 2006).

set of personal attributes and underlined the importance for physicians-to-be to acquire self-knowledge. The specific set of attributes is captured in a Venn diagram; this representational figure is reproduced in Chapter 1 (Figure 1.3). The diagram identifies the personal characteristics unique to the healer and to the professional as well as those that are common to both roles. It also includes a description of the behavioral concomitants for the various attributes.

The flagship course for the Physicianship Program has been a longitudinal four-year course called Physician Apprenticeship. It, too, was first rolled out in 2005. Its goals are to (1) assist students in their transition from layperson to physician; (2) guide them in becoming reflective and patient-centered; and (3) provide a safe environment where they are encouraged to discuss issues arising out of their educational experiences. The apprenticeship provides opportunities for discussing the cognitive base of physicianship in addition to practicing the medical interview within clinically relevant settings. Although teachers in the apprenticeship are invited to teach certain clinical knowledge and skills, their raison d'être was, and continues to be, personal mentorship.

The Physician Apprenticeship (PA) groups, which are formed in the students' first year, consist of six students, two senior medical students, and a clinical teacher. Given the size of McGill's medical classes

(approximately 180 students), this means that each cohort has twenty apprenticeship groups. With the exception of the student co-leaders, who graduate halfway through the program, they remain a stable group for the duration of the four-year curriculum. They meet as a group five or six times per year. There are also occasional one-on-one meetings between teacher and student.

The teachers in the apprenticeship are all clinicians. They are selected based on their reputation for good teaching (e.g., recipients of teaching awards, peer recommendations, and nominations from the student body). The students are randomly assigned to their PA groups by the Dean's office. There is no attempt to match teacher and student according to age, sex, or ethnicity or to align students' career aspirations with teachers' specialties.

Based in the conviction that the teaching and learning of physicianship is inseparable from the transmission of values, the program emphasizes small-group discussions with prompts to stimulate personal reflections. It also aims to communicate its core values through symbols and rituals; this is illustrated in the following three design elements. First, the teachers in the Physician Apprenticeship are called Osler Fellows, named after Sir William Osler, important to the history of McGill, and a person who is universally recognized as the consummate and

The Physician as Healer and Professional

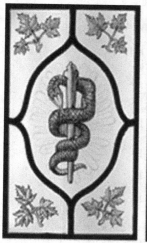 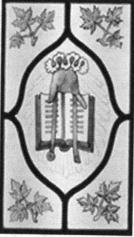

Epistēmē, Technē, Phronēsis

Figure 15.2. The logo of the Physicianship Program at McGill University. The frame on the left, the rod and serpent, originates from Greek mythology and is linked to Asklepios, the god of healing. The frame on the right, the "Heavenly Hand and Book," dates to medieval times and is the traditional symbol of universities; the book represents learning and scholarship, while the hand symbolizes transcendent sources of wisdom. The maple leaves are a reminder to the fact that McGill University is a modern Canadian institution. The three Greek words at the base of the frames represent the aspirations of the Physicianship Program – that its practitioner will acquire universal knowledge from nomothetic sciences, become skillful in clinical methods, and aspire to practical medical wisdom.

complete physician – a doctor to emulate. Second, to emphasize the healing mandate of medicine, the White Coat Ceremony is called Donning the Healer's Habit. Third, the program adopted a logo to represent its conception of the philosophical fundaments and the ontogeny of medicine (Figure 15.2). The logo consists of two pictorial frames: one represents the healing function and the other represents scholarship. The catchphrase at the bottom of the logo's pictorial frame is Epistēmē, Technē, Phronēsis. Those Greek words represent three different categories of intellectual thought, as per Aristotelian philosophy.

Episteme is scientific reasoning; it emphasizes demonstration in logic and conclusions of a theoretical or abstract nature. In contrast, techne and phronesis both describe practical reasoning. The precise difference between these two modes of thinking is often debated. Suffice it to point out that the former is generally translated as craftsmanship and the latter as practical wisdom or prudent decision-making. Techne describes a process, the quintessence of

which is in making or producing, during which there is the recognition of relevant generalizations (such as protocols or methods previously agreed upon by a community of practice). It culminates in an end or outcome that is external to the agent. For example, in the case of the navigator, the outcome might be a safe journey. Phronesis is a process with deliberation as its vital core. Combined with a disposition to act in a particular manner, deliberation culminates in a correct (good and right) course of action. In doing so, it contributes iteratively and inductively to the continued moral and intellectual development of the person; in contrast to techne, the end is internal to the agent. Techne can be taught and learned explicitly and is finely honed through experience; phronesis is acquired solely through experience and guided reflection.

The physicianship logo suggests that medicine is a fusion of theory and practice, with practice predominating. The incorporation of phronesis in the curricular blueprint acknowledges that medical education must attend to the development of identity. It also signifies the aspiration of the program, i.e., that its graduates will embark on the life-long process of acquiring clinical judgment and medical wisdom.

Specific elements of the Physicianship Program

So far, a general outline of the Physicianship Program has been provided. The reader, especially if engaged in an "on-the-ground" delivery of similar courses, may wish to be acquainted with more specific details. That is the purpose of this section.

We have found it critically important to meet with the students from the very beginning of medical school. Actually, physicianship is introduced on day one; students are offered a plenary session in which we outline the historical roots of the healing traditions and the professions. We define "healing," "profession," and "professionalism." More recently, we have added the concepts of "identity," "professional identity," and "socialization" to that orientation session. Following the plenary, students are invited to a small group (sixteen students to a group) in which they have an opportunity to reflect on their personal motivations for medical practice and on their nascent professional identities (or "proto-professionalism").[26] Student feedback regarding these orientation sessions has been overwhelmingly positive; it helps them to set expectations – to calibrate their hopes and desires with the profession's expectations. It is a motivational experience and it is reassuring for them to have the faculty speak of issues such as healing. This is followed a few months later by a session in which the focus is on the personal attributes of the healer and professional; the Venn diagram (Figure 1.3) serves as the organizing framework. The Venn diagram has become a sort of leitmotif for the program. Students are provided with vignettes that illustrate specific professional behaviors-in-action; they are asked to refer to the Venn diagram in analyzing the events and in suggesting corrective measures or appropriate responses. Over the years of conducting this session, we have found three aspects that are important for educational leaders to consider:

- It is most effective to refer to contexts that are germane to students' actual experiences; for example, it is better to discuss a hypothetical case of cheating in the classroom than an instance of disrespectful interpersonal interactions by team members during a hemodialysis treatment.
- There is a tendency to focus on examples of unprofessional behaviors; it is wise to balance this with cases of exemplary behaviors (such as an illustration of a student initiative with the local indigenous population).
- It is prudent to avoid stereotyping, such as, for example, overplaying the narrative of the arrogant surgeon in the operating room.

Recently, we have introduced a new module, with lecture and small group, on identity formation and socialization. Two sets of discussion prompts that we have found particularly useful are those that deal with "a first experience" (e.g., first time being with a dying patient; first time dissecting a cadaver) and those that invite reflections on perceived changes in one's persona (e.g., an incident when one felt like a doctor or when one was treated as if they were a doctor). This session remains a work in progress.

In the second-year class, we introduce the social contract and discuss, again in small groups, reciprocal obligations and expectations of society and the medical profession. There are also interactive sessions on health advocacy. It is also at this juncture that the students gather to craft their class pledge. Each class creates its own pledge (an example of which can be found in Chapter 2). They read it aloud in front of their peers, faculty, family members, and loved ones at the White Coat Ceremony. This represents a public acknowledgement of a personal acceptance of professional values.

Later on, the ceremony and its impact on personal meanings are explored in the context of meetings of the Physician Apprenticeship groups.

For the third-year class, the focus is on communication in teams. There is a preliminary whole-class interactive meeting followed by a conflict negotiation scenario, organized at the Simulation Center. Each student interacts with a standardized physician, resident, or nurse; the students are challenged to recognize personal and contextual factors that initiate and perpetuate conflictual situations. There are also panel discussions, with student, physician, and patient, where the healing function is discussed.

In their final year, the students revisit the social contract with a focus on self-regulation. The small groups use a variety of strategies such as debates and role-plays. In a separate meeting, they are prompted to consider how they will deal with the tensions inherent in the profession: altruism versus self-interest; respect for duty-hour regulation versus service; meeting professional obligations versus maintaining a healthy personal life; professional autonomy versus accountability. Students are also invited to consider how they will reunite the professional and healer functions of the physician.

The longitudinal Physician Apprenticeship has its own set of educational activities. These are summarized in Table 15.1.

Many of the topics included in the curriculum for the students are mirrored in the faculty development program offered to the Osler Fellows. This targeted program, called the Osler Fellowship, prepares the teachers for their role as mentors. It is described in Table 15.2.

Aspects of the program focused on personal transformation

As previously noted, a key objective of the Physician Apprenticeship is to assist students in their "transition from layperson to physician." Initially, this aim was not described specifically using the term "identity." Nonetheless, there was an implicit understanding that achieving this goal involved paying attention to the evolution in students' personal growth and maturation. The program has consistently emphasized guided reflection, including reflections on self-knowledge. The Osler Fellows have reported that they are bearing witness to the changes in their mentees' outlooks and evolving conceptions of who they are. In

Table 15.1. Content of Physician Apprenticeship

Year	Number of group meetings	Discussion topics	Learning activities
1	8	– Issues of interest to the group* – Communication skills – The patient perspective – Professionalism issues	– Interactive small-group discussions** – 5 home visits to a patient*** – 3 clinical encounters – 2 medical interviews in the Simulation Center
2	6	– Issues of interest to the group* – Complementary and alternative medicine – Healing in medicine – Determinants of health – Cultural sensitivity	– Interactive small group discussions** – 1 medical interview in the Simulation Center – Reflective writing
3	5	– Issues of interest to the group* – Relief of suffering – Resilience in medical practice – Inter-professionalism – Career planning	– Interactive small group discussions** – 1 encounter in the Simulation Center – Case discussions – Visits to the Osler Fellows' clinical workplace
4	3	– Issues of interest to the group* – Advanced communication skills – The social contract – Self-regulation – Reuniting the healer and professional roles	– Interactive small group discussions** – 1 medical interview in the Simulation Center – Interactive lectures – Debates – Role plays

* Student-generated issues have priority over all planned activities as agenda items for group discussions.

** The group meetings often take place in informal settings (e.g., restaurant or Osler Fellow's home); in first year, it includes a dialogue triggered by reflections following the *Commemorative Service for Donors of Bodies*.

*** The purpose is to provide an opportunity for students to appreciate patients' perspectives on illness; the patients are called *My First-Year Patient*; students conduct the home visits in pairs and they are expected to submit written reports based on these visits.

retrospect, identity formation might have provided a fruitful conceptual framework with which to organize educational activities and understand their impact. In the most recent iterations of the program, including core-learning modules and the Physician Apprenticeship, there has been a shift toward an explicit discussion and consideration of professional identity formation.

An undergraduate medical education program is replete with many opportunities for examining one's personal growth. Medical practice, by virtue of its very nature (e.g., its complexity, inescapable ambiguities, limitations, high stakes, need for discernment), represents a potent context for character development.

Important way-stations in maturation can include experiences with any or all of the following: sickness, misery, plight, vulnerability, end of life, death, cadavers, responsibility, abandonment, dignity, fear, hope, blame, uncertainty, disagreement, disappointment, privacy, power, privilege, prestige, pride, poetry, mystery, and majesty. It can be said that medical education is able to provide the conditions for personal development in an accelerated fashion. The implication here is that medical schools are not required to create artificial situations in order to promote identity transformation; their responsibility is to harness and channel the ample opportunities that exist for spontaneous and guided reflection.

Table 15.2. Content of the Osler Fellowship

Year	Number of workshops	Topics	Learning activities
1	4	– Introduction to concepts related to the "Physician as Healer and Professional" and identity formation – Small-group facilitation skills – Introduction to narrative medicine – Diversity and social justice	– Interactive plenary and small-group discussions – Case vignettes – Role plays – Reflective writing and close reading
2	2	– Introduction to the Calgary-Cambridge Guide and the Simulation Center – The learning environment and the hidden curriculum – Erosion of empathy*	– Interactive plenary and small-group discussions – Case discussions – Interviews with standardized patients – Reviews of videotapes
3	2	– Special topics** – The physician as healer – Career planning	– Interactive plenary and small-group discussions – Role plays – Dialogues triggered by portfolio entries – Group exercises related to career planning
4	2	– The social contract – Celebration of the Osler Fellows	– Interactive plenary and small-group discussions – Debates – Closing ceremony with student and Osler Fellow testimonials

* The session on ethical erosion will be changed to one focused on identity formation.
** The special topics vary from year to year and generally involve visiting professors; past topics have included narrative medicine, medical students as agents of change, mindfulness, and critical consciousness.

With respect to this latter point, cadaver-dissection programs are particularly illustrative. I find it unfortunate that some schools are abandoning them. The first day in the anatomy laboratory is indelible in the memories of generations of physicians. The first few hours of anatomy teaching around the cadaver are invariably imbued with anxiety. That anxiety is often transformed later on, once students leave the laboratory and return home (often with a residual smell of formaldehyde on the hands and flickers of body parts in the mind's eye), into a sense of awe and a feeling that they have crossed the threshold into a new world – the world of medicine. They exit the anatomy lab as different people than they had been going in. This transformative event, as many others that occur during medical school, should not be left unexamined. Ideally, the learning that begins in the anatomy lab should continue into small groups and a commemorative service for the donors of bodies. Some experts have even explored the effects of cadaver dissection on learners' evolving conceptions of self by inviting students into a dialogue about their dreams. Psychiatrist Eric Marcus has analyzed medical students' dreams; he has found that nightmares of cadavers are prominent.[27] His outcome data suggest that dreams can reveal salient aspects of students' identification with patients and doctors in unique and distinct phases of professionalization.

Medical teachers can use a variety of theoretical anchors in structuring their conversations with students about critical events such as cadaver dissection or the first contact with death. The concept of *liminality* may be useful. Liminality relates to the phases that a person traverses in rites of passage, in transitions from one state, position, or status to another.[28,29] The three phases are separation, transition (or limen), and incorporation. The liminal phase is marked by intense demands on the emotional state and, if traversed successfully, culminates in the incorporation of new personae. The concept may be applicable to undergraduate medical education, particularly when students are faced with new and emotionally charged situations, such as finding themselves in the antechamber of a sickroom with a person at the end of life, in the birthing room, with a person undergoing a cardiac arrest, or at the White Coat Ceremony. It has guided the selection of events we consider ripe for conversations focused on the "self." There is a focus on experiences, particularly "first-time" events that may include a transitional (liminal) phase and that have an inherent potential for the incorporation of new personae. Students frequently recount instances in which they catch themselves acting like a doctor, feeling like a doctor, thinking like a doctor, talking like a doctor, or seeing like a doctor. Discussion prompts intended to elicit such reflections are presented in Table 15.3.

During the decade that the Physicianship Program has been in existence, understandings of professionalism and professional identity formation have continued to evolve. The influence of the Carnegie Foundation series has already been noted. There have been other important developments. In a commentary on the perceived erosion of professional ethics, Jack Coulehan and Peter Williams lay blame on tensions existing between values espoused by educational blueprints and those expressed in actual educational and clinical activities.[30] They refer to the espousal–expression gap and capture it using the term "hidden" curriculum. This notion is now thoroughly ensconced in the vernacular idiom of our day-to-day practices. Although it is more than fifty years old, its first in-depth exploration is more recent, originating in the work of Fred Hafferty and Ronald Franks.[31] While some of the effects of the hidden curriculum may be harmless, the accepted belief is that it is generally negative and undesirable. Unfortunately, the byproducts of the "hidden" curriculum are far from inconspicuous. Many educational leaders, including accreditation bodies, have recommended that professional schools address the hidden curriculum and reflect on its impact on students, particularly on character and moral development.

Over the past three decades, there has been a resurgence of interest in moral philosophy. The concept of phronesis has triggered a profound reflection on the fundamental nature of teaching.[32,33] Many philosophers regard medical practice and education as primarily (although not exclusively) a "phronetic" type of activity.[34,35,36,37] Phronesis has been proposed as a model to understand the evolution from proto-professionalism to complete professionalism[26] and as a concept that can describe the process of moral development.[38] It has potential to be a useful concept because it combines disposition, reason, and action. As noted previously, in phronesis, sometimes translated as "doing well," dispositions to choose in a particular way become incorporated in a person's character through repeated and incremental use. It is said that phronesis is self-constituting. For example, in the case of a physician, a particular outcome of a deliberation may be an act of altruism, but the process does not stop there; that physician also develops a penchant for altruism, i.e., a reinforced inclination toward that moral quality. The notion of the acquisition of a moral compass – of becoming through doing – is captured in this chapter's epigram. Shakespeare also expressed it in Hamlet: "Assume the virtue if you have it not ... For use almost can change the stamp of nature." Since phronesis deals with the process whereby settled character traits are developed, it may have immediate relevance for understanding professional identity formation. The applicability of phronesis in representing and guiding the characterological and behavioral outcomes of an undergraduate medical program is increasingly apparent, even though much remains to be understood in contemporary terms.

It is noteworthy that the original article in which the impact of the hidden curriculum in medical education was elucidated also highlighted the importance of identity formation. Hafferty and Franks contrasted the developmental and instrumental roles of ethics teaching, stating: "[We] believe that there is a fundamental distinction between a pedagogical approach that highlights ethical principles as residing squarely within the physician's professional *identity* and a view of ethics that frames ethical principles as *tools* to be employed in the course of clinical work."[31] When the authors cautioned against teaching ethics as an entity "external both to the situation and the actors involved" they were invoking a distinction between phronesis and techne, and they were lining up behind the concept of practical wisdom (without, however, referring to the original Greek term).

Table 15.3. Triggers useful for initiating dialogues focused on personal change

Triggers given to students	Comments
Describe yourself: your "self"; your "identity"; your "persona"; your "character."	This trigger is useful as a baseline.
What do you think doctors do in their encounters with patients? When you create a mental image of yourself as a physician 10 years from now, what do you see yourself doing? Prompt: Make believe that you are in charge of recruiting doctors for a country that has never had any; write a short (e.g., 4 sentences) job description that will appear in the national newspaper.	These triggers are particularly useful at the beginning of a program.
How are you hoping to learn medicine? When you think of a patient who would be ideal for you in terms of your future learning, what does that patient look like?	
Tell us about a doctor who made you want to emulate them or with whom you felt "taken care of" in the manner you would like to take care of others.	
Do you feel yourself becoming a physician? If so, please recount an experience that has contributed to that feeling or perspective. Tell us about an activity or event that made you feel more or less like a doctor.	
Describe your first experience of "X," where X = you took care of a dying patient; participated in dissecting a cadaver; got angry at a patient; felt incompetent; assisted at a cardiac arrest; cried in a clinical setting; felt like throwing in the towel; were on-call; were required to physically hurt a patient (e.g., performed an invasive procedure); felt proud of one of your actions as a medical student; made a clinical mistake; felt you had earned the privilege of being called "doctor."	These triggers are particularly useful in engaging students who are now well-engaged in the program.
Tell us about an event where others treated you like a doctor or treated you differently than before.	
Have you found yourself talking like a doctor? Tell us about that.	
Polonius in Hamlet says: "To thine own self be true." Is there an incident when you felt that you succeeded or did not succeed in this? Prompts: Are there times that you feel like an imposter?	These are particularly useful toward the end of the program (e.g., during clerkship rotations) or at times when students have ample opportunity to reflect.
As you find yourself becoming more like a doctor, what have been the gains and losses in terms of your self-image? What aspects of yourself (e.g., activities, characteristics, roles) have you had to let go, neglect, or reinforce? What aspects are you trying to project or avoid projecting to the world or your peers?	

Lessons learned

As would be expected with any major curricular revision, physicianship has been subject to ongoing monitoring and review.[39,40] Important insights were gained from one particular component of the overall program-evaluation protocol: a study, called the Physician Apprenticeship Case Study, conducted over one four-year curricular cycle, from 2008 to

2012.[41] The case consisted of three Physician Apprenticeship groups (for a total of twenty-four students and three teachers). There were four main findings. The students and teachers began the apprenticeship experience with expectations that were somewhat divergent; the students were expecting faculty members to deliver extensive, authentic, "first-hand" clinical experience while, in contrast, the teachers seemed to be more attuned to a contemplative aspect of students' experiences. The apprenticeship succeeded in ensuring a safe space for reflection, and the teachers were adept at catalyzing and guiding critical reflection. The interpersonal bonds and relationships that developed between student and teacher were strong, intimate, and highly meaningful. The apprenticeship experience succeeded in supporting students' identity formation and in reaffirming the Osler Fellows' powerful attachments to core professional values. The latter finding – teachers themselves vicariously reconnecting with a professional ethos – was also seen in a previous cross-sectional study of the program.[42] Findings from both of these studies provide evidence that a longitudinal apprenticeship can contribute to the formation of a professional identity. They also permitted the construction of a provisional conceptual model for explicating key features of the apprenticeship learning process. This model emphasizes two points: (1) the contributions made by the teachers to their students' identities and evolving sense of belonging to a new community are channeled through relationships; and (2) a successful apprenticeship is characterized by an ability to create a "safe space" for dialogue with the use of educational strategies that promote and guide reflection. Although mentorships and apprenticeships are generally conceived of as educational strategies, educators must not lose sight of the fact that they also provide critically important opportunities for relationship building that can activate and reinforce a novice's identification with a new kinship – in our context, the medical profession.

A lesson that we learned in the first iteration of the Physicianship Program may be useful for others. One of the instruments we used to promote reflection was a portfolio. This is a tool familiar to many educationalists; it generally constitutes a compilation of students' documented accomplishments, particularly in their reflective abilities. It often includes solicited reflective writings. Called the "Physicianship Portfolio," it was designed to be a developmental rather than an assessment tool. It included formal and informal elements, some of which were intended to be shared with Osler Fellows and fellow students in the context of the Physician Apprenticeship groups. Others were meant to be strictly confidential. The portfolio template proposed a total of twenty-six possible entries. A selection of six of these is presented in Table 15.4.

Although the portfolio was intended to be adaptable, flexible, and a means to an end, it was not uniformly perceived as such by students and teachers. Some students experienced the portfolio as an imposition, a sort of "paper chase" representing extra work for little gain. A few expressed the belief that they possessed innate abilities in self-reflection and that the school neither could nor should attempt to teach these skills. Others perceived that the program was unduly emphasizing creative writing as a privileged entry for reflection, arguing that other avenues such as singing, or even cooking and exercising, were just as effective. Faculty members also expressed reservations, particularly with respect to a perception that they were expected to critically review the portfolio entries. Even though it had been made clear that the locus of control and access to the portfolio belonged to the students and that any assessment was to be formative rather than summative, teachers felt inadequate to the task of providing feedback. The portfolio was subsequently made entirely optional. Nonetheless, it is hoped that it can soon be revised and updated with specific attention to reflections on professional identity formation.

Another lesson learned, which may be reassuring to many, is that the modifications we have recently made to our program, with the aim of bolstering identity formation, were relatively easy to implement. We were not required to turn the entire educational blueprint topsy-turvy. We introduced modifications to the modules on professionalism and healing that had been previously delivered. We altered several scenarios, vignettes, or discussion prompts by including issues related to socialization. We presented, discussed, and distributed the schematic representation of socialization (Figures 1.4 and 1.5 in Chapter 1) to both students and teachers. We were gratified to see that the language of identity formation was not considered foreign or intimidating. The topic resonated deeply with students. For example, in one of our recent introductory lectures on the topic, several

Table 15.4. Examples of submissions for the Physicianship Portfolio

Portfolio entry as described in the instructions given to students	Nature of entry	Comments
Write a reflection that speaks to any of your hopes, aspirations, fears or insights concerning anything at this important transition point in your life. Put this secret personal message into a sealed envelope.	Mandatory entry; beginning of the program.	This entry is a sort of "reflective time capsule."* It was to remain sealed until prior to graduation when it was to be read by the Osler Fellow in the presence of the student.
Write a reflection on the White Coat Ceremony. "How realistic is the class pledge? Are there any negative aspects to the symbol of the white coat?"	Mandatory entry; end of second year.	To be reviewed by the Osler Fellow at the invitation of the student.
Describe a "healing moment" that you experienced or observed or describe a situation where an opportunity to promote healing was missed.	An optional entry.	This entry was considered confidential to the student.
Write a "Dear Me" letter which addresses any of the following: In what aspects do I feel most and/or least prepared to begin clerkships? What aspects of clerkships are most exciting and/or most worrisome to me? What features of my personality do I want to be most evident to my patients? What kind of impression do I want to give my supervisors? What are my personal goals for the first rotation of the next 12 months?	Mandatory entry; beginning of clerkships (i.e., third year).	This entry is another "reflective time capsule." Students were asked to think of it as an autobiographical letter, similar to the one they submitted as a requirement for admission to medical school, except that in this instance it is a letter for "admission" to clerkships. It was intended to be reviewed by the Osler Fellow midway during clerkships.
Write a reflection on how a particular clinical encounter (e.g., a specific core or elective rotation, a patient or a physician) turned you "on" or "off" a specific discipline.	An optional entry.	This entry was confidential to the student. The Osler Fellow may have invited students to share in a group meeting with a focus on career planning.
If you wrote a note of condolences to a family following the death of a patient or if you were ever named in an official obituary in the newspaper, please include a copy in your portfolio.	Optional entry.	This entry was considered confidential to the student.

* A detailed description of the "reflective time capsules" will be available in a soon-to-be published book, edited by Alan Peterkin and Pamela Brett-MacLean, on reflection in health professional education.[45] The book, a compendium of novel strategies that aim to promote reflection, may be helpful to others who wish to increase their focus on personal transformations.

students were comfortable enough to make highly appropriate suggestions for adding elements to the schema. Another recommendation originating from the student body was that, when discussing identity formation, it is important for the faculty to recognize generational differences. It may be beneficial to have residents and recent graduates participate in future panel or small group discussions. The Osler Fellows have also recognized the value of the concept of identity transformation in their work as mentors.

The successful implementation of a program designed to teach and foster professional identity formation requires several critical ingredients: a vision anchored in a coherent and overarching conceptual framework, clear learning objectives, support from the educational leadership, local champions, an organizational structure that is supple, adaptable, and responsive to ongoing teacher and student feedback, resources for faculty development, and a collective sense of duty that is infused with passion.

Future directions

The major target of future developments at McGill University's undergraduate medical program is expected to be in evaluation and research. The medical education community has an obligation to better understand the underlying processes of professional identity formation and to delineate the impact and outcomes of specific educational interventions. I believe that the concept of practical wisdom (phronesis) holds the promise of opening several avenues for research. The following ideas, tentative and conjectural in nature, may represent catalysts for further discussion among colleagues with a shared interest in this domain.

Practical wisdom acknowledges the existence of personal dispositions, i.e., innate penchants for certain kinds of thoughts and understandings. This means that medical school education and enculturation does not start with students as *tabula rasa*; the professional identity that germinates and unfolds has a strong resonance with a person's past being. Emergent new self-conceptions must be able to incorporate a person's past without damaging the enduring core of self or interfering with attempts at creating new self-representations (e.g., the adoption of new roles). The idea of "disposition" reinforces the need for constant attention to the fact that students accepted to medical school already have a particular way of being in and seeing their world. It would be intriguing to conduct longitudinal studies exploring how self-definition evolves and how tightly it remains anchored to a sense of an enduring self. It may therefore be beneficial at some point to examine the predispositions (including baseline ethical values) of entering students.

The most important aspect of practical wisdom is "deliberation." Deliberation (particularly in nontechnical contexts) is not concerned about a search for the optimal means to accomplish a desired end; rather, it is a search for the best way of specifying a problem, that is, the quest to identify all the relevant factors that have a bearing on the issue(s) at hand. In classical moral philosophy the excellence of someone's character is better judged by the quality of the complete process of deliberation than by the choice(s) in which it culminates.[43] In medical education, research on moral development has tended to emphasize the examination of ethical decisions taken in specific contexts, followed by inferences on the ethical character of the decision-maker, rather than examining the decision-making process per se. The important

thing, however, is how well the person understands what makes up the problem. An interesting research question would be: How do students arrive at the "best specification" in clinical cases and how do these changes in understanding (if they occur) correlate with evolving self-conceptions?

It is generally believed that the development of practical medical wisdom is most efficient when a student is challenged with increasingly ambiguous and complex cases. Development of a physician persona is incremental and requires a series of "step-ups." This provides a rationale for the strategy of providing our learners with progressive and graded responsibilities. It would be interesting to explore how identity formation is affected by the multitude of factors that currently isolate students from the realities of clinical work and that shield them from ambiguity and uncertainty. Students are increasingly learning medicine at a distance from the hospital and other clinical sites. They learn more and more of the clinical method from standardized patients rather than real, in-the-flesh, sick persons. They are extricated from patient care responsibility by duty-hour regulations. They learn pediatrics in well-baby clinics rather than pediatric emergency rooms. They are offered "shadowing experiences" rather than authentic experiences that would demand that they demonstrate responsibility, show that that they know their limits, and can be safe and trustworthy. It makes one wonder whether experiences of a passive nature (e.g., shadowing) as a substitute for active, on-duty, in the thick-of-things, clinical work negatively influences learners' emergent identities.

Conclusion

The attainment of medical practical wisdom is an aspirational goal. Any individual medical student, junior resident, chief resident, newly minted physician, or senior attending physician might never attain the goal. This realization may be of benefit to the collectivity of physicians by urging us to continue to aspire to something noble. It may also serve as a buffer against professional hubris.

Most clinician–teachers will agree with the idea that the ultimate aim of medical education is the production of the "good doctor" and will endorse philosopher John Dewey's belief that "the self is not something ready-made, but something in continuous formation through choice of action."[44] Ancient concepts from Hellenistic Greece are likely to be helpful in proposing underlying mechanisms.

It would be beneficial for all of us to articulate an image of the "good doctor" as well as the "ideal doctor" and to keep that image uppermost in our minds. The ideal doctor is a *phronimos* – a person with an appropriate medical savoir, consummate savoir-faire, and an effective yet humble savoir-être. Since conceptions of this ideal are bound up in notions of professionalism, it is heartening that the contemporary discourse on professionalism has increasingly come to incorporate identity formation as a critical and inescapable feature. The medical student who asks, "How can I do that and still be *me*?" must be helped to understand two fundamental things: that the "me" *will* inevitably change during medical school and that the "new me" *must* incorporate conceptions of the "good" and "ideal" doctor.

References

1. Harper, G. Breaking taboos and steadying the self in medical school. *Lancet*. 1993; 342(8876):913–15.

2. Bryan, CS. *Teaching Character: Why, How, and by Whom?* Calhoun Lectureship. Clemson, SC: Strom Thurmond Institute of Government and Public Affairs, Clemson University; 2006.

3. Pellegrino, ED, Siegler, M, Singer, PA. Teaching clinical ethics. *J Clin Ethics*. 1990; 1(3):175–80.

4. Tauber, AI. Medicine and the call for a moral epistemology, part II: constructing a synthesis of values. *Perspect Biol Med*. 2008; 51(3):450–63.

5. Cohen, JJ. Viewpoint: linking professionalism to humanism: what it means, why it matters. *Acad Med*. 2007; 82(11):29–32.

6. Stern, DT, Papadakis, M. The developing physician – becoming a professional. *N Engl J Med*. 2006; 355(17):1794–99.

7. Monrouxe, LV. Identity, identification and medical education: why should we care? *Med Educ*. 2009; 44(1):40–49.

8. Merton, RK, Reader, GG, Kendall, P, eds. *The Student-Physician: Introductory Studies in the Sociology of Medical Education*. Cambridge, MA: Harvard University Press; 1957.

9. Foster, CR, Dahill, L, Golemon, L, Wang Tolentino, B. *Educating Clergy: Teaching Practices and Pastoral Imagination*. San Francisco, CA: Jossey-Bass; 2005.

10. Benner, P, Sutphen, M, Leonard, V, Day, L. *Educating Nurses: A Call for Radical Transformation*. San Francisco, CA: Jossey-Bass; 2010.

11. Cooke, M, Irby, DM, O'Brien, BC. *Educating Physicians: A Call for Reform of Medical School and Residency*. San Francisco, CA: Jossey-Bass; 2010.

12. Jarvis-Selinger, S, Pratt, DD, Regher, G. Competency is not enough: integrating identity formation into medical education discourse. *Acad Med*. 2012; 87(9):1185–90.

13. Cruess, RL, Cruess, SR, Boudreau, JD, Snell, L, Steinert, Y. Reframing medical education to support professional identity formation. *Acad Med*. 2014; 89(11):1446–51.

14. Brubaker, R, Cooper, F. Beyond "identity." *Theory Soc*. 2000; 29:1–47.

15. Cruess, SR, Cruess, RL. Professionalism must be taught. *BMJ*. 1997; 315(7123):1674–77.

16. Fuks, A, Brawer, J, Boudreau, JD. The foundation of physicianship. *Perspect Biol Med*. 2012; 55(1):114–26.

17. Steinert, Y, Cruess, S, Cruess, R, Snell, L. Faculty development for teaching and evaluating professionalism: from programme design to curriculum change. *Med Educ*. 2005; 39(2):127–36.

18. Boudreau, JD, Jagosh, J, Slee, R, Macdonald, ME, Steinert, Y. Patients' perspectives on physicians' roles: implications for curricular reform. *Acad Med*. 2008; 83(8):744–53.

19. Boudreau, JD, Cruess, SR, Cruess, RL. Physicianship: educating for professionalism in the post-Flexnerian era. *Perspect Biol Med*. 2011; 54(1):89–105.

20. McNamara, H, Boudreau, JD. Teaching whole person care in medical school. In Hutchinson, TA, ed. *Whole Person Care: A New Paradigm for the 21st Century*. New York, NY: Springer; 2011:183–200.

21. Boudreau, JD, Cassell, EJ, Fuks, A. Preparing medical students to become skilled at clinical observation. *Med Teach*. 2008; 39(9–10):857–62.

22. Boudreau, JD, Cassell, EJ, Fuks, A. Preparing medical students to become attentive listeners. *Med Teach*. 2009; 31(1):22–29.

23. Fuks, A, Boudreau, JD, Cassell, EJ. Teaching clinical thinking to first-year medical students. *Med Teach*. 2009; 31(2):105–11.

24. Cruess, R, McIllroy, JH, Cruess, S, Ginsburg, S, Steinert, Y. The Professionalism Mini-Evaluation Exercise: a preliminary investigation. *Acad Med*. 2006; 81 (10 Suppl):S74–S78.

25. Young, ME, Cruess, SR, Cruess, RL, Steinert, Y. The Professionalism Assessment of Clinical Teachers (PACT): the reliability and validity of a novel tool to evaluate professional and clinical teaching behaviors. *Adv Health Sci Educ Theory Pract*. 2014; 19(1):99–113.

26. Hilton, SR, Slotnick, HB. Proto-professionalism: how professionalisation occurs across the continuum of medical education. *Med Educ*. 2005; 39(1):58–65.

27. Marcus, ER. Psychodynamic social science and medical education. *J Psychother Pract Res*. 1999; 8(3):191–94.

28. van Gennep, A. *The Rites of Passage.* Chicago, IL: University of Chicago Press; 1961.

29. Turner, V. *The Ritual Process: Structure and Anti-Structure.* London, UK: Aldine Transaction; 1969.

30. Coulehan, J, Williams, PC. Vanquishing virtue: the impact of medical education. *Acad Med.* 2001; **76**(6):598–605.

31. Hafferty, FW, Franks, R. The hidden curriculum, ethics teaching, and the structure of medical education. *Acad Med.* 1994; **69**(11):861–71.

32. Kristjánsson, K. *Aristotle, Emotions, and Education.* Hampshire, UK: Ashgate; 2007.

33. Eisner, EW. From episteme to phronesis to artistry in the study and improvement of teaching. *Teaching and Teacher Education.* 2002; **18**(4):375–85.

34. Toulmin, S. On the nature of physicians' understanding. *J Med Philos.* 1976; **1**(1):32–50.

35. Davis, FD. Phronesis, clinical reasoning, and Pellegrino's philosophy of medicine. *Theor Med.* 1997; **18**(1–2):173–95.

36. Frank, AW. Asking the right question about pain: narrative and phronesis. *Lit Med.* 2004; **23**(2): 209–25.

37. Kaldjian, LC. Teaching practical wisdom in medicine through clinical judgement, goals of care, and ethical reasoning. *J Med Ethics.* 2010; **36**:558–62.

38. Kinghorn, WA. Medical education as moral formation: an Aristotelian account of medical professionalism. *Perspect Biol Med.* 2010; **53**(1):87–105.

39. Ruhe, V, Boudreau, JD. The 2011 Program Evaluation Standards: a framework for quality in medical education programme evaluations. *J Eval Clin Pract.* 2013; **19**(5):925–32.

40. Ruhe, V, Boudreau, JD. Curricular innovation in an undergraduate medical program: what is "appropriate" assessment? *Educ Asse Eval Acc.* 2011; **23**(3):187–200.

41. Boudreau, JD, Macdonald, ME, Steinert, Y. Affirming professional identities through an apprenticeship: insights from a four-year longitudinal case study. *Acad Med.* 2014; **89**(7):1038–45.

42. Steinert, Y, Boudreau, JD, Boillat, M, Slapcoff, B, Dawson, D, Briggs, A, Macdonald, ME. The Osler Fellowship: an apprenticeship for medical educators. *Acad Med.* 2010; **85**(7):1242–49.

43. Wiggins, D. Deliberation and practical reason. In *Proceedings of the Aristotelian Society.* London, UK: The Aristotelian Society; 1975:29–51.

44. Dewey, J. *Education and Experience: The 60th Anniversary Edition.* West Lafayette, IN: Kappa Delta Pi; 1998.

45. Boudreau, JD. Reflective time capsules. In Peterkin, A, Brett-MacLean, P, eds. *Keeping Reflection Fresh.* Kent, IN: Kent State University Press; 2016. In press.

Chapter 6

Developing and implementing an undergraduate curriculum

Mark D. Holden, Era Buck, and John Luk

Texas has a reputation comparable to its size, for doing things in a big way and for being individualistic. This chapter presents a Texas-sized pilot study that includes six undergraduate institutions and four medical schools engaged in an initiative to transform medical education. A fundamental part of the transformation is the authentic integration of professional identity formation into premedical and undergraduate medical education.

Time initiative

In 2007, the University of Texas (UT) System launched Transformation in Medical Education (TIME), a broad initiative to redesign the continuum of premedical to undergraduate medical education. This ambitious project, funded by the UT Regents and championed by the Executive Vice Chancellor for Health Affairs, aimed to reform the content, methods, and timeline of the attainment of the medical degree, based on the belief that current methods are inefficient, outdated, and unnecessarily long and expensive. The TIME steering committee identified four foundational elements for the initiative: (1) instituting a pre-health-professions program; (2) implementing competency-based education; (3) incorporating nontraditional topics; and (4) intentionally focusing on professional identity formation.

Within the TIME initiative, six undergraduate campuses and four medical schools across the UT System created four pilot program partnerships. Each partnership included one to three undergraduate campuses and one or two medical schools, with the goal of developing and implementing a pilot that incorporates all four foundational elements. The heterogeneity of the partnerships and their pilots provided the opportunity to identify successful designs and strategies as well as lessons learned. This heterogeneity also extended to methods of student selection, number of institutions, curriculum design, and geographic spread, which ranges from eight to 800 miles between partner institutions.

As the first TIME initiative element, each undergraduate campus established a pre-health-professions program. By including students interested in a variety of health professions, these programs allow students to share experiences and learn collaboratively, with the goal of fostering teamwork and interprofessional professionalism. These programs also provide a structure for developing and managing educational activities and tracking student progress.

The second TIME initiative element, competency-based education, grew from the work of the Accreditation Council on Graduate Medical Education (ACGME) and the Royal College of Physicians and Surgeons of Canada to incorporate competency-based principles into postgraduate medical education.[1,2] Undergraduate medical education has since adopted competency-based medical education, including the development of graduation competencies. Incorporating elements from the ACGME and CanMEDS (Canadian Medical Education Directives for Specialists) schemas, the TIME initiative developed a competency-based framework appropriate for the learner from matriculation into the undergraduate campus through graduation from medical school. This framework includes six domains: (1) communication skills and collaboration; (2) professionalism; (3) medical knowledge and scholarship; (4) patient care; (5) practice-based learning and improvement; and (6) systems-based practice and management.[3] The TIME initiative utilizes competency-based medical education to provide

Teaching Medical Professionalism, 2nd Edition, ed. Richard L. Cruess, Sylvia R. Cruess and Yvonne Steinert.
Published by Cambridge University Press. © Cambridge University Press 2016.

consistent targets for learners and educators across the diverse schools and partnerships and to identify appropriate transition milestones from the undergraduate to the medical school campuses.

The third TIME initiative element is the incorporation of nontraditional fields, such as public health, languages, music, arts, humanities, philosophy, psychology, and sociology. These important nontraditional topics facilitate the development of well-rounded students with diverse experiences beyond the biological and physical sciences, with the resilience to effectively manage the rigors of medical training, and with the ultimate goal to become humanistic physicians with diverse interests and skills.[4]

The fourth TIME initiative element is the intentional focus on the promotion and assessment of professional identity formation (PIF). The initiative anticipates that students will arrive on the medical school campuses at a younger age and encounter the intense academic and personal challenges of medical school with fewer life experiences and less maturity. Some faculty members voiced concerns over the potential for professionalism issues and questioned whether these younger students would be emotionally prepared for the demands of graduate medical education.

The medical schools within the TIME partnerships have substantial expertise and experience in the incorporation of professionalism within their curricula. All UT System medical schools have institutes, centers, or departments of medical ethics and humanities and well-established curricula that include traditional medical ethics and professionalism topics. However, the concept of PIF in medical education is not as well defined and is much less established.[5] Consequently, the TIME steering committee called for the creation of a UT System TIME PIF Task Force to explore PIF within the context of undergraduate medical education.

PIF Task Force and framework

In 2011, the TIME steering committee solicited applications from faculties across the UT System for the UT TIME PIF Task Force charged with defining professional identity formation as it relates to medical education, identifying activities to promote professional identity formation, and recommending strategies for the assessment of identity formation. After selection of a chair, the task force was populated to achieve a breadth of background disciplines,

representation from all four pilot program partnerships, inclusion from both undergraduate and health science campuses, and geographic diversity from across the UT System. Designated as UT Health Professionalism Scholars, the fourteen members represented seven institutions, the four pilot program partnerships, and multiple disciplines: anesthesiology, anthropology, education, ethics, internal medicine, medical humanities, obstetrics/gynecology, pediatrics, philosophy, physician assistant studies, psychiatry, psychology, student admissions, and student affairs.

After reviewing pertinent theory and background on identity development, PIF in other professions, and literature exhorting the expansion of PIF in medical education,[6,7] the task force developed a consensus definition of PIF as it relates to undergraduate medical education:

> Professional Identity Formation is the transformative journey through which one integrates the knowledge, skills, values, and behaviors of a competent, humanistic physician with one's own unique identity and core values. This continuous process fosters personal and professional growth through mentorship, reflection, and experiences that affirm the best practices, traditions, and ethics of the medical profession. The education of all medical students is founded on PIF.[3]

This definition and perspective of PIF facilitated the task force's efforts to explore activities to promote students' PIF and strategies to assess their PIF. However, the group was unable to identify a published conceptual framework upon which to arrange these activities and strategies to construct a potential curriculum for PIF. The task force looked to the outcome of the educational process – the practicing physician – to identify the essential features, activities, and characteristics required to function as a competent, humanistic physician. Through a highly iterative process influenced by the diverse backgrounds and experiences of the task force members, the group identified six domains with thirty subdomains describing physician professional identity (outlined in Figure 16.1).[8]

While these domains and subdomains provided categories on which to focus educational activities and assessment methods, they lacked a developmental perspective necessary to encompass the timeframe of the TIME initiative, spanning from high school graduation to medical school graduation. The task force adapted developmental descriptions from the

Domain	Subdomains
Attitudes	Humanism Cultural competence Service orientation
Habits	Self-directed learning Critical thinking Self-care Empathic labor Reflection Self-awareness
Perception & recognition	Biostructure and function Observational skills Cultural sensitivity Discernment Emotional intelligence Ethics competence Narrative competence

Domain	Subdomains
Duties & responsibilities	Confidentiality Appropriate disclosure Honoring commitments
Personal characteristics	Leadership Interest and curiosity Resilience and adaptability Capacity for improvement Discernment
Relationships	Collegiality Appropriate boundaries Effective relationships Effective communication Patient-centered autonomy Selection of role models

Figure 16.1. Professional identity formation domains and subdomains

professionalism competencies of the Pediatrics Milestone Project, which include five levels of professional identity milestones.[9] The first three levels are relevant to learners in the TIME initiative:

Phase I: Transition – participates as an interested but passive observer

Phase II: Early developing professional identity – appreciates the professional role but does not take primary responsibility

Phase III: Developed professional identity – understands the professional role with a genuine sense of duty and responsibility

The fourth and fifth phases (mature professional identity and broadened professional identity) are relevant to graduate medical education and professional practice, indicating that PIF continues to evolve following medical school graduation.[10]

Incorporating this longitudinal trajectory, the task force constructed a framework of educational activities and assessment strategies for each domain and subdomain across the three developmental phases. The framework also includes phase-specific objectives, definitions, background references, and resources for educators and learners (Figure 16.2). To enhance the utility of the framework, the task force worked with technology experts to convert the contents into a searchable web-based tool configurable by domain, subdomain, phase, and key word.[3,8]

While the framework does not incorporate competency-based education, it does map many of the subdomains to the TIME initiative competencies.

The PIF framework serves as a longitudinal thread alongside the TIME competencies, as advocated by Jarvis-Selinger.[11] This parallel construction is particularly important because the institutions in the TIME pilot program partnerships vary significantly in their individual academic curricula and approaches. The PIF framework provides a menu of options for each subdomain along the three-phase continuum, allowing individual institutions to incorporate the most appropriate, useful, and efficient aspects as they focus on PIF within their curricula.

Rationale for recommended methods to promote professional identity formation

Convergent with the writings of others, four guiding principles informed the development of recommendations for educational activities to foster and support PIF.[7,11,12,25] First, activities targeting PIF should encompass existing pedagogical strategies when possible and have an explicit focus on PIF. Second, activities should promote a way of being, not only a way of doing. Third, activities should target psychological growth at the individual level and socialization at the collective level. Lastly, the curricular approach should be longitudinal and build increasing responsibility for patient care.

Educators will recognize most of the activities listed on the task force framework website in support of each phase of PIF.[3] Grounding the framework and its phases in existing activities provided concrete references to the domains, drawing everyday

Domain: Perceptions and recognition		
Subdomain: Clinical observational skills		
Definition: The ability to recognize the clinical significance of normal and abnormal appearances of the body, of nonverbal and verbal communication, and the display of human emotions.		
Objectives	**Activities**	**Assessments**
Phase 1: Transition		
Recognize normal and abnormal appearance of people in art, photography, and film	Film studies, art history and art appreciation courses, faculty-led museum visits	Journaling, reflective essays, participation in museum visits
Phase 2: Early developing professional identity		
Link physical and observational findings to disease mechanisms and manifestations	Practice histories and physicals with standardized and real patients Small group PBL sessions and case conferences	OSCEs Grading of history/physical Write-ups Faculty and peer evaluations in small group exercises
Phase 3: Developed professional identity		
Recognize signs of physical disease and abnormalities in neuropsychological function	Working with patients in clinical clerkship and elective settings	OSCEs Clinical performance assessments by faculty
References: Bardes, CL, Gillers, D, Herman, AF. Learning to look: developing clinical observation skills at an art museum. *Med Educ.* 2001;35(12):1157–1161. Cox, K Teaching and learning clinical perception. *Med Educ.* 2009;30(2):90–96. Shapiro, J, Rucker, L Beck, J. Training the clinical eye and mind: using the arts to develop medical students' observational and pattern recognition skills. *Med Educ.* 2006;40(3):263–268.		

Figure 16.2. Example of professional identity formation framework

relevance to potentially elusive identity constructs. This approach facilitated application of the PIF framework to curricular and extracurricular development. In addition to being familiar and integral to medical education, many activities span multiple domains and subdomains in the framework, allowing for efficient integration of students' PIF with existing formal and informal curricula.[13–15] The framework includes extracurricular activities in recognition that identity formation is a complex process encompassing learning in the formal, informal, and hidden curricula. The recommended activities utilize existing pedagogical strategies with an explicit emphasis on PIF, thus facilitating integration with other components of the curricula.

The recommended activities target deep personal transformation associated with identity change. The progression of activities includes adopting professional behaviors and practicing being in the role of physician while the underlying principles are internalized. Changes in behavior can influence attitudes as well as the reverse.[16] Instruction regarding professionalism is an essential and logical starting point and can be integrated with instruction regarding humanism.

The progression of PIF activities from transition to developed phases complements students' progression from the curious observer exploring professional opportunities to the engaged learner internalizing the knowledge and values of the profession consistent with other frameworks for personal and professional development.[17–20] The PIF phases of transition, early developing, and developed identities may require changes in attitudes, habits, and relationships. Psychological growth and professional socialization must be fostered in ways that emphasize their comparable importance to the mastery of scientific content and clinical skills.

Educational activities fostering the deep transformation associated with PIF should be longitudinal and cumulative in nature and include a clear focus on the patient as PIF occurs primarily in the context of patient care. The framework recommends engagement in authentic, situated learning early in the educational process. Transformation through PIF experiences arises from feedback and self-reflection, leading to insight into the potential congruence of personal and professional identities.[22–25] The PIF experiences listed in the framework derive from the practices, standards, and ethics of medicine as a science, an art, a profession, and a culture.[25] For PIF experiences to be relevant, students' work should relate closely to patients and patient care.[24,26] More broadly stated, PIF experiences appear grounded in the human condition, human interactions, humanism, and, ultimately, humanity.

Recommended pedagogic strategies

Reflection

For experiences to inform students' core values, self-reflection, especially regarding dissonances, provides necessary respite to discern the personal relevance.[22,27–32] Reflective writing as well as discussions of books and movies are included in the PIF framework as recommended activities. Both introspection and consideration of the reflections of others can foster personal growth.[33–35] Reflective writing may take the form of assigned essays with specific topics or routine personal journaling regarding the impact of experiences on personal growth. Recommended topics for reflection include critical incidents, clinical encounters, and ethical dilemmas.

Clinical experiences and clinical skills training

Patient-centered experiences can enhance students' PIF.[36] In the context of the framework described above, student experiences provide increasing proximity to patient care, for the patient encounter represents the epicenter of physician practice, as described by Verghese.[37] A physician must also effectively present explanations to patients and peers to effect high quality, compassionate, and safe patient care.[38–41] The necessary communication skills develop through a variety of simulated and authentic interactions in formal and informal curricula.[26,42,43] Early clinical experiences may occur through shadowing, volunteering, and longitudinal clerkship experiences to support developing PIF.[44]

Experiences of the profession

Professional standards, statutes, and credentialing regulate a physician's practice. PIF experiences relative to this realm enable students to gain insight into the official parameters of practice.[45–47] Medical student education in professionalism, including e-professionalism, remains a tenet of physicianhood.[48] Brody and Doukas point out that professionalism education for medical students falls under two precepts: trust-generating promise from physician to patient and application of virtue to practice.[49] The Physicianship curriculum at the McGill University Faculty of Medicine provides an exemplar of such education.[50] Such experiences may mitigate factors

that result in future impairment and disruptive conduct.[51–53]

Experiences in the arts, history, and wellness

The academic separation of sciences and humanities in medical education arose from historical roots resulting in greater emphasis on scientific equanimity over humanistic practice.[54] In the mid twentieth century, the introduction of humanities into American medical education came in response to a growing need to train holistic physicians with broad backgrounds and experiences.[54–55] Elective humanities experiences provide medical students with creative, reflective, and safe media to explore the human condition and to hone observational skills as well as metacognitive skills.[55–56] Examples of such opportunities include medicine in literature, cinema, history, and arts. Deliberately created to weave mindfulness, humanism, and healing, Remen's "Healer's Art" elective allows medical students and faculty to connect their education and practice with their humanity and to develop resilience against professional identity deformation.[57–60]

Mentoring and advising

Guidance provided by mentors, teachers, and role models, including peers, enables students to consider their personal growth with relative safety[24] exerting powerful influence on students' perception of the profession and the professional[61–62] often within the context of the hidden curriculum.[25] Opportunities for positive role modeling and mentorship may be established via learning communities and programs, including student organizations, for career exploration and formal advising opportunities.

Additional pedagogies

Learning communities harness the collective expertise, experiences, and energy of students to create and sustain an active culture of education and life on and off campus[63] offering longitudinal and regular touchpoints for PIF through experiences that bring together faculty and students.[64] Learning communities serve as a tool for teaching and learning professionalism[65] and may provide a focus on student career counseling and wellness in synergy with formal curricula.[66]

Interprofessional experiences positively support students' individual PIF and may give rise to tension in team dynamics when individuals strongly identify with their profession over the team.[67] Strategies to mitigate such tension include awareness of affective conflict emergence, commitment to shared goals, and exploration of shared values.[67] Interprofessional experiences focusing on common patient-care goals are effective.[67–69] Key ingredients for programmatic success include administrative support, faculty and student commitment, and interprofessional infrastructure.[70]

Extracurricular opportunities such as summer camps for children with medical conditions, student organizations and government, community service, and global health electives enrich students' education and better prepare them for practice in a multicultural, interprofessional, and patient-centered environment advancing their PIF through contextual exploration and application.[71] Students calibrate their moral compasses and affirm their future role in society through service learning experiences.[71] International medical missions and global health experiences immerse medical students in cross-cultural settings that can strengthen and challenge their PIF.[72,73]

The societal expectation that physicians will serve as leaders has been the subject primarily of informal, extra-, and hidden curricula.[74–76] Formal leadership training in the medical curriculum, including dual-degree programs, could more effectively prepare medical students to be positive change agents in the healthcare environment.[76–80] Research opportunities for medical students, including quality improvement studies, introduce them to scholarly aspects of the profession, hone their scientific literacy and critical thinking skills,[81–82] and can integrate reflection, self-improvement, and mentorship necessary to support PIF.[83]

Rationale for recommended strategies to assess professional identity formation

The complex nature of PIF presents formidable challenges to the assessment of students. Contemporary understanding of the process as multifaceted, nonlinear, and largely noncognitive led to careful examination of the assumptions and frameworks the task force employed to develop strategies for assessment.

The first consideration was the purpose of assessing PIF. The approach of the task force was to construct assessments *for* learning rather than assessments *of* learning.[84] Assessment for development (formative) identifies current status of students for the purpose of

planning a future course of action. Assessment of development (summative) identifies current status in order to identify progress from a past position or to compare to standards. Different domains or subdomains may develop at different rates as a result of experience. In addition, new identities arise cyclically throughout the educational process, e.g., from student observer of care to student provider of care to upper-level-student role modeling provision of care. The lack of an expectation of common trajectories or benchmarks renders an achievement paradigm associated with summative assessment rarely applicable. The process of PIF currently has insufficient explication to allow standard setting.[8] Assessments of PIF are information to be utilized by learners, mentors, and advisors to select and shape next steps in students' personal and professional growth and learning. The recommendation of the task force to the TIME partnerships is that assessment be designed and implemented formatively.

A second broad principle guiding the strategies for assessment of PIF is that such assessment should be programmatic by design.[85,86] This approach strengthens the validity of assessment by employing multiple methods from multiple perspectives over multiple occasions. Assessments specifically targeting development within subdomains are important building blocks to a broader view of PIF. No single assessment sufficiently captures the breadth and depth of PIF. For example, within a given time period, students might engage in reflective writing providing insight about their service orientation; participate in an objective structured clinical examination (OSCE) in which the standardized patients evaluate their professionalism; and be evaluated by preceptors on cultural competence in their patient encounters. Such a combination of assessments would provide a rich descriptive quilt of students' development within the attitudes domain in the framework. Careful planning or blueprinting facilitates programmatic assessment that encompasses the complexity of PIF. The task force recommends that responsibility for planning programmatic assessment be explicitly incorporated into curriculum design for PIF. Portfolios are also recommended for capturing the combined assessments and providing a longitudinal perspective.

The third guiding principle of the task force in approaching assessment of PIF was that it is a form of learning primarily in the affective domain as identified in Bloom's taxonomy of affective learning, rather than the more commonly used cognitive taxonomy.[87]

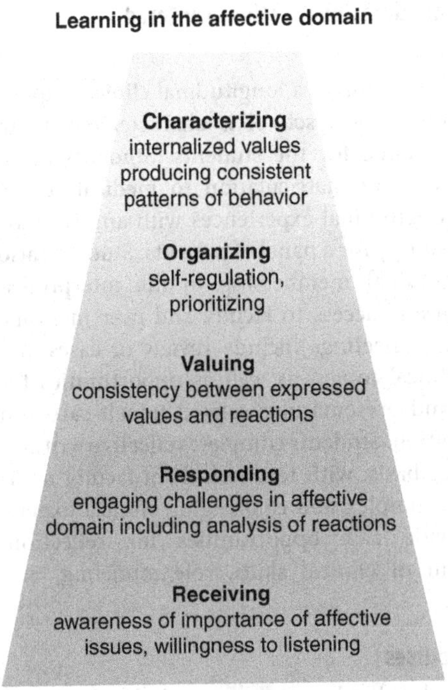

Learning in the affective domain

Characterizing
internalized values
producing consistent
patterns of behavior

Organizing
self-regulation,
prioritizing

Valuing
consistency between expressed
values and reactions

Responding
engaging challenges in affective
domain including analysis of reactions

Receiving
awareness of importance of affective
issues, willingness to listening

Figure 16.3. Assessment of professional identity formation development may consider levels attained in Bloom's taxonomy[87]

Bloom's levels of learning in the affective domain, as outlined in Figure 16.3, provide a useful framework for planning formative, contextual assessment of the domains and subdomains of PIF.

Students in the transition and early developing identity phases may be expected to exhibit an awareness of the importance of the values and habits of the profession. Through their continued PIF development, students would likely be able to respond critically to cases or literary representations of physicians facing challenging situations. Eventually, students would develop a consistency between their perception of who a physician should be and the reality of who they actually are. For example, students may believe that physicians should be empathic and, therefore, practice empathy with patients and colleagues. Eventually, they are able to self-regulate in ways that allow them to behave consistently with their physicianhood in the face of competing emotions or values. At this level, students would demonstrate empathy even as they process feelings such as anger or dislike that might otherwise be directed at the patient. Eventually students achieve a level of consistency across domains to serve as role models for the attitudes, habits, and values fundamental to being humanistic physicians.

An assessment system for PIF requires sufficient flexibility to accommodate development at different rates across subdomains. Students may respond to a sense of duty and value cultural competency in their acceptance of peers with different backgrounds, thus attaining different levels on Bloom's affective taxonomy. Considering the progression of development in Figure 16.3 helps move assessments away from dichotomous approaches toward more complex strategies examining the quality of development in a domain or subdomain. Such information can then become the focus of mentoring sessions or personal growth plans.

Because PIF develops within the context of learning and practicing, assessment also needs to be contextual. Therefore the task force recommended, where possible, to embed assessment of identity formation within existing assessments, adding elements specifically targeting PIF. Such opportunities are present in the application of reflective writing, OSCEs, faculty evaluations, peer evaluations, surveys, and portfolios. Reflective writing is a curricular activity thought to deepen the learning experience and promote PIF.[33-35] Adding an assessment element may range from having the written products as a topic of discussion with mentors to having students answer essay questions about what they need to facilitate their growth into the next phase of development. OSCEs and faculty evaluations as well as peer evaluations provide external formative touchpoints for learners. Adaptation of existing assessments may include adding questions regarding perceived development in a specific subdomain or more broadly about areas of strength or challenge in developing identity. Similarly, medical students regularly complete surveys for a variety of purposes. Inclusion of questions about professional identity in course evaluations or standardized survey instruments targeting specific subdomains can yield rich PIF information for learners and mentors. Portfolios designed to capture evidence of competency attainment can include a section for information about identity development. The aggregation of information into a portfolio would provide a longitudinal perspective allowing for a broader view of students' developmental trajectory not readily available from more narrow or discrete pieces of information.

The triangulated strategies described thus far constitute an overall approach to the assessment of PIF, measuring multiple aspects from multiple perspectives at multiple points in time. Development of assessment blueprints, at least at the pilot program partnership level, was endorsed by the task force as a strategy to ensure that all domains are assessed across time. This raises the question of whether there is a gestalt to PIF that will be missed by such a granular approach. The task force encouraged medical educators at all partnerships to explore opportunities for global assessment, having found no well-developed approaches for global assessment of professional identity to recommend prior to implementation of the TIME initiative.

Implementation of the recommendations

Promotion of professional identity formation

The TIME initiative institutions have incorporated multiple methods to enhance the development of professional identity, based on the rationale previously discussed. These methods include early, authentic clinical and immersion experiences, reflection, community service learning, learning communities, and mentoring and advising, in addition to structured courses incorporating foundational concepts in ethics, humanities, and professionalism. Undergraduate and medical school campuses of the four pilot program partnerships incorporate these strategies for different levels of students in various ways based on local curricula, resources, and preferences. We will summarize several examples in which these strategies have been integrated into curricula at undergraduate and medical school campuses.

Summer experiences

At many undergraduate campuses, students enter the TIME initiative in the summer immediately following high school graduation. During the initial summer, students are introduced to the program, expectations, active learning modalities, competency-based education, and the concept of PIF. Subsequent summer sessions include community service learning, clinical skills development, preceptorships with community practitioners, global health immersion experiences, and travel to medical school campuses. These diverse experiences integrate reflection, role modeling, mentorship, teamwork, and authentic clinical encounters, all of which are reinforced throughout their fall and spring semester courses and extracurricular activities, in part by medical school faculty who conduct workshops at the undergraduate campuses.

Longitudinal educational patient-centered medical home

The implementation of a longitudinal clinical experience in one medical school is characterized as an educational home for the students. Students begin this experience at matriculation to medical school and have longitudinal experiences with and increasing responsibility for a panel of patients. Students also have longitudinal membership in the interprofessional team and access to faculty and peer mentors. Weekly team meetings include review of cases and relevant clinical topics, as well as opportunities for reflection and presentations related to self-care and communication. Students complete reflective writings on a regular basis, with feedback from faculty mentors. These complex and challenging clinical experiences provide rich opportunities for reflection, development of clinical skills, role modeling, and mentoring.

Doctoring courses

The medical school campuses include doctoring courses of various designs. At one school, students participate in doctoring courses across all four years. These courses, taught mainly in small groups by clinical faculty, incorporate clinical skills development, simulated and real clinical encounters, ethics, professionalism, medical humanities, theater, reflective writing and discussions, and mentoring and advising. Students also discuss topics such as self-care, burnout, impairment, professional dilemmas, awe in medicine, career options, and humanism.

These activities and content topics are very pertinent to the development of professional identity and are included in the PIF framework.

Courses at another pilot partnership medical school and some undergraduate campuses use *The Brewsters: An Interactive Adventure in Ethics for the Health Professions*.[88] As students work through this fictional story, they select characters and make decisions in ethically and professionally charged situations, while incorporating the foundations of professionalism and ethics. Other programs incorporate art observation experiences or creative expressions projects. Integrated into these various activities are multiple opportunities for reflection and feedback.

Student learning communities

Several UT System medical schools have developed learning communities. At one school, all students are placed into learning communities on entry into medical school. These groupings are utilized for small-group class assignments during the first two years. The learning communities promote community service learning, socialization, social support, role modeling, and faculty and peer mentoring.[65] Some undergraduate campuses have also developed learning communities for their TIME students, promoting teamwork, mentoring, and social support.

Scholarly concentrations

Medical school curricula routinely provide students with opportunities for concentrated study in an area of interest. These are integrated over the duration of medical school and include elective courses and extracurricular experiences. They include learning communities, meetings of faculty and students with similar interests, opportunities for mentoring, and professional socialization. Some areas of concentration are specialty-related, e.g., aerospace medicine or geriatrics. Others allow students to deepen their exploration of subjects that receive minimal attention within traditional medical curricula, e.g., medical humanities or translational research. A third category of concentrations relates to cultivating the values of a competent, humanistic physician. These include programs in global, rural, and bilingual health in which students' experiences prepare them to address the needs of patients who often experience barriers to healthcare.

At one pilot partnership medical school, a scholarly concentration has been designed and implemented with the explicit purpose of supporting students' PIF. Small groups of six to eight students and two faculty members meet for dinner throughout medical school. These meetings include reflective discussions of assigned experiences as well as regular written reflections including journaling and essays. The small groups and eight-week preceptorship after the first year of study provide sustained mentoring within a learning community. The first year of the track focuses on personal development topics, e.g., stress management and mindfulness. The second year focuses on being authentic in interactions with others, e.g., experiencing and expressing empathy, cultural understanding, and delivering bad news. In the third and fourth years, these topics are revisited with an emphasis on application in a clinical context. Elements of this cohesive, longitudinal program are being adapted for use with all students.

Extracurricular activities

Students at medical and undergraduate campuses have access to a variety of extracurricular activities that promote PIF. These include clinical shadowing, research projects, student-run free clinics, partnerships with local schools for health education and coaching, faith-based volunteering, and community services. These diverse experiences provide rich opportunities for personal and professional growth.

Assessment of professional identity formation

Assessment activities vary widely across pilot program partnerships. Integration into other assessment activities has been challenging on the undergraduate campuses where there is little to no precedent for assessing professionalism or identity development. Appropriately for learners in the initial phases of identity development, most assessments focus on the receiving and responding levels of Bloom's hierarchy of affective learning.

One common activity among partnerships is reflective writing about movies or literature, highlighting the affective qualities that impact the success of physicians, or writing about the emotional impact of early clinical experiences, such as volunteering with health providers in resource-limited regions. Through these activities, mentors are able to assess the extent to which students develop an awareness of the importance of affective issues in physician identity and are willing to analyze their own affective reactions. For many students in this phase, learning the science necessary for entry into medical school overshadows the importance of affective development. Feedback on required reflections provides an important mechanism for introducing students to the importance and need for continuing development.[89,90] Integration of reflective writing is both a curricular strategy for developing reflective practice and an assessment strategy for assessing students' ability to critically reflect and their development in other content-dependent domains. For example, students' reflections on volunteer experiences provide insight about students' reflective capacity and about the nature of the volunteering activities and their contribution to students' PIF.

All campuses have developed some mechanism for identifying lapses in professionalism and providing feedback to students as issues arise. This type of assessment increases student awareness of the importance of affective issues and helps them engage in the process of identifying and addressing challenges. It is necessary to identify student lapses in professional development in order to identify students' needs for support and opportunities for remediation.[91] It may be challenging to maintain a culture of positive, constructive feedback necessary for growth if this is the primary form of assessment.

Another common strategy is the inclusion of PIF in end-of-semester or end-of-year evaluation meetings. These meetings between students and mentors or advisors include consideration of both competency achievement and PIF. During undergraduate years, the discussion around PIF at these meetings centers on issues of self-direction, self-assessment, ability to use feedback, and accepting responsibility for meeting obligations.

Peer evaluation has been identified in some partnerships as a transformational assessment strategy. Students who are trained to give specific, constructive feedback can communicate effectively with peers about their perceptions of one another's development in domains of interest. Students could discern whether and how the habits of their peers are those that would contribute to the effectiveness of being a physician, e.g., critical thinking, self-care, or self-directed learning. Such items can be included alongside more traditional evaluations of team members, e.g., punctuality, cooperation, or listening skills. For example, one summer course uses a team professionalism contract in which student teams agree to abide by professionalism principles in the course. Students are held accountable for the professional conduct and actions of the entire team. Thus, students learn to observe peer behavior, provide feedback, and devise corrective strategies. This moves the learning from the *responding* level of Bloom's affective taxonomy, in which students would analyze cases presented to the class, into the *valuing* level, in which they examine their own and others' behavior for consistency with clearly articulated values.

Several partnerships use individual professionalism contracts. These have been used as learning strategies as well as assessment tools. These contracts provide clear expectations, structure experiential learning of professional habits, and serve as a basis for self-assessment to be compared with the perspectives of other assessments as a topic for discussions with mentors, advisors, and peers.

Surveys designed specifically for students in the TIME program as well as standardized instruments have been used as part of programmatic assessment. One partnership has adapted a professionalism self-assessment originally designed for students in physician-assistant training. Standardized instruments of empathy that we have used include the Interpersonal Reactivity Index (IRI) and the Jefferson Scale of Empathy.[92,93]

Data from numerous sources appear in portfolios and can be considered as indicative of PIF. Cognitive assessments of the fundamentals of professionalism and ethics also serve as formative assessments of development when used as the basis for discussion of the implications for the process of becoming a physician. Evaluations and letters from clinical faculty whom students shadow and supervisors at sites where students volunteer often contain comments about responsibility, professionalism, and opportunities for addressing additional domains and subdomains of the PIF framework.

Management of assessment information provides significant additional challenges. The need for longitudinal assessment that reflects growth over time requires accumulation and coordination of assessment data. Some partnerships maintain databases dedicated to track all PIF information and feedback for students. Others utilize portfolios to compile evidence of PIF in addition to targeting evidence of competency-based achievement. Integrated approaches of combining curricular experiences and formative assessment, e.g., reflection, professionalism contracts, and self-assessments, including aspects of the learner's identity development, ease the management and implementation burdens. At the UT System level, an effort is underway to develop a common database format to serve as both portfolio and data repository.

Challenges in the development and implementation of a curriculum on professional identity formation

The TIME partnership campuses encountered a variety of challenges as they developed and implemented curricula incorporating the promotion and assessment of PIF. These challenges fall into three main categories: (1) working across undergraduate and medical campuses; (2) working across diverse partnerships; and (3) working across UT System institutions.

A number of the challenges encountered relate to gaps at the undergraduate and medical school campus level, such as differences in language and terminology, educational methods, curricular calendars, goals, priorities, and accreditation requirements. Undergraduate campuses work with a wide variety of students with diverse career goals, while medical schools focus primarily on preparing physicians. Medical campuses have access to large clinical faculties for teaching and mentoring, while undergraduate campuses may depend on local practitioners and visiting clinicians.

These underlying differences contribute substantially to communication challenges. Terminology often requires translation and explanation. Differences in context, scope, and scale hinder understanding across the undergraduate–medical school chasm. Face-to-face meetings are sometimes limited by geographic separation between campuses and differences in time zones across Texas. Communication challenges limit the ability to share information about existing programs, strengths, needs, and planning. Undergraduate and medical campuses express uncertainty about sharing student information in a feed-forward process.

Other areas of challenge include the faculties on the undergraduate and medical campuses. Recruiting and engaging interested faculty and acquiring buy-in require significant time and effort. Undergraduate campuses without clinical programs must recruit community clinicians and partner with medical school faculties. Faculty development across all campuses requires substantial investment of resources.

These issues involving communication and faculty make the process of setting and applying standards across undergraduate and medical campuses challenging, especially as they relate to PIF and professionalism. What are the professionalism expectations? How are they established? How are they incorporated in curricula? What are the policies for their application? PIF is a less developed and established construct with no established assessments with proven validity or reliability in medical education. This context makes building a curriculum, securing buy-in, and providing faculty development related to PIF challenging.

In addition to the challenges that affect undergraduate medical school campus interactions, several other issues affect PIF curriculum development and implementation at the pilot program partnership level. The four partnerships (which include a variable number of undergraduate and medical school campuses) and their component institutions may have different goals and priorities. For one partnership, the geographic separation between campuses makes communication, coordination, and faculty development more difficult, time consuming, and expensive. For partnerships with multiple undergraduate campuses, variations in programs or learners can impact curriculum implementation, especially when setting standards for content, processes, and metrics. Changes in campus leadership can affect partnership dynamics.

Moving up to the perspective of the UT System TIME initiative level, additional challenges have influenced the development and implementation of a PIF curriculum. As the PIF Task Force worked to explore the construct of PIF and to develop the framework and recommendations, the need for ongoing leadership and faculty development increased. Dissemination and communication about the PIF framework, website, and content required regular communication, especially as the number of people involved across the TIME initiative increased. As implementation continues, identification and dissemination of best practices will require data collection, management, and analytics. This system-level approach necessitates central support and oversight along with campus-level support and coordination. Finally, important changes in the UT System that will impact this work include reorganization of some partnership undergraduate campuses and the introduction of two new medical schools.

Strategies for overcoming challenges

The TIME initiative has utilized a number of strategies to overcome the challenges summarized above. Early identification of the need to establish a UT System-wide PIF Task Force was very helpful in exploring PIF and developing a curricular framework for PIF, including strategies for its promotion and assessment. This process fostered collaboration and a common language for the task force members distributed across the TIME partnership campuses. Individually and as a group, task force members communicated with TIME partnership leaders and faculty, cultivated local buy-in, and provided faculty development. The group has also been successful in disseminating academic scholarship from their collaborations. All of these outcomes promoted communication about PIF across the institutions and faculties involved in the TIME initiative.

The conversion of the PIF framework and menu-oriented recommendations into a web-based format has been very helpful in addressing the dispersed nature of the TIME partnership campuses and variations in pilot partnership programs.[3] This tool provides campus programs with a variety of options to assist in their incorporation of PIF within their curricula. The task force members also provide local expertise and resources for the campuses.

Additional strategies utilized to improve communications include joint meetings of the TIME initiative groups with imbedded faculty development workshops, updates from the PIF task force, demonstrations of the PIF website, and presentations about local innovations with elements of PIF. Open, frequent discussions fostered improved understanding of language, awareness of campus and partnership variations, faculty buy-in, and creation of a shared vision.

Pilot program partnership meetings include many of these same features. Partnerships with geographically dispersed campuses plan meetings in tandem with the larger TIME initiative conferences for better efficiency and use of resources. Those partnerships also utilize technological solutions for virtual meetings and rotate meetings across campuses to promote familiarity and engagement with local faculty and learners. Campuses with limited access to clinical faculty established relationships with local clinicians and community healthcare resources to provide students with opportunities for mentoring, clinical exposure, and reflection.

Some pilot program partnerships utilize traveling educational activities to enhance faculty development, to provide structured educational activities for learners, and to establish common standards across campuses. Selected leaders and faculty conduct these educational offerings that reinforce the TIME competencies, set common ground rules and expectations, provide more exposure to clinicians, and incorporate PIF and professionalism. Members from the PIF task force also travel to partnership campuses to engage learners in activities devoted to medical ethics, professionalism, and PIF.

Other key strategies for overcoming challenges benefit from consistent support and funding from the UT System, including the Regents and the Executive Vice Chancellor for Health Affairs. This support strengthens the vision and goals of the TIME initiative and the importance of PIF. The TIME steering committee has approved the PIF task force's recommendations for a central PIF director and a PIF faculty leader on each local campus. These dedicated champions will ensure further adoption and expansion of PIF within curricula across the TIME pilot program partnerships.

Lessons learned and next steps

PIF curriculum

Early clinical experiences have proved very powerful for students. The ability to see role models in action and engage in legitimate peripheral participation[94] with patient contact provide opportunities for students to assume identities beyond that of typical undergraduate students. The early practice of habits and attitudes integral to PIF allows those aspects to be incorporated into students' identities such that they can be retained, even as the cognitive load of learning clinical skills increases. Maintaining a balance of course content fosters students' development and may mitigate the impact of the hidden curriculum. At the undergraduate level, pre-professional curricula have traditionally focused on achievement in science courses in ways that inhibited students' development in other areas. The deliberate inclusion of education about professionalism coupled with increased emphasis on courses in the humanities and social sciences may counteract the impression students often develop that only biophysical sciences and clinical skills are important for becoming a physician.

One of the ongoing lessons is that de novo curriculum development requires more time and energy than most educators can envision. It is important to have a realistic timeline that allows for inevitable missteps and a scholarly approach to developing curricular goals and materials. Because there are no extant PIF curricula from which to draw models, passionate, dedicated faculty have invested a tremendous effort to realize the implementation of curricular activities to support and cultivate PIF. It is imperative that these initial curricula remain flexible and be dynamic and responsive to feedback and student needs.

PIF assessment

Systematic formative assessment that aggregates into potentially summative assessment decisions has been achieved through mentoring and advising programs. An important lesson has been that faculty development is necessary to achieve implementation of a system in which faculty provide and document effective feedback to learners regarding PIF. The culture of higher education may value formative assessment in theory more than in practice. For both faculty and students, there seems to be a strong preference for assessments to directly impact grades.

The PIF framework explicates many complex components of PIF well. It could be used to blueprint programmatic assessment for a partnership. This will be among the next steps for the PIF director and leaders at the campus, partnership, and system levels.

An additional important next step in assessing PIF is the exploration of options for global assessment of PIF. A common global assessment of PIF is attractive for a number of reasons. It would be comparable across settings, would help elucidate developmental trajectories among students, and would ease the assessment burden on students and programs. Kegan's work has been applied to written essays in other professions and presents an opportunity to adapt that work to medicine.[18,95–97] This will require basic psychometric studies and additional faculty development for effective implementation.

PIF coordination

As a curricular topic that is integrated into many courses and experiences, PIF is at risk of becoming fragmented or an afterthought. To circumvent this, the task force recommended that explicit responsibility be assigned and supported at the campus, partnership, and system levels. That recommendation has been approved, and next steps include identifying the appropriate leaders and champions and planning for coordination of efforts. Planning will include both curriculum and assessments.

Now that programs have begun, program evaluation will be an important next step. The TIME initiative approach of having several pilot programs from which to choose best practices will require that the program outcomes be comparable in terms of strengths and weaknesses of each approach. Additionally, approaches will need to be assessed for scalability and generalizability. Will programs be as effective in a different institutional context or with larger groups of students? Answering these questions will require continued dedication and effort from all involved with TIME.

Acknowledgements

The authors gratefully acknowledge the contributions and support of the following groups and individuals without whom this endeavor would not have been possible: The Professional Identity Formation Task Force (Mark D. Holden, M.D., Era Buck, Ph.D., John Luk, M.D., Frank Ambriz, M.P.A.S., PA-C, Eugene V. Boisaubin, M.D., Mark A. Clark, Ph.D., Angela P. Mihalic, M.D., John Z. Sadler, M.D., Kenneth Sapire, M.D., Jeffrey Spike, Ph.D., Alan Vince, Ph.D., John L. Dalrymple, M.D., J. Scott Wright, Ed.D., and David Henzi, Ed.D.); the TIME Initiative Steering Committee; the leaders and faculty of the TIME partnerships; the University of Texas System and, specifically, Kenneth Shine, M.D., Raymond Greenberg, M.D., Ph.D., Pedro Reyes, Ph.D., and Steve Lieberman, M.D.; Laura Rampy, M.S.; and the amazing students in the TIME partnerships.

References

1. Englander, R, Cameron, T, Ballard, AJ, Dodge, J, Bull, J, Aschenbrener, CA. Toward a common taxonomy of competency domains for the health professions and competencies for physicians. *Acad Med.* 2013; **88**(8):1088–94.

2. Frank, JR, Danoff, D. The CanMEDS initiative: implementing and outcomes-based framework of physician competencies. *Med Teach.* 2007; **29**(7):642–47.

3. The University of Texas Professional Identity Formation Task Force. Galveston, TX: University of Texas Medical Branch; 2013. [Accessed Jan. 30, 2015.] Available from http://ar.utmb.edu/timepif/home.

4. Dyrbye, LN, Harper, W, Moutier, C, Durning, SJ, Power, DV, Massie, FS, Eacker, A, Thomas, MR, Satele, D, Sloan, JA, Shanafelt, TD. A multi-institutional study exploring the impact of positive mental health on medical students' professionalism in an era of high burnout. *Acad Med.* 2012; **87**(8):1024–31.

5. Holden, M, Buck, E, Clark, M, Szauter, K, Trumble, J. Professional identity formation in medical education: the convergence of multiple domains. *HEC Forum.* 2012; **24**(4):245–55.

6. Inui, TS. *A Flag in the Wind: Educating for Professionalism in Medicine.* Washington, DC: Association of American Medical Colleges; 2003.

7. Cooke, M, Irby, DM, O'Brien, BC. *Educating Physicians: A Call for Reform of Medical School and Residency.* San Francisco, CA: Jossey-Bass; 2010.

8. Holden, MD, Buck, E, Luk, J, Ambriz, F, Boisaubin, EV, Clark, MA, Mihalic, AP, Sadler, JZ, Sapire, KJ, Spike, JP, Vince, A, Dalrymple, JL. Professional identity formation: creating a longitudinal framework through TIME (Transformation in Medical Education). *Acad Med.* 2015; **90**(6):761–67.

9. The Pediatrics Milestone Working Group. *The Pediatrics Milestone Project.* Chicago, IL: Accreditation Council for Graduate Medical Education and the American Board of Pediatrics; 2012. [Accessed Jan. 27, 2015.] Available from www.acgme.org/acgmeweb/Port als/0/PDFs/Milestones/320_PedsMilestonesProject.pdf.

10. Hicks, PJ, Schumacher, DJ, Benson, BJ, Burke, AE, Englander, R, Guralnick, S, Ludwig, S, Carraccio, C. The Pediatrics Milestones: conceptual framework, guiding principles, and approach to development. *J Grad Med Educ.* 2010; **2**(23):410–18.

11. Jarvis-Selinger, S, Pratt, DD, Regehr, G. Competency is not enough: integrating identity development into the medical education discourse. *Acad Med.* 2012; **87**(9):1185–90.

12. Cruess, RL, Cruess, SR, Boudreau, JD, Snell, L, Steinert, Y. Reframing medical education to support professional identity formation. *Acad Med.* 2014; **89**(11):1446–51.

13. Astin, AW. Student involvement: a development theory for higher education. *J Coll Stud Dev.* 1999; **40**(5):518–29.

14. Speirs Neumeister, KL, Rinker, J. An emerging professional identity: influences on the achievement of high ability first-generation college females. *Journal for the Education of the Gifted.* 2006; **29**(3):305–38.

15. Gyer, J. *Development of Adolescent Identity Formation through Extracurricular Activities.* Master's thesis. Dallas, TX: Southern Methodist University; 2014.

16. Albarracín, D, Wyer, RS Jr. The cognitive impact of past behavior: influences on beliefs, attitudes, and future behavioral decisions. *J Pers Soc Psychol.* 2000; **79**(1):5–22.

17. Chávez, AF, Guido-DiBrito, F, Mallory, SL. Learning to value the "other": a framework of individual diversity development. *J Coll Stud Dev.* 2003; **44**(4):453–69.

18. Kegan, R. *In Over Our Heads: The Mental Demands of Modern Life.* Cambridge, MA: Harvard University Press; 1994.

19. Baxter Magolda, MB. Three elements of self-authorship. *J Coll Stud Dev.* 2008; **49**(4):269–84.

20. Johnson, JL. Self-authorship in pharmacy education. *Am J Pharm Educ.* 2013; **77**(4):69.

21. Nadelson, LS, McGuire, S, McAdams, K, Farid, A, Davis, K, Nagarajan, R, Wang, S, Kaiser, U, Hsu, Y-C. *Am I a STEM Professional? Self-Authorship and Student Professional Identity Development.* Poster presentation.

NSF Improving the Undergraduate STEM Experience Conference. Washington, DC: National Academy of Sciences; 2014. [Accessed Jan. 30, 2015.] Available from http://stem.boisestate.edu/wp-content/uploads/2014/02/SA-and-LP-Poster.pdf.

22. Naudé, L. On (un)common ground: transforming from dissonance to commitment in a service learning class. *J Coll Stud Dev.* 2015; **56**(1):84–102.

23. Moss, JM, Gibson, DM, Dollarhide, CT. Professional identity development: a grounded theory of transformational tasks of counselors. *J Couns Dev.* 2014; **92**(1):3–12.

24. Ryynänen, K. *Constructing Physician's Professional Identity – Explorations of Students' Critical Experiences in Medical Education.* Helsinki, FI: Oulu University Press; 2001.

25. Goldie, J. The formation of professional identity in medical students: considerations for educators. *Med Teach.* 2012; **34**(9):e641–e648.

26. Graungaard, AH, Andersen, JS. Meeting real patients: a qualitative study of medical students' experiences of early patient contact. *Educ Prim Care.* 2014; **25**(3):132–39.

27. Phillips, D, Fawns, R, Hayes, B. From personal reflection to social positioning: the development of a transformational model of professional education in midwifery. *Nurs Inq.* 2002; **9**(4):239–49.

28. Wald, HS, Borkan, JM, Taylor, JS, Anthony, D, Reis, SP. Fostering and evaluating reflective capacity in medical education: developing the REFLECT rubric for assessing reflective writing. *Acad Med.* 2012; **87**(1):41–50.

29. Niemi, PM. Medical students' professional identity: self-reflection during the preclinical years. *Med Educ.* 1997; **31**(6):408–15.

30. Mann, K, Gordon, J, MacLeod, A. Reflection and reflective practice in health professions education: a systemic review. *Adv Health Sci Educ Theory Pract.* 2009; **14**(4):595–621.

31. Thompson, BM, Teal, CR, Rogers, JC, Paterniti, DA, Haidet, P. Ideals, activities, dissonance, and processing: a conceptual model to guide educators' efforts to stimulate student reflection. *Acad Med.* 2010; **85**(5):902–08.

32. Shapiro, J, Kasman, D, Shafer, A. Words and wards: a model of reflective writing and its uses in medical education. *J Med Humanit.* 2006; **27**(4):231–44.

33. Nothnagle, M, Reis, S, Goldman, RE, Anandarajah, G. Fostering professional formation in residency: development and evaluation of the "forum" seminar series. *Teach Learn Med.* 2014; **26**(3):230–38.

34. Song, P, Stewart, R. Reflective writing in medical education. *Med Teach.* 2012; **34**(11):955–56.

35. Travers, CJ, Morisano, D, Locke, EA. Self-reflection, growth goals, and academic outcomes: a qualitative study. *Br J Educ Psychol.* 2015; **85**(2):224–41.

36. Noble, C, O'Brien, M, Coombes, I, Shaw, PN, Nissen, L, Clavarino, A. Becoming a pharmacist: students' perception of their curricular experience and professional identity formation. *Curr Pharm Teach Learn*. 2014; **6**(3):327–39.

37. Verghese, A. *Bedside Manners*. Austin, TX: Texas Monthly; Feb. 2007. [Accessed Jan. 30, 2015]. Available from www.texasmonthly.com/content/bedside-manners.

38. Shivji, FS, Ramoutar, DN, Bailey, C, Hunter, JB. Improving communication with primary care to ensure patient safety post-hospital discharge. *Br J Hosp Med (Lond)*. 2015; **76**(1):46–49.

39. Scalise, D. Clinical communication and patient safety. *Hosp Health News*. 2006; **80**(8):49–54.

40. American College of Obstetricians and Gynecologists. ACOG Committee Opinion No. 587: effective patient-physician communication. *Obstet Gynecol*. 2014; **123**(2 Pt 1):389–93.

41. Travaline, JM, Ruchinskas, R, D'Alonzo, GE Jr. Patient-physician communication: why and how. *J Am Osteopath Assoc*. 2005; **105**(1):13–18.

42. Eisenberg, A, Rosenthal, S, Schlussel, YR. Medicine as a performing art: what we can learn about empathic communication from theater arts. *Acad Med*. 2015; **90**(3):272–76.

43. Mills, JKA, Dalleywater, WJ, Tischler, V. An assessment of student satisfaction with peer teaching of clinical communication skills. *BMC Med Educ*. 2014; **14**:217.

44. Konkin, J, Suddards, C. Creating stories to live by: caring and professional identity formation in a longitudinal integrated clerkship. *Adv Health Sci Educ Theory Pract*. 2012; **17**(4):585–96.

45. Roh, H, Park, SJ, Kim, T. Patient safety education to change medical students' attitudes and sense of responsibility. *Med Teach*. 2015; **37**(10):908–14.

46. Kenyon, CF, Brown, JB. Mission Statement Day: the impact on medical students of an early exercise in professionalism. *Med Teach*. 2007; **29**(6):606–10.

47. Cork, N, Llewellyn, O, Glasbey, J, Khatri, C; Royal Society of Medicine Student Members Group; STARSurg Collaborative. Bridging medical education and clinical practice. *Lancet*. 2014; **384**(9954):1575.

48. Kaczmarczyk, JM, Chuang, A, Dugoff, L, Abbott, JF, Cullimore, AJ, Dalrymple, J, Davis, KR, Hueppchen, NA, Katz, NT, Nuthalapaty, FS, Pradhan, A, Wolf, A, Casey, PM. e-Professionalism: a new frontier in medical education. *Teach Learn Med*. 2013; **25**(2):165–70.

49. Brody, H, Doukas, D. Professionalism: a framework to guide medical education. *Med Educ*. 2014; **48**(10):980–87.

50. Boudreau, JD, Cruess, SR, Cruess, RL. Physicianship: educating for professionalism in the post-Flexnarian era. *Perspect Biol Med*. 2011; **54**(1):89–105.

51. Lipsitt, DR. Developmental life of the medical student: curriculum considerations. *Acad Psychiatry*. 2015; **39**(1):63–69.

52. Rawson, JV, Thompson, N, Sostre, G, Deitte, L. The cost of disruptive and unprofessional behaviors in health care. *Acad Radiol*. 2013; **20**(9):1074–76.

53. Graves, L. Teaching the wounded healer. *Med Teach*. 2008; **30**(2):217–19.

54. Boudreau, JD, Fuks, A. The humanities in medical education: ways of knowing, doing and being. *J Med Humanit*. Apr. 8, 2014. ['Online first': DOI 10.1007/s10912-014-9285-5]

55. Eichbaum, QG. Thinking about thinking and emotion: the metacognitive approach to the medical humanities that integrates the humanities with the basic and clinical sciences. *Perm J*. 2014; **18**(4):64–75.

56. Rodenhauser, P, Strickland, MA, Gambala, CT. Arts-related activities across U.S. medical schools: a follow-up study. *Teach Learn Med*. 2004; **16**(3):233–39.

57. Remen, RN, Rabow, MW. The Healer's Art: professionalism, service and mission. *Med Educ*. 2005; **39**(11):1167–68.

58. Rabow, MW, Evans, CN, Remen, RN. Professional formation and deformation: repression of personal values and qualities in medical education. *Fam Med*. 2013; **45**(1):13–18.

59. Rabow, MW, Wrubel, J, Remen, RN. Authentic community as an educational strategy for advancing professionalism: a national evaluation of the Healer's Art course. *J Gen Intern Med*. 2007; **22**(10):1422–28.

60. Rabow, MW, Newman, M, Remen, RN. Teaching in relationship: the impact on faculty of teaching "the Healer's Art." *Teach Learn Med*. 2014; **26**(2):121–28.

61. Felstead, I. Role modelling and students' professional development. *Br J Nurs*. 2013; **22**(4):223–27.

62. Cohen, MJ, Kay, A, Youakim, JM, Balaicuis, JM. Identity transformation in medical students. *Am J Psychoanal*. 2009; **69**(1):43–52.

63. Learning Communities Institute. Boston, MA: LCI. [Accessed May 4, 2015.] Available from http://sites.tufts.edu/lci.

64. Smith, S, Shochet, R, Keeley, M, Fleming, A, Moynahan, K. The growth of learning communities in undergraduate medical education. *Acad Med*. 2014; **89**(6):928–33.

65. Malloy, MH. The Osler Student Societies of the University of Texas Medical Branch: a medical professionalism translational tool. *HEC Forum*. 2012; **24**(4):273–78.

66. Fleming, A, Cutrer, W, Moutsios, S, Heavrin, B, Pilla, M, Eichbaum, Q, Rodgers, S. Building learning

communities: evolution of the colleges at Vanderbilt University School of Medicine. *Acad Med.* 2013; **88**(9):1246–51.

67. Mitchell, R, Parker, V, Giles, M, Boyle, B. The ABC of health care team dynamics: understanding complex affective, behavioral, and cognitive dynamics in interprofessional teams. *Health Care Manage Rev.* 2012; **39**(1):1–9.

68. Arenson, C, Umland, E, Collins, L, Kern, SB, Hewston, LA, Jerpbak, C, Antony, R, Rose, M, Lyons, K. The health mentors program: three years experience with longitudinal, patient-centered interprofessional education. *J Interprof Care.* 2015; **29**(2):138–43.

69. Towle, A, Brown, H, Hofley, C, Kerston, RP, Lyons, H, Walsh, C. The expert patient as teacher: an interprofessional Health Mentors programme. *Clin Teach.* 2014; **11**(4):301–06.

70. Bridges, DR, Davidson, RA, Odegard, PS, Maki, IV, Tomkowiak, J. Interprofessional collaboration: three best practice models of interprofessional education. *Med Educ Online.* 2011; **16**:10.

71. Eckenfels, EJ. Contemporary medical students' quest for self-fulfillment through community service. *Acad Med.* 1997; **72**(12):1043–50.

72. Ramakrishna, J, Valani, R, Sriharan, A, Scolnik, D. Design and pilot implementation of an evaluation tool assessing professionalism, communication and collaboration during a unique global health elective. *Med Confl Surviv.* 2014; **30**(1):56–65.

73. Tannan, SC, Gampper, TJ. Resident participation in international surgical missions is predictive of future volunteerism in practice. *Arch Plast Surg.* 2015; **42**(2):159–63.

74. Veronesi, MC, Gunderman, RB. Perspective: the potential of student organizations for developing leadership: one school's experience. *Acad Med.* 2012; **87**(2):226–29.

75. Haq, C, Grosch, M, Carufe-Wert, D. Leadership opportunities with communities, the medically underserved, and special populations (LOCUS). *Acad Med.* 2002; **77**(7):740.

76. Chadi, N. Medical leadership: doctors at the helm of change. *Mcgill J Med.* 2009; **12**(1):52–57.

77. Sweigart, JR, Tad-Y, D, Pierce, R, Wagner, E, Glasheen, JJ. The Health Innovations Scholars Program: a model for accelerating preclinical medical students' mastery of skills for leading improvement of clinical systems. *Am J Med Qual.* Apr. 8, 2015. ['Online first': DOI 10.1177/1062860615580592]

78. Crites, GE, Ebert, JR, Schuster, RJ. Beyond the dual degree: development of a five-year program in leadership for medical undergraduates. *Acad Med.* 2008; **83**(1):52–58.

79. Sherrill, WW. Dual-degree MD-MBA students: a look at the future of medical leadership. *Acad Med.* 2000:**75**(10 Suppl):S37–S79.

80. Hojat, M, Michalec, B, Veloski, JJ, Tykocinski, ML. Can empathy, other personality attributes, and level of positive social influence in medical school identify potential leaders in medicine? *Acad Med.* 2015; **90**(4):505–10.

81. The Health Foundation. *Evidence Scan: Improvement Science.* London, UK: Health Foundation; 2011. [Accessed May 5, 2015.] Available from www.health.org.uk/sites/default/files/ImprovementScience.pdf.

82. Houlden, RL, Raja, JB, Collier, CP, Clark, AF, Waugh, JM. Medical students' perceptions of an undergraduate research elective. *Med Teach.* 2004; **26**(7):659–61.

83. Fishleder, AJ, Henson, LC, Hull, AL. Cleveland Clinic Lerner College of Medicine: an innovative approach to medical education and the training of physician investigators. *Acad Med.* 2007; **82**(4):390–96.

84. Schuwirth, L, Ash, J. Assessing tomorrow's learners: in competency-based education only a radically different holistic method of assessment will work. Six things we could forget. *Med Teach.* 2013; **35**(7):555–59.

85. Schuwirth, LW, van der Vleuten, CP. Programmatic assessment and Kane's validity perspective. *Med Educ.* 2012; **46**(1):38–48.

86. van der Vleuten, CP, Schuwirth, LW, Driessen, EW, Dijkstra, J, Tigelaar, D, Baartman, LK, van Tartwijk, J. A model for programmatic assessment fit for purpose. *Med Teach.* 2012; **34**(3):205–14.

87. Krathwohl, DR, Bloom, BS, Masia, BB. *Taxonomy of Educational Objectives: the Classification of Educational Goals. Handbook II: Affective Domain.* New York, NY: David McKay; 1964.

88. Spike, JP, Cole, TR, Buday, R. *The Brewsters: An Interactive Adventure in Ethics for the Health Professions.* Second edition. Houston, TX: University of Texas Health Science Center at Houston; 2011.

89. Wald, HS, Davis, SW, Reis, SP, Monroe, AD, Borkan, JM. Reflecting on reflections: enhancement of medical education curriculum with structured field notes and guided feedback. *Acad Med.* 2009; **84**(7):830–37.

90. Wald, HS, Anthony, D, Hutchinson, TA, Liben, S, Smilovitch, M, Donato, AA. Professional identity formation in medical education for humanistic, resilient physicians: pedagogic strategies for bridging theory to practice. *Acad Med.* 2015; **90**(6):753–60.

91. Hendelman, W, Byszewski, A. Formation of medical student professional identity: categorizing lapses of professionalism, and the learning environment. *BMC Med Educ.* 2014; **14**:139.

92. Davis, MH. Measuring individual differences in empathy: evidence for a multidimensional approach. *J Pers Soc Psychol.* 1983; **44**(1):113–26.

93. Hojat, M, Gonnella, JS, Nasca, TJ, Mangione, S, Veloksi, JJ, Magee, M. The Jefferson Scale of Physician Empathy: further psychometric data and differences by gender and specialty at item level. *Acad Med*. 2002; 77(10 Suppl):S58–S60.

94. Lave, J, Wenger, E. *Situated Learning: Legitimate Peripheral Participation*. Cambridge, UK: Cambridge University Press; 1991.

95. Forsythe, GB. Identity development in professional education. *Acad Med*. 2005; 80(10 Suppl):S112–S117.

96. Monson, VE, Roehrich, SA, Bebeau, MJ. *Developing Civic Capacity of Professionals: A Methodology for Assessing Identity*. Paper presented at the annual meeting of the American Educational Research Association. New York, NY; 2008.

97. Monson, VE, Hamilton, NW. Entering law students' conceptions of an ethical professional identity and the role of the lawyer in society. *Journal of the Legal Profession*. 2010; 35(1):1–28.

17

Supporting professionalism and professional identity formation at the postgraduate level

Linda Snell

It is during the … years that medical graduates spend as residents and clinical fellows that doctors come of professional age – acquiring the knowledge and skills of their specialties or subspecialties, forming professional identities, and developing habits, behaviors, attitudes, and values that last a professional lifetime.[1] (p. 2)

Postgraduate medical education is a unique educational environment, with its emphasis on work-based learning, clinical supervision as a predominant method of training, performance-based assessment, and the challenge of simultaneously delivering education, training, and service.[2] (p. 3)

Introduction

Learning how to be a professional is an essential part of residency – that period of time between end of medical school and unsupervised practice. Although professional socialization starts in medical school, professional values and behaviors are internalized and a physician's identity is formed to a great extent during residency. Despite this, there are few publications on teaching or assessing professionalism in residency or on how to influence the development of a professional identity at the postgraduate level. This chapter incorporates what has been learned at the undergraduate level and from the literature on identity formation to discuss the context, theory, and practice of how professionalism can be taught and assessed at the residency level. It also links learning, assessment, and institutional strategies to the development of a professional identity as a physician during residency education. The importance of producing professional physicians, and the central importance of residency education in this process, is underscored by both positive and negative examples. Papadakis et al.[3] correlate poor performance on professionalism measures during postgraduate education

with more disciplinary actions in practice. On the other hand, Wright[4] underlines the importance of identifying and emulating positive role models, and their particular influence at the residency level. However, despite the calls for professional identity formation to be a foundational part of medical education during the residency years,[5] "traditional residency education has not attended to shepherding new physicians through this process."[6]

Residency: the context

Compared to medical school, the largest part of learning during residency is work based, with an emphasis on education situated primarily in clinical settings: the workplace. As such, there are characteristics of this setting that have a strong influence on learning professionalism and fostering identity development.

Work-based learning

Education in the workplace is primarily via informal learning, which has been described as "non-routine and tacit … occurring as part of everyday workplace interactions … predominantly unstructured, and experiential in nature. It is also often incidental and occurs without participants being consciously aware of it. Informal learning is not constrained by predetermined times, places, or content for learning. Instead, it generally happens spontaneously, through interactions with others outside formal classroom settings, and without a prescribed body of knowledge to be learned."[7] (p. 1221) This depiction of informal learning aptly describes the type of learning that residents do as part of their daily clinical activities. It applies equally to learning the knowledge and skills needed for medical expertise and to learning about professionalism and developing a professional identity.

Teaching Medical Professionalism, 2nd Edition, ed. Richard L. Cruess, Sylvia R. Cruess and Yvonne Steinert. Published by Cambridge University Press. © Cambridge University Press 2016.

Clinical experiences

Residents do most of their learning in the real world of patient care and clinical service. If this environment and the individuals within it model professionalism, the "product" (graduating resident) will be much more likely to develop an appropriate professional identity and professional behaviors.[8] Residents learn in large part from their interactions with patients, teachers, and colleagues. Specifically related to professionalism, residents learn the "rules of professional behavior" and then have the opportunity to apply them in multiple and more complex situations.[9]

Traditional residency curricula usually consist of a series of short "rotations" or "blocks" of a specified duration in a discipline or clinical setting, ordered sequentially as residents progress through their two to seven years of education. This implies multiple transitions before moving to the next stage or year. The learning that occurs on each rotation is highly contextual, random, and opportunistic, depending on the number and type of patients seen. Over time and with "graded responsibility," the resident has the opportunity to "practice with feedback" and eventually gains more autonomy and independence with less direct supervision. During this evolution, a resident's ability to self-reflect and to apply the knowledge base of professionalism increases as he or she internalizes attitudes and behaviors, as depicted in Figure 8.1 in Chapter 8. Holmboe et al.[10] suggest that spending longer time periods in one setting would likely provide better ongoing supervision and longitudinal relationships with faculty members, and more opportunities to engage fully in the different cultures of teams and varying contexts.

Presence of role models

The strongest influence in learning professionalism and developing a professional identity comes from role models.[11–13] Role modeling has been described as "a nuanced, deliberate learning strategy that provides residents with templates for interpersonal communication and clinical decision making that have both immediate and long-term relevance."[14] (p. 176) Residents learn from role models through two pathways: first, via active exploration of affect and values, and second, via incorporation of observed behaviors. In both cases, there is generalization and behavior change.[15] Residents can and do recognize good role models and their attributes.[4] As well, they appear to be aware of and explicitly use role modeling to learn clinical and interpersonal skills. They also identify role models for professionalism, yet often "the covert transmission of the attitudes, values, and beliefs that shape professional identity and influence professional behavior do not rise to the level of awareness."[14] (p. 180) Residents themselves are effective role models for their peers,[16] likely through the mechanism of near-peer learning. Residents model professional attributes such as respect, honesty, integrity, compassion, and teamwork for their peers as well as their junior learners.

However, although there are positive exemplars, there are also negative role models. Residents report observing various types of unethical conduct and unprofessional behaviors among their peers and teachers, which the authors propose might have a negative effect on their own ethical and professional development.[17] Similarly, Wright et al.[18] found that only half of residents' clinical teachers are perceived as positive role models.

Reflection, self-assessment

Self-reflection is an important part of professional development. A model of reflection has been described that breaks the process into developmental components that can be enabled and taught separately.[19] Residents are aware that they are passively absorbing the explicit and implicit culture of medicine, as well as actively seeking to assimilate (or to avoid assimilating) the medical culture.[20] The recognition of one's own personal lapses in professional behavior may be an early step in implementing change in these behaviors.[21]

Work-based assessment

Whether for the acquisition of knowledge or skills, or the demonstration of attitudes and values, assessment is a major driver of learning.[22] In residency, assessment is usually a combination of knowledge- and clinical skills-focused examinations and periodic end-of-stage global assessments, along with formative assessment or feedback provided throughout. Clearly, feedback as a trigger for reflection and behavior change can play a major role in learning professionalism and forming identity. Newer assessment strategies that foster self-assessment and reflection include learning portfolios, multisource feedback, and encounter cards.[23,24] A number of strategies that have been described at the medical student level to assess professionalism and identity have potential for use in postgraduate education.[25]

Gordon et al.[26] have suggested that resident assessment be divided into two separate systems. The first would be a faculty-controlled "quality control system" screening for minimum standards. The second is a resident-controlled system focusing on self-assessment that is linked to reflection and coaching. The latter, particularly a system incorporating narrative description, has the potential to facilitate the development of identity.[13]

Opportunities for identity development

From the sociological perspective, a residency can be conceived as a community of practice, as emphasized in Chapter 1. During residency, "social interaction between individuals promotes learning and a community is created when those who wish to share a common body of knowledge engage in activities whose aim is to become knowledgeable and skilled in a defined field. The learning takes place within the defined domain and thus is 'situated.' As a consequence, the individual [in this case the resident] moves from 'legitimate peripheral participation' to full participation in the community. An important aspect of full participation is the acquisition of the identity associated with the community."[13] (p. 720) Welcome programs and social events can also foster integration into a community of practice.

The resident is developing an identity as "being" a resident in parallel with one as "becoming" a physician.[27] Throughout residency, "competence and identity are both present, but they shift in relation to each other as residents move from primarily demonstrating competence through the performance of particular tasks, to eventually taking on the identity of a resident and ultimately a physician, something that can only be seen as identity overtakes competency as the primary indication of growth."[27] (p. 5) In other words, individual competencies are integrated into something more than the sum of the parts. The "transition from novice to early expertise – from *thinking as a student* to *thinking like a doctor* as preparation for *thinking as a doctor*"[28] (p. 380) occurs primarily in residency. Not only are "individual core competencies (e.g. ACGME;[29] CanMEDS[30]) more holistically rendered, they are also more integrated as residents move from junior levels of *doing* to senior levels of *being* a physician."[27] (p. 5) Pratt et al.[31] observed that changes

in professional identity occur when the residents' ideas about who they were as professionals (i.e., their professional identity) did not match the work that they did. This led to stress, and to a resident response that either enriched (deepened their understanding of identity), "patched" (used a previous identity to "patch" holes in a future one), or "splinted" (protected an underdeveloped identity). The dissonance between the complex tasks required, increased responsibilities, and autonomy on one side, and an unformed identity as a resident on the other, is more acute during the residents' initial months of training.[32]

A number of factors influence identity formation in the workplace, the major ones discussed above and expanded on in Chapter 1 being role modeling, mentors, and learning from experiences.[13] Other elements that influence the identity development of residents are stress, input from family and friends, increasing competence, relationships with patients and colleagues, the healthcare system, and the learning environment. Stress is a very present factor in residency. Pressures experienced by residents can negatively impact their development, yet positive experiences, either challenging or powerful, may foster personal growth and development.[33] Specific sources of stress and satisfaction have been identified.[34] These include on the one hand a lack of confidence, a sense of incompetence, worry about hurting patients, and a feeling of not being respected, and on the other hand satisfaction with patient care, teamwork, and having opinions listened to. When they are not working or sleeping, residents still spend time with family and friends, so the influence of these individuals on identity formation remains throughout residency.[35]

Health systems changes

The context in which residents work, and changes in academic and healthcare systems, can produce effects on both education programs and individual learners' professional development. Patient load and acuity, noneducational tasks, emotional stress, emphasis on research over teaching, emphasis on quantity not quality, and the perspective by health institutions that residents are workers and not learners negatively influence curriculum design and may send messages that negatively affect the development of residents' professional values.[36] The healthcare system and the learning environment form part of the informal and hidden curriculum for both learning professionalism and forming a professional identity; both must be addressed. Specifically, "the incentives and disincentives built into any institutional culture may require changes, along with other factors including economic and structural policies established at the institutional level."[37] (p. 207)

Regulatory and education standards about professionalism

Professionalism and "being professional" is a standard of accreditation for postgraduate programs in many countries, as found, for example, in the CanMEDS roles[30] used in more than fifty jurisdictions around the world, and in the Accreditation Council for Graduate Medical Education's competencies in the United States.[29] Other countries use the Charter on Professionalism to outline appropriate professional behaviors for physicians at all levels.[38] In all these documents, the curricular content for a residency program is broadly outlined and there is an expectation that residents' professional behaviors will be assessed. More recently, there have been allusions to the formation of a professional identity in some of these standard-setting documents.[30]

Residency: the learning process, with specific examples

This section discusses what can be done to facilitate learning professionalism and foster the development of a professional identity in residency, using specific examples from the McGill University residency programs and elsewhere. This is an evolving area and many of the examples build on what has been learned about teaching and assessing professionalism and developing a professional identity at the undergraduate level.

The selection and admission process

"If the objective of medical education is to provide society with individuals who have internalized the values and norms of medicine, the process can certainly be facilitated if those selected already possess many of these attributes."[12] (p. 1449) In many residency programs at McGill, the role of the resident as professional is addressed during the residency selection interview. In pediatrics, for example, candidates are asked to describe their role models and their influence on the resident, to discuss the "larger meaning of professionalism" (e.g., "What does it mean to

you to be a professional, beyond being a good person?"), and to analyze their own experiences with lapses in professionalism that they have observed. In internal medicine, prospective residents are asked to discuss challenging professionalism scenarios provided during their interviews.

The technique of multiple-mini interviews (MMIs) has been used at the postgraduate level to select residents. This method seems well suited for contributing to decisions about admissions.[39] In some disciplines at McGill, MMIs have specifically been used to assess attributes associated with professionalism. Elsewhere, Hofmeister et al.[40] have used MMIs to assess teamwork, disclosure of error, ethical behavior, ability to accept feedback, ability to accept self-limitations, caring, taking responsibility, time management, ability to accept professional limitations and cultural sensitivity.

Learning core content and concepts (the "cognitive base")

Just as there is a scientific knowledge base that residents apply to their clinical practice of medicine, there is a base of knowledge about professionalism and identity formation that can be applied to their professional practice; this must be taught explicitly. The cognitive base of professionalism is described in Chapter 1. This should include "an institutionally agreed-upon definition of medical professionalism, a list of its attributes and the concept of the social contract"[41] (p. 8), "the nature of professionalism, the reasons why society supports the privileged position of professionals, the history and evolution of professionalism, the nature and reasons for the existence of their obligations as professionals"[41] (p. 4), and an understanding of professional identity and the processes through which it is formed. In our institution, the cognitive base is the same in undergraduate and postgraduate education, and for all faculty members within the academic community. We hope that this provides a common structure for all learners and a shared vocabulary for teachers and residents to discuss professional issues in the workplace. On a broader level, shared core content establishes the norms of a community of practice, thereby influencing the nature of the desired identity needed for entry into the community. This was aptly stated by Sklar: "How do I figure out what I want to do if I don't know who I am supposed to be?"[42] (p. 695)

The knowledge portion of this cognitive base can most efficiently be taught using traditional didactic strategies such as freestanding lectures, grand rounds, or didactic presentations at departmental resident half-days, as well as with readings and online learning. As residents have limited time compared to medical students, the use of self-study packages or asynchronous learning methods to increase efficiency and accessibility should be considered. At McGill, an example of online learning is the multimedia self-study package that has been developed to teach key concepts of professionalism. This includes a brief plenary lecture that has to be completed before attending a simulation session used to apply the concepts.[43] The concepts include many of the elements of the cognitive base described above. Specific learning goals of the session are to define professionalism, recognizes the attributes of professionalism in clinical contexts, describe the social contract between physicians and society, and understand how the faculty of medicine's codes of conduct link with professionalism.

In our institution, a number of other formal didactic and skill-building sessions are provided for residents. Although not formally "labeled" as a professionalism curriculum, these activities address many of the factors influencing identity formation in residency. A resident wellness day provides resources and presentations on "coping with stress" and "work-life balance." Half-day sessions on "finding a mentor" and "being an effective role model" are given in some departments.

Elsewhere, Klein et al.[44] describe a curriculum for first-year residents, introducing various components of professionalism during a five-day resident retreat, with the topics being "revisited" at noon conferences throughout the year. This type of learning format provides a basic introduction to professionalism principles, which might best be complemented with strategies to encourage ongoing reflection and application. In a good example of this, Markakis et al.[45] describe a longitudinal, multifaceted curriculum to foster the development of professionalism and humanism. The components include formal learning strategies such as workshops and retreats, as well as providing support systems and mentoring, with explicit attention paid to development of values. They state that the program has "enabled its trainees to develop the requisite excellent diagnostic and technical tools and skills and also the humane and professional attributes of the fully competent physician."[45] (p. 141)

Goold and Stern[46] found that the professionalism content needed by residents includes basic concepts of ethics, interprofessional relationships, communication skills, self-monitoring, the learning environment, and resident–attending interactions. The authors suggest lectures, workshops, or standardized patient simulations as potential learning strategies. As well, resident reflection on these topics can contribute to identity development. Grewal and Davidson[47] and Taylor et al.[48] suggest that training in emotional intelligence (EI) could help the teaching of professionalism. Curricular topics proposed by these authors include identifying your ideal self, coping strategies, stress management, and developing a vision for yourself; many of these could also foster the formation of a new identity.

Application of formal learning: "professionalism scenarios"

Residents must have multiple opportunities to apply the concepts of professionalism relevant to their context and to internalize them into attitudes that are expressed in professional behaviors and in their developing identity.

The use of case studies or vignettes may prompt the resident to think about professionalism in their own practice. In half-day sessions at McGill, following a short didactic session about the cognitive base of professionalism, residents discuss vignettes in small groups led by a trained faculty member or senior resident. The goal of the activity is to let the residents identify attributes of professionalism and solve professionalism dilemmas. Vignettes are likely more powerful if derived from the institution's experience; many of our vignettes are adapted from "real" cases. Examples of professionalism vignettes which can be used to promote reflection can be found in Snell[49] (pp. 288–89) and Borrero et al.[50] (pp. 16–17)

Another way of using case studies is with simulation-based scenarios. A formative "Ethics and Professionalism OSCE" (Objective Structure Clinical Experience) has been used by at least one department in our setting, where residents in small groups participate in simulated professionalism dilemmas, followed by a debriefing and discussion of the principles exhibited.

A "flipped classroom" format and simulation, which focuses on the application of professionalism principles to contemporary real-life scenarios, has also been implemented in our setting.[43] In this activity, the multimedia self-study package about key concepts of professionalism described above is completed before a simulation session. Residents then participate in a half-day simulation consisting of five simulated professionalism scenarios addressing common issues seen by residents. Two scenarios focus on the role of social media, and three focus on professionalism in the hospital setting. The cases used as the basis for the scenarios are based on real incidents. Specific professionalism concepts addressed include breach of confidentiality on Facebook, dishonesty discovered on social media, reliability and trust in clinical presentations, addressing poor interprofessional communication, and tackling unprofessional behavior in a supervisor. The goal is to apply the concepts learned and acquire practical tools that address professionalism situations faced in the clinical environment. Debriefing provides feedback by team leaders and peers and the opportunity for reflection. Although the residents who have participated found the scenarios realistic, they suggested that they be less "blatant," and that they express more subtle professionalism challenges. Overall, the activity is well received by residents, who have had a significant improvement in their understanding of professionalism.

Work-based learning

Reed et al. have pointed out that "didactic instruction alone is insufficient to instill professionalism among learners. Additional strategies, such as explicit and consistent role modeling of professional behaviors, reflection, and self-assessment, are needed to encourage the development of mindful, professional practitioners."[51] (p. 1332) Other work-based learning occurs during practice with feedback and by informal discussions with colleagues.[52] Whatever learning method is used, we must recognize the dual role of the resident as "apprentice (learner) and practitioner," and directly relate the method to the residents' rapidly expanding experience in the clinical setting. As in most other residency programs, in our setting clinical supervisors work side-by-side with residents, and have opportunities to observe both the resident behavior and what is going on in the environment in which they both work. As such, faculty members are encouraged to specifically address issues of professionalism and identity formation that arise in the patient-care setting, and to promote reflection in a safe environment. They must

learn to do so effectively and safely; this is a major goal of the McGill faculty development programs, discussed below and in Chapter 9. The residents' experience of concrete professional behaviors (e.g., punctuality, accurate charting, truth telling, and self-regulation) should be accompanied by open discussion and contemplation of professionalism issues, using a vocabulary and framework that the teachers and learners share.

Specific attention should be paid to ensuring that residents are exposed to positive role models, to making mentors available, and to providing opportunities for self-assessment and reflection. As Larkin has said, "Inside or outside the hospital, actions always speak louder than words, and thus modeling is a very powerful way to impart to residents the importance of professional behavior. The actions of our opinion leaders and teaching faculty are certainly more instructive to students learning humanistic skills than all the books and learned journals of an entire medical library."[53] (p. 171) Role models who explicitly discuss their own behaviors with residents in a way that allows reflection are likely to be more effective,[15] and this has been built into the McGill faculty development program on role modeling. "Faculty members serve as role models for resident professionalism; we cannot expect residents to perform in a more professional manner than their superiors."[53] (p. 172) In Canadian Family Medicine programs, clinical preceptors have been described as "competency coaches" who "facilitate the learner in taking ownership of personal lifelong learning and career development, with an intentional focus on developing the resident's professional identity."[54] (p. 6) Providing opportunities to reflect, and training residents (and faculty) about reflection, allows residents to process their observations and experiences in a way that fosters identity formation and the development of professionalism.

Being "welcomed" into both the community of learners (residency program) and the community of practice (the specialty, department, or practice group) as a junior member also fosters the development of the desired identity. Formal welcome and recognition events are held in most disciplines within our teaching hospitals. In some specialties, exemplary professional behaviors of residents are recognized.

Elsewhere, Nothnagle et al. report an innovative seminar series for senior residents specifically aimed at supporting resident identity formation through reflection.[6] The ninety-minute sessions include time for individual reflection, small- and large-group discussion, and reflection and skills development on topics related to professional identity. They explicitly address elements of the hidden curriculum.

Ratanawongsa et al.[55] note that resident well-being has a significant influence on identity formation. Increased professional satisfaction and accomplishment, a positive "sense of self," and coping strategies are important factors to promote well-being. In our setting, at both the program and the university level, systems exist to provide support and facilitate coping with the unavoidable stressors of residency. The expectation is that this will positively affect the development of a professional identity.

Assessment in the workplace

One global tool that can holistically assess all of professionalism does not exist; however, a few valid and reliable instruments exist to assess specific behaviors.[56] Work-based assessment modalities that have been used to evaluate or to promote reflection on professional behaviors include encounter cards, OSCEs such as the one described above, multisource feedback, in-training evaluation reports (ITERs), and portfolios. Currently, there are only a few tools available in medicine to assess the development of a professional identity,[25] and while valid and feasible, these have not been used on a large scale. Therefore, for the foreseeable future, professional behaviors may have to be used as a surrogate for following identity formation.

One example is the professionalism mini-evaluation exercise (P-MEX), developed at McGill University.[57] Patterned on the Mini-CEX, the P-MEX is a type of encounter card that has been used at the postgraduate level. This tool is specifically designed to assess professionalism and provide formative assessment to residents based on observation during authentic clinical encounters. The P-MEX assesses twenty-one observable professional behaviors during a brief, real clinical encounter, and has shown good construct validity. In our setting, there has not been complete acceptance of this means of evaluation at the resident level by either the residents or their teachers. However, a modified version has been used effectively in other contexts.[58] Nonetheless, the behaviors described in the P-MEX serve as the foundation of the assessment of professionalism at all levels, including the assessment of faculty members described below.

The standard ITER, usually used at the end of a clinical rotation, can also be used to assess professional behaviors and provide feedback for reflection. For example, the following criteria are found on the internal medicine residency in-training assessments at McGill: "integrity and honesty; sensitivity and respect for diversity; responsible and self-disciplined; recognition of own limitations, seeking advice when needed; understands the principles of ethics applied to clinical situations; communicates with patients with compassion and empathy." Narrative comments on the ITER have been shown to be particularly important in describing professional attributes and values such as work ethic and skills, discerning limits, response to feedback, and professional conduct.[59] Narrative comments can also predict issues in professionalism.[60] Gordon's resident-driven assessment system described above has the potential to facilitate a resident's professional development.[20]

Elsewhere, Gauger et al.[61] describe a tool used to assess professionalism in surgical residents. This tool describes behaviors for fifteen domains of professionalism, with descriptors in the continuous ordinal scale to discourage "inflated ratings." The domains include behaviors and attributes such as punctuality, appearance, honesty/accountability/response to error, responsibility/sense of duty, response to criticism, ability to assess oneself, respect for others, self-regulation, altruism, inter-professional relationships, trustworthiness/confidentiality, moral and ethical standards, and attitude toward the medical profession. Results of assessments such as this can be used to provide formative assessment and feedback and to facilitate reflection.

Larkin et al.[62] describe the use of multisource feedback (MSF) methods focused on professional behaviors as defined in emergency medicine. The MSF is an assessment tool that is completed by multiple persons within a learner's sphere of influence. Multi-rater assessments are ideally completed by students, peers, nurses, faculty supervisors, patients, families, and the residents themselves. The authors note that the criteria used must be described in such a way that they model exemplary or unprofessional behaviors. Examples of specific positive behaviors include the following: arrives on time and is prepared for work; appropriate dress; completes medical records honestly and punctually; treats patients, family, staff, and paraprofessional personnel with respect; protects confidentiality; actively seeks feedback and immediately self-corrects; accepts responsibility and accountability; and participates in a peer-review process. Examples of unprofessional behaviors include the following: substance abuse or dependence; lying, cheating, stealing; unwilling to learn from past mistakes; discriminates against others; falsifies medical records or research data; unkempt appearance. The authors propose that the results of an MSF be fed back to residents to aid in development of professionalism.

Other programs use learning portfolios for professional issues: they hold great promise for formative assessment, facilitating self-assessment, and reflection. Portfolios provide a flexible, multifaceted means of collecting qualitative and quantitative evidence of achievement of competence or demonstration of progression over time. Portfolio entries can be linked with self-assessment or guided reflection and thus become an effective tool to support identity formation. Acquiring a professional identity thus becomes an active rather than a passive experience.[52]

Many of these assessment tools have been described in detail in Chapter 11. However, despite the development of residency-specific tools or the adoption of assessment instruments used at other levels of medical education, it is unlikely that one assessment tool can capture all aspects of professionalism or identity formation. The "rule of multiples" would thus apply: to effectively measure professionalism, one needs multiple tools and multiple observers, used multiple times.

Residents within systems: needs and requirements

Faculty development

One cannot expect residents to learn to be professional without faculty members knowledgeable in the concepts and skilled in the teaching and role modeling of professional behaviors and values.[44] Faculty development is needed to ensure that clinical supervisors know and use the same cognitive base as their residents, to enhance skills to teach and assess professionalism and support identity formation, and to build skills in explicit role modeling and encouraging of reflection.

The faculty development program at McGill includes workshops to aid in the development of an institutional approach to the teaching and evaluation of professionalism, as well as a definition that is understood and agreed upon by faculty members. The participants in these faculty development sessions usually teach at both the medical student and the postgraduate level, so a coherent "message" is given across the continuum of medical education.[63] As well, in half-day workshops on role modeling and reflection, clinical teachers use group discussion, video vignettes, and a guided reflection of their own role modeling, to address issues of professionalism that arise during clinical practice and to learn how to encourage reflection in a safe environment.

Faculty development should also "serve as an important foundational basis for the introduction of educational programs aimed at understanding the factors involved in the process of socialization and in the promotion of identity formation."[12] (p. 1450) As stated by Gordon et al., "Faculty development programmes might benefit from paying explicit attention to the process of enculturation and its influence on learning and practice."[26] (p. 894) As detailed in Chapter 9, faculty workshops on professional identity formation in our own setting have included individuals involved in postgraduate education. These sessions address the nature of identity formation and the actions that clinical teachers can take to foster this social process.

Institutional and organizational changes

In addition to teaching, factors such as institutional culture and practice characteristics influence professionalism, leading Reed et al.[51] to suggest that organizational cultures must evolve to encourage professionalism and identity formation. Leach[9] also links good resident education and good patient care to a system designed to enable, ensure, and improve both. Simple things, such as changing a program's educational objectives or competencies to include explicit mention of all aspects of professionalism and of identity, will help.[12,13]

The structure and context of medicine's organizations where residents work can affect residents' ethical behavior and professionalization and are an important part of their socialization.[64] Although essential for patient safety, restrictions of work hours may afford residents a "moral dilemma" as they are forced to choose between providing adequate care and adherence to time rules.[65] At McGill, restricted-work-hour rules have had both positive and negative impacts on professionalism.[66] The emergence of "shift worker mentality" around sign-over has been counterbalanced by residents who are less tired, more consistent interactions with patients, and more stable team structures, thus improving teamwork, patient ownership, quality of work performed, and empathy. Interventions regarding effective team-based care may further improve the positive professionalism aspects while decreasing the negatives. Similarly, Ratanawongsa et al.[67] found that duty-hour restrictions were perceived by residents as a barrier to practicing professionally at the same time as they promoted professionalism by improving resident well-being. Lopez suggests that work-hour limits alone are not enough and that other organizational changes such as extra staffing are needed to ensure that residents can develop empathy and make a "safe and ethical choice."[64] (p. 318) As Ludmerer[36] (p. 1083) has stated, "The overarching theme is that what matters in residency training is not the hours of work alone but what residents do during those hours." The learning environment and organizational culture must be changed so that identity formation and professionalism is enabled.

Assessment of faculty members' professionalism by learners may also lead to an improved learning environment. Learners at all levels within our institution are asked to rate their teaching faculty (and the residents who teach them) on a number of criteria related to professionalism, and to provide comments. These ratings and comments are collated and fed back to teachers annually, with, in some cases, significant changes in professionalism behaviors of faculty members.[68]

Practical guidelines

A residency program director wishing to ensure the appropriate development of identity of postgraduate learners could consider education and systems interventions at a number of levels. The aim for individuals should be to convey core content and provide opportunities to understand and apply it, participate in professional practice and model their own behaviors on positive exemplars, and develop self-assessment and reflective capacity. At the systems level, the goal is to select residents for professionalism, attend to the hidden curriculum, promote a positive learning environment, and foster a community of practice. Specific strategies are outlined in Table 17.1, linked to individual learning or organizational interventions.

Lessons learned: teaching professionalism and supporting professional identity formation at the residency level

Learning to be a professional is a sequential and progressive activity that occurs throughout the continuum of medical education and is a vital part of postgraduate education. Much of the formation of a professional identity occurs during the residency years. In this period, residents spend the majority of their time in the clinical workplace, so learning professional attitudes and behaviors must occur there.

Much of residents' learning is informal and occurs by reflection on experience and with exposure to role models. Reflection and self-assessment can be enabled through explicit teaching and formative assessment. Residents should be explicitly engaged in reflecting on identity and their own development.

Core concepts and the vocabulary of professionalism must also be taught; frequent opportunities must be provided to apply this cognitive base to the residents' context. However, it is more difficult to establish structured programs at the residency level than it is in medical school. The emphasis on work-based learning and the dual role of service and education are in part responsible for this. The necessity to have specific programs for specific disciplines means that core material must be generic, yet adaptable to different programs, allowing for differences in identity.

Formal instruction of the core concepts of professionalism must occur for teachers and learners alike. Faculty teachers must be comfortable with these concepts and be able to apply and discuss them in the clinical context. Residents must learn and use the same vocabulary and framework as their mentors. Faculty development is therefore essential. Attitude development and behavior change demand less used learning strategies: teachers must be comfortable with, among other strategies, explicit role modeling, debriefing on experiences, and encouraging reflection.

Attending to the structure and function of organizations and systems is essential: residents work within these systems that strongly influence their professional values and identity. The hidden curriculum must be addressed.

Table 17.1. Strategies to enhance professionalism and promote professional identity formation in residents at the individual and organizational level

Aim of intervention	Goal of learning	Sample strategy
Impart core content	Knowledge acquisition	Lectures, grand rounds Academic half-days Directed reading Web-based learning
Provide opportunity to apply knowledge	Understanding	Group discussions Cases, vignettes, scenarios Workshops Flipped classroom Web-based learning
	Model or practice behavior in a "safe" setting	Simulation, e.g., OSCE Role play Video review
Encourage professional behaviors and support identity formation	Observation Participation Application	Role modeling Clinical experiences with focused teaching Guided reflection
Assess formatively to foster professional behaviors and develop identity	Self-evaluation Reflection	Portfolios Multisource feedback Narratives Encounter cards P-MEX

	Goal	Sample interventions
Act at the organization or system level	Select for professionalism	Multiple-mini interview: professionalism stations Traditional interview: professionalism questions or scenarios
	Attend to the learning environment and hidden curriculum	Faculty development programs Wellness programs Resident support systems Mentoring Assessing faculty members' professionalism
	Foster a community of practice	Welcome programs Recognition of exemplary professionalism, e.g., awards

Conclusion

A major goal of the period between graduating from medical school and entering unsupervised practice is the development of a professional identity. Explicit teaching of professionalism and emphasis on professional behaviors supports this process. However, both "learning professionalism" and forming a professional identity call for explicit teaching, learning, and assessment strategies, as well as systems changes.

> Residency is an intense experience. The learning curve is steeper than at any other time in a physician's life. It is also a time in which the habits of a lifetime are developed.[9] (p. 97)

References

1. Ludmerer, KM. *Let Me Heal: The Opportunity to Preserve Excellence in American Medicine.* Oxford, UK: Oxford University Press; 2015.

2. Steinert, Y. *Faculty Development for Postgraduate Education – The Road Ahead.* Members of the FMEC PG consortium; 2011. [Accessed June 25, 2015.] Available from www.afmc.ca/pdf/fmec/21_Steinert_Faculty%20 Development.pdf.

3. Papadakis, MA, Arnold, GK, Blank, LL, Holmboe, ES, Lipner, RS. Performance during internal medicine residency training and subsequent disciplinary action by state licensing boards. *Ann Intern Med.* 2008; **148**(11):869–76.

4. Wright, S. Examining what residents look for in their role models. *Acad Med*. 1996; **71**(3):290–92.

5. Cooke, M, Irby, DM, O'Brien, BC. *Educating Physicians: A Call for Reform of Medical School and Residency*. San Francisco, CA: Jossey-Bass; 2010.

6. Nothnagle, M, Reis, S, Goldman, RE, Anandarajah, G. Fostering professional formation in residency: development and evaluation of the "forum" seminar series. *Teach Learn Med*. 2014; **26**(3):230–38.

7. Varpio, L, Bidlake, E, Casimiro, L, Hall, P, Kuziemsky, C, Brajtman, S, Humphrey-Murto, S. Resident experiences of informal education: how often, from whom, about what and how. *Med Educ*. 2014; **48**(12):1220–34.

8. Ludmerer, KM. The history of calls for reform in graduate medical education and why we are still waiting for the right kind of change. *Acad Med*. 2012; **87**(1):34–40.

9. Leach, DC. Resident formation – a journey to authenticity: designing a residency program that educes professionalism. In Cruess, R, Cruess, S, Steinert, Y, eds. *Teaching Medical Professionalism*. New York, NY: Cambridge University Press; 2009:93–107.

10. Holmboe, E, Ginsburg, S, Bernabeo, E. The rotational approach to medical education: time to confront our assumptions? *Med Educ*. 2011; **45**(1):69–80.

11. Brownell, AK, Côté, L. Senior residents' views on the meaning of professionalism and how they learn about it. *Acad Med*. 2001; **76**(7):734–37.

12. Cruess, RL, Cruess, SR, Boudreau, JD, Snell, L, Steinert, Y. Reframing medical education to support professional identity formation. *Acad Med*. 2014; **89**(11):1446–51.

13. Cruess, RL, Cruess, SR, Boudreau, JD, Snell, L, Steinert, Y. A schematic representation of the professional identity formation and socialization of medical students and residents: a guide for medical educators. *Acad Med*. 2015; **90**(6):718–25.

14. Balmer, D, Serwint, JR, Ruzek, SB, Ludwig, S, Giardino, AP. Learning behind the scenes: perceptions and observations of role modeling in pediatric residents' continuity experience. *Ambul Pediatr*. 2007; **7**(2):176–81.

15. Cruess, SR, Cruess, RL, Steinert, Y. Role modelling– making the most of a powerful teaching strategy. *BMJ*. 2008; **336**(7646):718–21.

16. Sternszus, R, Cruess, S, Cruess, R, Young, M, Steinert, Y. Residents as role models: impact on undergraduate trainees. *Acad Med*. 2012; **87**(9):1282–87.

17. Baldwin, DC Jr, Daugherty, SR, Rowley, BD. Unethical and unprofessional conduct observed by residents during their first year of training. *Acad Med*. 1998; **73**(11):1195–1200.

18. Wright, SM, Kern, DE, Kolodner, K, Howard, DM, Brancati, FL. Attributes of excellent attending-physician role models. *N Engl J Med*. 1998; **339**(27):1986–93.

19. Nguyen, QD, Fernandez, N, Karsenti, T, Charlin, B. What is reflection? A conceptual analysis of major definitions and a proposal of a five-component model. *Med Educ*. 2014; **48**(12):1176–89.

20. Gordon, MJ. Cutting the Gordian knot: a two-part approach to the evaluation and professional development of residents. *Acad Med*. 1997; **72**(10):876–80.

21. Forgeron, MP. A resident's perspective on professionalism. *Annals RCPSC*. 2001; **35**(1):45–47.

22. Stern, DT, ed. *Measuring Medical Professionalism*. New York, NY: Oxford University Press; 2006.

23. Epstein, RM. Assessment in medical education. *N Engl J Med*. 2007; **356**(4):387–96.

24. Sherbino, J, Bandiera, G, Frank, JR. Assessing competence in emergency medicine trainees: an overview of effective methodologies. *CJEM*. 2008; **10**(4):365–71.

25. Cruess, R, Cruess, S, Steinert, Y. Amending Miller's Pyramid to include professional identity formation. *Acad Med*. 2015. In press.

26. Gordon, J, Markham, P, Lipworth, W, Kerridge, I, Little, M. The dual nature of medical enculturation in postgraduate medical training and practice. *Med Educ*. 2012; **46**(9):894–902.

27. Jarvis-Selinger, S, Pratt, DD, Regehr, G. Competency is not enough: integrating identity formation into the medical education discourse. *Acad Med*. 2012; **87**(9):1185–90.

28. Corrigan, O, Ellis, K, Bleakley, A, Brice, J. Quality in medical education. In Swanwick, T, ed. *Understanding Medical Education: Evidence, Theory and Practice*. Oxford, UK: Wiley-Blackwell; 2010:379–91.

29. Swing, SR. The ACGME outcome project: retrospective and prospective. *Med Teach*. 2007; **29**(7):648–54.

30. Frank, JR, Snell, L, Sherbino, J, eds. *Draft CanMEDS 2015 Physician Competency Framework*. Ottawa, ON: Royal College of Physicians and Surgeons of Canada; 2015. [Accessed June 25, 2015.] Available from www .royalcollege.ca/portal/page/portal/rc/common/docu ments/canmeds/framework/canmeds2015_framework_ series_IV_e.pdf.

31. Pratt, MG, Rockmann, KW, Kaufmann, JB. Constructing professional identity: the role of work and identity learning cycles in the customization of identity among medical residents. *Acad Manage J*. 2006; **49**(2):235–62.

32. Raymond, MR, Mee, J, King, A, Haist, SA, Winward, ML. What a new residents do during their initial months of training. *Acad Med.* 2011; **86**(10 Suppl): S59–S62.

33. Wright, SM, Levine, RB, Beasley, B, Haidet, P, Gress, TW, Caccamese, S, Brady, D, Marwaha, A, Kern, DE. Personal growth and its correlates during residency training. *Med Educ.* 2006; **40**(8):737–45.

34. Yeo, H, Viola, K, Berg, D, Lin, Z, Nunez-Smith, M, Cammann, C, Bell, RH Jr, Sosa, JA, Krumholz, HM, Curry, LA. Attitudes, training experiences, and professional expectations of US surgery residents: a national survey. *JAMA.* 2009; **302**(12):1301–08.

35. Baldwin, DC Jr, Daugherty, SR, Ryan, PM, Yaghmour, NA. What do residents do when not working or sleeping? A multispecialty survey of 36 residency programs. *Acad Med.* 2012; **87**(4):395–402.

36. Ludmerer, KM, Johns, MM. Reforming graduate medical education. *JAMA.* 2005; **294**(9):1083–87.

37. Cruess, RL, Cruess, SR. Teaching professionalism: general principles. *Med Teach.* 2006; **28**(3):205–08.

38. ABIM Foundation, American Board of Internal Medicine; ACP-ASIM Foundation, American College of Physicians-American Society of Internal Medicine; European Federation of Internal Medicine. Medical professionalism in the new millennium: a physician charter. *Ann Intern Med.* 2002; **136**(3):243–46.

39. Dore, KL, Kreuger, S, Ladhani, M, Rolfson, D, Kurtz, D, Kulasegaram, K, Cullimore, AJ, Norman, GR, Eva, KW, Bates, S, Reiter, HI. The reliability and acceptability of the Multiple Mini-Interview as a selection instrument for postgraduate admissions. *Acad Med.* 2010; **85**(10 Suppl):S60–S63.

40. Hofmeister, M, Lockyer, J, Crutcher, R. The multiple mini-interview for selection of international medical graduates into family medicine residency education. *Med Educ.* 2009; **43**(6):573–79.

41. Cruess, RL, Cruess, SR, Snell, L, Ginsburg, S, Kearney, R, Ruhe, V, Ducharme, S, Sternszus, R. *Teaching, Learning and Assessing Professionalism at the Post Graduate Level.* Members of the FMEC PG consortium; 2011. [Accessed June 25, 2015.] Available from www.afmc.ca/pdf/fmec/20_Cruess_ Professionalism.pdf.

42. Sklar, DP. How do I figure out what I want to do if I don't know who I am supposed to be? *Acad Med.* 2015; **90**(6):695–96.

43. Khandelwal, A, Nugus, P, Elkoushy, MA, Cruess, RL, Cruess, SR, Smilovitch, M, Andonian, S. How we made professionalism relevant to twenty-first century residents. *Med Teach.* 2015; **37**(6):538–42.

44. Klein, EJ, Jackson, JC, Kratz, L, Marcuse, EK, McPhillips, HA, Shugerman, RP, Watkins, S, Stapleton, FB. Teaching professionalism to residents. *Acad Med.* 2003; **78**(1):26–34.

45. Markakis, KM, Beckman, HB, Suchman, AL, Frankel, RM. The path to professionalism: cultivating humanistic values and attitudes in residency training. *Acad Med.* 2000; **75**(2):141–50.

46. Goold, SD, Stern, DT. Ethics and professionalism: what does a resident need to learn? *Am J Bioeth.* 2006; **6**(4):9–17.

47. Grewal, D, Davidson, HA. Emotional intelligence and graduate medical education. *JAMA.* 2008; **300**(10):1200–02.

48. Taylor, C, Farver, C, Stoller, JK. Perspective: Can emotional intelligence training serve as an alternative approach to teaching professionalism to residents? *Acad Med.* 2011; **86**(12):1551–54.

49. Snell, L. Teaching professionalism and fostering professional values during residency: the McGill experience. In Cruess, R, Cruess, S, Steinert, Y, eds. *Teaching Medical Professionalism.* New York, NY: Cambridge University Press; 2009:246–62.

50. Borrero, S, McGinnis, KA, McNeil, M, Frank, J, Conigliaro, RL. Professionalism in residency training: is there a generation gap? *Teach Learn Med.* 2008; **20**(1):11–17.

51. Reed, DA, West, CP, Mueller, PS, Ficalora, RD, Engstler, GJ, Beckman, TJ. Behaviors of highly professional resident physicians. *JAMA.* 2008; **300**(11):1326–33.

52. Branch, WT Jr, Kern, D, Haidet, P, Weissmann, P, Gracey, CF, Mitchell, G, Inui, T. The patient-physician relationship. Teaching the human dimensions of care in clinical settings. *JAMA.* 2001; **286**(9):1067–74.

53. Larkin, GL. Mapping, modeling, and mentoring: charting a course for professionalism in graduate medical education. *Camb Q Healthc Ethics.* 2003; **12**(2):167–77.

54. Walsh, A, Antao, V, Bethune, C, Cameron, S, Cavett, T, Clavet, D, Dove, M, Koppula, S. *Fundamental Teaching Activities in Family Medicine: A Framework for Faculty Development.* Mississauga, ON: College of Family Physicians of Canada; 2015. [Accessed June 25, 2015.] Available from www.cfpc.ca/uploadedFiles/ Education/_PDFs/FTA_GUIDE_TM_ENG_Apr15_ REV.pdf.

55. Ratanawongsa, N, Wright, SM, Carrese, JA. Well-being in residency: a time for temporary imbalance? *Med Educ.* 2007; **41**(3):273–80.

56. Lurie, SJ, Mooney, CJ, Lyness, JM. Measurement of the general competencies of the accreditation council for graduate medical education: a systematic review. *Acad Med.* 2009; **84**(3):301–09.

57. Cruess, R, McIlroy, JH, Cruess, S, Ginsburg, S, Steinert, Y. The Professionalism Mini-Evaluation Exercise: a

preliminary investigation. *Acad Med*. 2006; **81** (10 Suppl):S74–S78.

58. Tsugawa, Y, Tokuda, Y, Ohbu, S, Okubo, T, Cruess, R, Cruess, S, Ohde, S, Okada, S, Hayashida, N, Fukui, T. Professionalism Mini-Evaluation Exercise for medical residents in Japan: a pilot study. *Med Educ*. 2009; **43**(10):968–78.

59. Ginsburg, S, Gold, W, Cavalcanti, RB, Kurabi, B, McDonald-Blumer, H. Competencies "plus": the nature of written comments on internal medicine residents' evaluation forms. *Acad Med*. 2011; **86**(10 Suppl):S30–S34.

60. Frohna, A, Stern, D. The nature of qualitative comments in evaluating professionalism. *Med Educ*. 2005; **39**(8):763–68.

61. Gauger, PG, Gruppen, LD, Minter, RM, Colletti, LM, Stern, DT. Initial use of a novel instrument to measure professionalism in surgical residents. *Am J Surg*. 2005; **189**(4):479–87.

62. Larkin, GL, Binder, L, Houry, D, Adams, J. Defining and evaluating professionalism: a core competency for graduate emergency medicine education. *Acad Emerg Med*. 2002; **9**(11):1249–56.

63. Steinert, Y, Cruess, S, Cruess, R, Snell, L. Faculty development for teaching and evaluating professionalism: from programme design to curriculum change. *Med Educ*. 2005; **39**(2): 127–36.

64. Lopez, L, Katz, JT. Perspective: creating an ethical workplace: reverberations of resident work hours reform. *Acad Med*. 2009; **84**(3):315–19.

65. Taylor, TS, Nisker, J, Lingard, L. To stay or not to stay? A grounded theory study of residents' postcall behaviors and their rationalizations for those behaviors. *Acad Med*. 2013; **88**(10):1529–33.

66. Sun, NZ, Gan, R, Snell, L, Dolmans, D. Resident duty hour reform – erosion of professionalism or catalyst for evolution? *Acad Med*. 2015. In press.

67. Ratanawongsa, N, Bolen, S, Howell, EE, Kern, DE, Sisson, SD, Larriviere, D. Residents' perceptions of professionalism in training and practice: barriers, promoters, and duty hours requirements. *J Gen Intern Med*. 2006; **21**(7):758–63.

68. Young, ME, Cruess, SR, Cruess, RL, Steinert, Y. The Professionalism Assessment of Clinical Teachers (PACT): the reliability and validity of a novel tool to evaluate professional and clinical teaching behaviors. *Adv Health Sci Educ Theory Pract*. 2014; **19**(1):99–113.

Chapter 1

Changing the educational environment to better support professionalism and professional identity formation

Mark J. DiCorcia and Lee A. Learman

Increasing attention to the impact of the hidden curriculum on the formation of professional identity has spurred medical schools to focus on the professional behaviors of faculty and the healthcare team. However, medical schools are complex organizations, and so are the health systems with which they partner to train the next generation of physicians. Beyond achieving short-term improvements in specific areas, can a medical school actually change its culture to promote the development of professionalism? In 2000, undaunted by the potential challenges, leaders at Indiana University School of Medicine (IUSM) launched a set of initiatives to explicitly incorporate professionalism into the culture of the school. After providing a synopsis of the approach used to achieve culture change at IUSM, we describe the initiatives subsequently undertaken between 2008 and 2015 to improve the learning climate and support the formation of professionalism in IUSM's learners at a departmental level.

Changing the culture of a medical school

As described in published reports by the Dean and other leaders at IUSM, there was no one event that ignited the desire to implement a change. Rather, there was growing awareness that graduating students were less satisfied than national norms, felt their learning climate to be more adverse than students from other schools, and hesitated to bring their concerns forward because they felt it unsafe and believed that nothing would be done to improve the situation. The Dean was also concerned that a new focus on the business of medicine would detract from the core values of the profession.[1–3]

The key elements of the culture change at IUSM included affirmation of core organizational values, implementation of appreciative and relational strategies as part of a relationship-centered care initiative (RCCI), revisions in admissions criteria, and alignment of compensation incentives with important qualitative aspects of faculty performance.[1–3]

The organizational change process at the medical school started with a small but meaningful narrative exercise based on appreciative inquiry and reflection. A "Discovery Team" was recruited to collect and analyze the stories shared at appreciative interviews, with eighty stakeholders describing examples of when the organizational culture of the school exemplified the standards of professionalism desired in the school's medical students. The themes and stories were subsequently shared at an open forum, after which a steering committee identified a cascade of additional change opportunities.[3]

In concordance with the principle of emergent design, the next steps were not pre-defined; the change rippled outward in unpredictable ways, and the steering committee responded by organizing opportunities to guide rather than dictate the process. Supportive interventions included student-organized publications, a redesigned admissions process, new relational practices at faculty meetings, changes to department-chair performance reviews, and mission-based management. As predicted by complexity theory, a small series of initiatives spread in a non-linear, transformative fashion to effect large-scale change. Among the qualitative and quantitative outcomes reported were a marked improvement in graduating students' overall satisfaction with their medical education (a change from below to above the national

Teaching Medical Professionalism, 2nd Edition, ed. Richard L. Cruess, Sylvia R. Cruess and Yvonne Steinert.
Published by Cambridge University Press. © Cambridge University Press 2016.

means) and a marked increase in the number of in-state and out-of-state applicants to IUSM.[3] Despite compelling evidence showing a positive impact at the school level, success of this initiative was uneven across the clinical departments, and a leadership opportunity became available in the Department of Obstetrics and Gynecology (OBGYN).

The story of change in this department follows in the sections below. During his first year of service, the new OBGYN chair implemented a set of initiatives to establish the departmental vision and values, align recruitment practices and incentives, and lay the framework of a relational culture. In the second year, the department recruited a vice chair for education who accelerated the pace of change, and created, as well as implemented, training in communication skills and behavior grounded in impression-management theory. Some of the strategies described in the remainder of this chapter resemble those that were used successfully for the school as a whole. Other strategies, particularly those related to skill development, were unique to the Department of OBGYN. This chapter culminates with future plans under consideration in early 2015, before the authors departed Indiana University for leadership positions at a new medical school.

Recruitment of a new chair: A departmental needs assessment

Recruitment of a new OBGYN chair was identified by the Dean as an opportunity to help the department achieve the same level of success evident for the school as a whole. RCCI faculty leaders were included in the recruitment process, which ultimately recruited a new chair (LAL) to Indiana University in August 2008. Several months after his arrival, the chair was invited to join the formation team, a multidisciplinary group of campus RCCI leaders looking to sustain and grow the positive impact of the initiative. Many leaders of the medical school's change process were regular participants. The formation team provided a forum for sharing, vetting, planning, and implementing ideas on how to improve the educational environment and promote a greater culture of humanism. Importantly, with an awareness that change strategies are more likely to succeed when they are created from within the group, formation team members did not propose any specific approaches or initiatives for the department to follow. Instead, they provided support and shared their experiences.

The new chair possessed a doctorate in social psychology, which provided an invaluable lens through which to appraise the department's current culture and identify strategies for implementing improvements to the learning environment. He was aware of the informal curriculum and its importance to the formation of professional identity in medical students,[4] and had spent fourteen years at a medical school that prioritized formation of professionalism in undergraduate and graduate medical education.[5,6]

While promoting professionalism through positive strategies is critical for optimizing the informal curriculum, it was equally important to address unprofessional or disruptive behaviors.[7] When the chair arrived in Indianapolis, he found a cadre of dedicated and like-minded faculty members and also observed and heard about several senior faculty role models referring to patients by their chief complaint, expressing anger to patients, or creating a negative environment for learners. In response to these events, difficult conversations were conducted in which the faculty members' positive contributions to the department were acknowledged, individuals' accounts of events were listened to, and the chair sought to understand the behavior from their perspective. He explained the impression it created, set very clear expectations for the future, and described the consequences for any subsequent infractions. Two of these interventions resulted in immediate and sustained improvements in the faculty members' behavior. Those few who did not embrace the renewed focus on fostering humanism in medicine went on to pursue other opportunities.

Co-creating the future and harnessing faculty passions

It was clear that the majority of the faculty strongly valued teaching and patient care. These longstanding departmental priorities created a strong foundation that could be appreciated together, and from which an even stronger vision for the future could grow. With the help of RCCI leaders at IUSM, organized faculty development retreats, moderated by local and national RCCI leaders, were held in January and June 2009, with interim small work groups meeting between retreats to improve momentum and effectiveness. At the beginning of the January retreat, faculty members were asked to close their eyes and envision their most fulfilling professional environment imaginable. After

Our Vision and Values

In the Indiana University Department of Obstetrics and Gynecology, we are leaders and advocates for women's healthcare, education and research in the state, with a strong regional and national presence. We provide a positive role model for other departments within the Indiana University School of Medicine. We exemplify our values by:

- Honoring the diverse contributions of faculty and staff to our various missions.
- Being a place where learners and teachers want to come and stay.
- Possessing a collaborative, respectful and trusting work environment.
- Fostering a rich mentorship system.
- Having fiscally sound, responsible, and transparent economic and decision-making policies.
- Having a patient-centered focus in which patients are engaged as active partners in all aspects of care.
- Using an evidence-based approach to patient care and teaching and conducting "cutting edge" basic, clinical and translational research.
- Having a robust and comprehensive quality improvement system to continuously improve patient care.

Figure 18.1. Vision and Values Statement (October 2009)

describing what they pictured and felt in this aspirational setting, the faculty generated topics that served as the focus for a series of small-work-group discussions on how to move closer to the aspirational vision. The small work groups continued to meet over the next several months. As pre-work for the second retreat, each group was asked to harvest specific ideas, and to then place them in an action priority matrix – a 2 × 2 grid of high and low impact and high and low effort and complexity. The June retreat was committed to implementing the low-hanging fruit (high impact, low effort and complexity) and prioritizing which farther-reaching goals (high impact, high effort and complexity) to implement.

A variety of tangible outcomes resulted, most importantly a shared "Vision and Values Statement" (described in Figure 18.1), woven together from multiple small groups into one document and endorsed by the entire faculty. The statement appears on every faculty meeting agenda and is distributed to faculty and resident recruits as a statement of shared expectations and aspirations.

The faculty members also developed ideas to help the department move closer to the vision. The working groups harvested several dozen ideas for improving relationships with other departments, enhancing faculty cohesion and respect for the diverse contributions of our colleagues, improving formal and informal mentoring, creating equity in night-call duty, and fostering and modeling humanism in and for medical students and residents. The prioritization process

yielded six specific initiatives for implementation. The following three initiatives focused directly or indirectly on development of humanism and formation of professional identity:

(1) The department will implement faculty development programs (a) for mentors and mentees, (b) to improve skills in teaching, rounding, and communication, and (c) to prepare faculty to perform and utilize 360° assessments.

(2) Faculty will make a commitment to model respect in communications about each other across sites and specialty niches, and to provide ongoing feedback to each other to improve the consistency of respectful behavior.

(3) Faculty and residents at all sites will value and showcase patient care activities that medical students are capable of contributing to the team, and medical students will follow patients all the way through the hospital course.

The remaining initiatives addressed issues such as transparency in financial goals and decisions, subspecialist recruitment, development of academic niches, and development of evidence-based-medicine skills. Rather than receiving these initiatives as top-down marching orders, the faculty themselves authored every idea that was harvested, vetted, and selected for implementation. This included the recruiting and selection process of residents and faculty.

Recruiting with care and rigor

As in many clinical departments, residents are key instructors and role models for each other and for medical students. The program director and other educational leaders identified the need to change the residency interview procedures to better evaluate the "goodness of fit" between the candidates and our core values. We implemented behavioral interviewing (BI), a method developed by industrial psychologists to elicit individuals' prior behavior to better predict future performance. Despite studies in the 1980s showing BI to be more predictive than traditional interviews,[8] BI was only introduced in OBGYN residency program selection very recently.[9,10]

A key step in developing behavioral interviewing questions was to identify the key attributes the department was seeking in residents. The faculty members, charged with developing the next generation of OBGYN specialists, sought to recruit residents who shared their core values as a professional practice community and who would also help realize the department's vision.

As each resident continued his or her personal journey of professional formation, we appreciated that they were also making a critically important impact on the informal curriculum and formation of the medical students. We created a series of questions to elicit each candidate's experiences with stress management, peer respect, altruism, self-reflection, commitment to teaching and learning, enthusiasm, resiliency, leadership, tolerance of interpersonal differences, pursuit of excellence, and values supporting ethical decision-making. The questions were bundled together into five interview stations, each staffed by the same one or two faculty interviewers for all interview sessions, with additional stations for interviews with the program director and chief residents. Following each session, the faculty and resident interviewers discussed each candidate's answers to the questions, which were scored and carried weight equal to or greater than the candidate's academic record in the final ranking decisions. Since implementing behavioral interviewing in 2009, we have noticed qualitative differences in the humanism, self-reflection, resilience, and orientation to teaching and learning demonstrated by the residents.

For faculty, the departmental executive committee, which consisted of departmental division directors and mission-based vice chairs, reflected on the recruitment procedures and identified areas for improvement. Humanism and a relational approach to leadership were sought in all faculty candidates, but the procedures were insufficient for selection of faculty leaders. We subsequently introduced a formal appraisal of leadership characteristics and skills for all finalists for faculty leadership positions. This evaluation was outsourced to a company that conducts a two- to three-hour interview with the candidate, provides a summary and debriefing to the chair, and prepares a confidential summary for the new faculty leader and a personal development plan building on strengths to enhance performance. This formal appraisal process helped identify leadership challenges in finalists that the interview and vetting process had not identified and that could have led to discord among the faculty had the individual been recruited. Allowing time to fully vet candidates helped identify those who could help move initiatives forward and collectively build the department we all envisioned.

Aligning faculty recognition

To further engage faculty and help them reconnect with their individual passions and goals, a program of "mission grants" was implemented (and named after a beloved former faculty member who embodied humanism and compassion). The grant program was funded using the chair's start-up funds to cover up to twenty percent of faculty time to pursue an academic project that served the department's vision and values. The several grants awarded annually focused primarily on curriculum development. The criteria for annual teaching recognition was also revised. The 4.0 Award had been given to faculty and residents with sufficient student contact who exceeded a threshold of overall teaching effectiveness scores (i.e., between a 4.0 and 5.0 for eight out of nine rotations), given by the medical students on end-of-clerkship evaluations. To further align the award with the department's high expectation for professional behavior, a criterion requiring an equally high score on a measure evaluating professionalism and humanism was created. The newly defined 4.0 Award was added to the criteria listed in a departmental academic incentive program, which distributes a small bonus payment annually to faculty who exceed a threshold of expected performance in education, research, or service.

Leadership development: recruiting a catalyst

Pivotal to implementing improvements in the educational environment was the recruitment of a Vice Chair for Education, to support the educational programs in administrative ways and in the further development of our culture of humanism. In 2009, after the initial retreats had been conducted and the vision and values statement was created, we sought a leader for this role who would bring both experience and formal training in education and be credible to clinically oriented faculty and learners. The typical phenotype for this kind of role would be an obstetrician–gynecologist with a master's degree in education or a non-physician with a doctoral degree in education. We were fortunate to recruit a vice chair (MJD) with a uniquely fitting set of experiences and expertise: a master's degree in education focused on curriculum development, a Ph.D. in health communication, and many years of experience practicing as an occupational therapist and hospital administrator in mental health. The vice chair's unique combination of formal training and clinical capabilities made him a highly effective catalyst for accelerating the development of humanism in the department. His ability to translate principles of communication and education to the real world of clinical teaching and learning further supported the formation of professional identity for students, residents, and faculty members.

The disconnect between reality and expectation: doctors are made, not born

Not long after the new vice chair (MJD) was hired, a chief resident came to his office with a litany of legitimate professionalism concerns regarding medical student performance on the obstetrics and gynecology clerkship. It was the second clinical rotation of the third year, and the extensive list encompassed everything from inappropriate attire to the lack of preparation before a surgical case. As a newly graduated, nonphysician educator, the vice chair was shocked, and in an attempt to gain a deeper understanding of the issue, he asked a seemingly rhetorical question, "Has anyone explicitly told the students what is expected of them?" The equally shocked and perplexed resident responded, "They should just know what is expected of them. This is a surgical rotation."

This encounter was nothing short of a revelation for the vice chair. It illustrated a fundamental flaw: not preparing learners with a clear understanding of the professional behavior expected in the clinical learning and practice milieu as well as the role of the medical student–doctor on practice teams that include more advanced learners (residents) and attending physicians. It also highlighted the lack of focused resident and faculty development in recognizing and promoting the role that clinical preceptors and teams play in the development of these professional behaviors and identities. It is just as much a faculty's role and responsibility to understand the reality that "doctors are made, not born" in relationship to the behavioral aspect of medicine as it is to teach students to create a differential diagnosis.[11] However, addressing professional expectations and promoting professional identity was clearly a more unfamiliar task than providing biomedical training, and therefore not in line with resident and faculty expectations of themselves as clinical preceptors. Ironically, at times the developing learner was faulted for not being fully formed at the onset of his or her training.

What then became the key task was to identify which philosophical and pragmatic issues lay at the heart of the matter for both the learners and the preceptors, in order to develop and implement a process of change. Cognizant that reality is co-constructed,[12] the vice chair set out to understand and address this issue from the learner and preceptor perspectives, in order to create a cohesive intervention that recognized the role that each member of the learning dyad played in professional identity formation. The ultimate goal was to change the culture of the department and the experience for both learners and clinical preceptors, so as to support professionalism and professional identity formation, as well as foster the department's vision and values related to education for all stakeholders.

What resulted was an intervention that encompassed a series of educational practice changes, theoretical lectures, and training in giving and receiving feedback, which has narrowed the chasm between preceptors' and learners' expectations and understanding of clinical medical education, professional expectations, and professional identity formation. The program, which is based upon the subsequent topic areas covered in this chapter, has been used to train residents and faculty and is part of a school-wide student orientation before the start of all third-year clerkships. An OBGYN-focused version is presented at the clerkship-specific orientation. The program has greatly reduced the incidence of unprofessional behaviors and expectancy violations, making it nearly a nonissue in the OBGYN clerkship.

The change in learner identity: from the classroom to the clinic

One of the initial questions we asked ourselves as educators was, "What changes are fundamental from the pre-clinical years in medical school to the clinical years?" After all, students should be prepared for the rigors of clinical training, especially given what they have had to accomplish, and in some cases overcome, in the pre-clinical years of medical school. However, what became apparent is that there were several fundamental shifts in learning processes, foci, and assessment that proved students were ill-prepared despite their previous experiences.

First and foremost is the learning environment itself. The standard classroom setting, where most students received the vast majority of their education, creates a teacher-centered approach based on the behaviorist tradition.[13,14] The instructor is solely responsible for the structure and content of the learning and outcomes, and the focus is the learners' needs, understanding, control, and schedule.[15] In sharp contrast, during the clinical years, a completely different educational paradigm is introduced: a patient-centered approach based on constructivism, without much prior preparation or training, at a time when the stakes are very high for the learner.

In the clinical years, the patient is the focus of not only the preceptor but also the learner, who is no longer the central focus in the learning paradigm and must assume ownership and control over his or her own education.[13,14] Education happens through and as a result of providing excellent patient care and integrating knowledge with practice. For many learners, this transition is challenging. If the proper foundation is not created prior to the start of the clinical experience, and if the preceptors are less conscious of the paradigm change, they are less likely to facilitate the shift in learner and professional identity. This is

moving the learner from "student head," whose hallmark is often a focus on a singular issue, process, or outcome, to "doctor head," which requires higher order, system-level thinking.[16] For example, if a student will be preparing for a case in the operating room for the following day and asks his or her preceptor if the only needed preparation is to read about the procedure, the preceptor could say, "That's student head. What else would a doctor want to know about prior to a surgery besides the basic steps of the procedure?" Hopefully, the student will identify independently, or with prompting, the need to be familiar with the patient's history, diagnosis, co-morbidities, and basic anatomy.

Second, the student is unable to develop for any sustained period of time a singular sense of learner or professional expectation, behavior, and identity because the clinical experiences in the various medical specialties can be short lived (e.g., two to five weeks in traditional block clerkships). Even for those clinical experiences that are integrated, there can be great variations in the experiences and roles students are asked to assume. In each specialty and setting, what the student is exposed to via the specialty or departmental culture, and the resulting hidden curriculum, can vary greatly.[16] The key to success in both types of clinical education is not merely a question of form, but that learners have the opportunities to actively engage in patient care in an environment that is structured, fosters interaction, and invites participation in cultural practices.[17] This is because medicine is not monolithic, and each specialty, department, and institution has its own culture and worldview. Therefore, the clinical experience is not unlike visiting a foreign country: students are told they are merely visiting "OBGYN world" or "Pediatrics world" and "Hospital X or Y." One should expect to encounter differences in language, customs, cultural norms, and identity expectations, but both the visitor and the "natives" will need to navigate these differences with mutual respect, reflection, and understanding in order to promote mutual growth. However, for someone who is in the process of transformation, there is not one sense of emerging, consistent identity or set of behaviors and expectations that can solidify over time. Instead, there is the continuous destabilization or reinventing of the self in each specialty, and the driving motivation is often survival based (i.e., to pass the clerkship), which is "student head" instead of the focus being on learning medicine and integrating a sense of professional behaviors, role, and identity.

Third, the assessment of performance during the clinical years is based far more on subjective assessment of skills and group-level behaviors (i.e., working in teams with the introduction of a new hierarchy and coordinating with other professions) than in the pre-clinical years, when assessment relies more heavily on individual objective performance, such as exams. Although there are still exams in the clinical years (e.g., National Board of Medical Examiners Subject Exams), the increased importance placed on communication and group process whereby constructive feedback can be given in real time and publicly adds to the difficulty in transitioning between learning milieus. In addition, learners are being asked to accept their lack of mastery over the skills and information in each clinical setting, at a time when the stakes regarding graded performance can be at its highest. This often breeds resistance to learning and feedback, which is then manifested as an external attribution instead of humility, acceptance, and taking responsibility for one's professional growth. In turn, this external attribution can breed resistance on the part of preceptors to give constructive feedback, especially for non-biomedical issues.

Attribution theory: interpreting behavior and attributing causality

Attribution theory[18] posits that when an individual must assign a reason or rationale for his or her own negative behavior (e.g., being late to work), the individual is inclined to find an external attribution (e.g., there was an accident on the highway) versus an internal attribution (e.g., I'm lazy) as the cause of the situation. In contrast, when an individual needs to assign a reason or rationale for someone else's negative behavior (e.g., being late to work), the individual is inclined to find an internal attribution (e.g., the other person is lazy) versus an external attribution (e.g., there was an accident on the highway) as the cause of the situation. When this feedback "attribution dance" unfolds between a preceptor (e.g., you were late to work and missed morning report) and learner (e.g., there was an accident on the highway), it can be interpreted that the learner is being (1) defensive, (2) not accepting responsibility for his or her actions, and (3) unwilling to learn. This perception

of not taking responsibility for one's own action as a professional in training can be seen as such an affront to professional identity that it can result in two common responses, which can have a negative impact on the mentor-mentee relationship.

The preceptor could invest scarce and limited time and energy in a struggle to make the learner take ownership of the learner's actions or could take the easier and more common approach, which is to just stop investing the effort to give the learner feedback. One of the telltale signs of the latter response is, when a learner asks a preceptor, "How am I doing?" and receives monosyllabic responses such as, "Fine." In such circumstances, it is not until the end-of-clerkship summative evaluation that the learner receives the preceptor's actual subjective assessment of the learner's skill-based and professionalism performance. Fortunately, it is easy to rectify this communicative misstep. Clinical preceptors and learners had to be trained to recognize this communication process, understand it, and be provided with a tool for both giving feedback and receiving it.

However, before embarking upon that process, a list of past patterns of learner behaviors consistent with the clerkship and the department's culture that the residents deemed violations of professional identity for the specialty was compiled, in order to make the learners explicitly aware of them. This then became the initial round of behaviors that we focused on in the educational intervention (described in Table 18.1). We then set forth to develop a two-pronged approach to change the learning environment, which required us to address both the structural impediments to learning and communication skills training.

Creating a climate for formative feedback

To promote humanism in medicine, we have to be willing to promote humanism in medical education. Unless an educational atmosphere is created that explicitly recognizes and rewards the behaviors being promoted, we cannot in good conscience expect there to be change on the part of the learners.[11] If we begin with the educational axiom that education is an expected process of growth and change through exposure, trial and error, and feedback, then we accept the natural learning curve and expect progression from adequacy to mastery. Any expectation of a learner to be more

Table 18.1. Residents' impressions of medical schools' failures to meet expectations

Resident impressions
"If I tell a student they have to come, see their patient and have their notes ready for me to review by 6:30 a.m. then I expect it to be done. It's a problem if I get there and the student isn't done and is saying, 'I didn't know the computer system because I'm new.' Well, you knew that so you needed to schedule more time and come in early. Now you can only review my notes and that's less effective for learning, plus I've lost the time I would have spent going over your notes with you. Students can't have excuses; this is about education and ultimately patient care."
"You have preparatory work to do before a surgery that is part of the experience. You need to read up on the patient, the surgery, diagnosis, why we're doing it, typical indications, so you can ask insightful questions. You can't just show up to the OR at 8 a.m. and think you get to scrub in, end of story."
"During one night we went in to the student call room and woke the student up, and told her we were going back to the O.R. to perform a c-section. I guess she must have reached the minimum number she needed for the rotation because she said, 'No thanks, I think I'll just sleep.'"
"Some don't show a lot of interest. They don't stimulate conversation by asking questions about their patients' diagnosis or treatment options. They never think to formulate a clinical question and then search the literature or bring in a research article to help us care for the patient."
"There have been times when a student needed their third vaginal delivery and forced their way into the room even though the resident determined it was best for the patient that the student not be involved. Just because something is a required experience students are not entitled to do it, like they paid for it, regardless of the situation. That's a human being, a patient we're treating. Required doesn't mean you are entitled to do it."
"Sometimes you get a feeling of entitlement like they shouldn't have to come to the hospital until a certain time or even at all. I had one student who just didn't show up for his shift. When I spoke to him about being a 'no show, no call,' he had never heard the term and didn't know what I was talking about. This isn't a class you're cutting, this is patient care."

"fully formed" than they are is unrealistic and bound to breed resistance to instruction, feedback and, most importantly, self-reflection, behaviors deemed integral to the formation of the professional role and identity of those entering a life in medicine.

Explicitly establishing this educational axiom with students as a departmental mantra has helped to foster a relationship with learners that has allowed them to more readily acknowledge their actions, take responsibility for them, and mutually construct a plan for improvement. Importantly, there are no "scarlet letters" for behaviors that are identified, accepted, and corrected. Corrected behaviors do not get documented on evaluations because they are considered "water under the bridge," provided that the behavior or infraction does not breach a legal or ethical boundary, which could require a greater response. The rationale is that in terms of the natural progression of skill building and professional formation, no health professional has "clean hands." All health professionals have, without malice or intention, erred in the pursuit of professional identity formation, skill acquisition, and

mastery, and at times under less than ideal circumstances. The goal of medical education has become increasingly focused on quality and performance improvement processes, which promote increased self-reflection and questioning: do you recognize it, do you take responsibility for it, and have you demonstrated progress toward correcting it?[19] But, to facilitate that process in medical education, the learning environment must be purposefully and consciously shaped and molded to address students' worries about documentation and grade implications, so that growth in skills, as well as professional identity, is fostered.

For example, in the department, no performance concern can be documented on the summative final evaluation (which is reflected in the student's Medical Student Performance Evaluation or Dean's letter) that was not documented on the formative mid-rotation evaluation, because it is assumed the learner was not given the feedback or the opportunity to improve before the final summative evaluation. However, this was not meant to place the sole expectation on the preceptor to provide constructive feedback and documentation. Instead, the institution developed a mid-rotation process that required the student to complete a narrative self-assessment of strengths and areas for improvement on each of the dimensions that the preceptor would evaluate, both at the formative mid-rotation and the end-of-clerkship summative evaluation (e.g., data acquisition, problem solving, communication, and professionalism). Then, at mid-rotation, the learner and the preceptor exchange evaluations in order to assess for any discrepancies in perception, discuss areas of strengths and concerns, and construct any plan for remediation, thereby creating a shared accountability for learning and outcomes. The department then took this process one step further by requiring each student to have a fifteen-minute, face-to-face meeting (in person or by videoconferencing) with the clerkship director or his or her designee, to review the learner-preceptor evaluations and discuss the learning environment, evaluate goals, and identify if any modifications or enhancements were required to assist with goal attainment. This model has proved effective, but only after a philosophical and communicative foundation was created.

Communication skills training to promote professional identity formation

All the world's a stage,
And all the men and women merely players;

They have their exits and their entrances, And one man in his time plays many parts, His acts being seven ages.
Shakespeare, As You Like It, Act 2, Scene 7

Given the lack of philosophical and pragmatic understanding that medical students appeared to have about the behavioral expectations of learning and working in a clinical milieu, a plan was formulated to address the findings and concerns we have outlined thus far in the chapter. Drawing inspiration from this famous Shakespeare quote, the vice chair designed a two-session lecture series utilizing impression management[20-22] and attribution theory[23] as the theoretical frameworks for promoting professional identity formation. In session one (ninety minutes), the goal is to set the stage for understanding and embracing the role that consciously managing an authentic impression synonymous with being a physician is important to foster the student doctor-patient relationship and the preceptor-student relationship. The second

session (sixty minutes) is designed to train students in communication skills grounded in impression management and attribution theory. The sessions train faculty and residents to provide feedback and train students to accept feedback using DiCorcia's 4-Part Impression Management Feedback Statement (outlined in Table 18.2). This communication tool was developed to address behavioral expectations that are specific to the OBGYN department, IUSM, and the health system.

Impression management: the lens for interpreting and judging professionalism

First, it is important to recognize that all human beings, including medical students, are actively involved in impression management on a daily basis. However, the driving question for medical educators becomes, "What level of awareness, purpose and flexibility do medical students exhibit over their behaviors as the learning milieu changes from the classroom to the clinic, and as their identities transform from medical student to student doctor?" Therefore, session one of the series was designed to illuminate the process and importance of impression management for both the actor (i.e., the message sender) and the audience (i.e., the receiver) and raise their awareness of the quandaries that the student will face on the clinical stage.

At its foundation, impression management is the process through which a person or group of people try to control the impressions or judgments that other people form of them (e.g., as a physician or learner), of an object (e.g., medical equipment), or of an event (e.g., medical intervention such as a test or surgery). What changes for the learner is that the impression drastically moves away from the learner as "John or Jane Doe" to solely "Dr. Doe." Despite all of the work that students have invested in making this transition a reality, they are slow to internalize that their patients and preceptors need and expect them not only to think like physicians, but to act and behave accordingly and with authenticity. To illustrate this point, we stated, tongue-in-cheek, that, "It is not enough to *be* a doctor but you have to play one on TV," for therapeutic, professional, and societal reasons.[24]

At this point in their training, medical students can become desensitized to the idea that the clinical transactions between the provider, treatment team, hospital environment, and patient violate many cultural and societal norms regarding corporal and information privacy.[25,26] This becomes especially compounded when introducing learners into the clinic setting, where the medical education community is asking the patient to allow a learner to "practice" skills on the patient's body, using the patient's personal and private information. Creating the impression of a "sacred space" for patients in this setting fulfills the need of the healthcare provider, and in this case, the medical student, to gain the patient's trust and participation in not only healthcare but also fulfillment of learning objectives.[25,26] Although this is a shared responsibility of the preceptor and the learner, the learner has not yet acquired the skills to manage this part of the doctor-patient relationship and clinical learning environment. Session one begins with helping medical students to understand impression management from the student's, or actor's, perspective.

Impression management: for the actor

Ultimately, people attempt to manage impressions because they are goal directed. Whether that goal is to pass the clerkship, or for the patient to allow the learner to participate in the patient's care and thus the learner's education, individuals are motivated in order to achieve a desired goal. There are many factors that the receiver (i.e., the audience) utilizes to form an impression of the actor, including self-presentation or self-image. Does the person exemplify the physical and behavioral representation, based on societal and professional expectations, of a physician?[24] Simply put, do you act and look like a doctor? Creating the desired impression takes more than donning a white coat, regardless of its length. For preceptors and patients, it is more important to be the embodiment of the ideals and behaviors that the white coat represents. For the student, it is therefore necessary to constantly be reflecting on and managing one's self-presentation or self-image to gauge how close one comes to the ideal and to evaluate the behaviors that promoted or interfered with constructing the desired impression[11,12] for the patient and the preceptor. Of course, there are other behaviors that influence the perception of professional identity, and many of them revolve around communication.

Verbal and nonverbal communication play an instrumental role in professional identity formation. After all, communication is the process that gives shape to reality through understanding and meaning; without it, there can be no doctor-patient interaction.[12] Nonverbal behavior holds the greatest sway on sense-making because of its tendency to be more unconscious, thereby believable, whereas verbal communication tends to be a more conscious process.[27] Ultimately, both forms of communication require conscious awareness and purposeful application in practice in order to facilitate the behaviors and impressions associated with professional identity.

Impression management: for the audience

The principal reason for teaching medical students to actively manage their behavior, grounded in the core values of medicine, is because the resulting impressions are the basis for building the doctor-patient relationship. Unlike health professionals, who might exact a different set of criteria for judging the competency of another health professional, the general public relies heavily on developing stereotypes of professional identity based almost entirely on interaction[24] (illustrated by Shakespeare's "entrances" and "exits" of the clinical encounter). In their current "part" or role, medical students are learning to navigate two very different worlds simultaneously. The first is the world of health professionals, and the second is the world of the patient. Each requires a distinct set of behaviors related to establishing a sense of professional identity and requires altering behaviors and communication in order to support the development of heuristics, so that each stakeholder can make sense of the encounters of everyday life.[27]

The process of developing simple heuristics or stereotypes is by definition fraught with errors, as individual differences are dismissed in favor of group generalizations to simplify a complex world.[27] Although "re-reading" of a person or situation is not only helpful but necessary for improving accuracy, rarely do individuals get a second chance to make a first impression. Nowhere is this clearer than for the medical student in the clinical setting, participating in a patient's care or being evaluated by the preceptor's impressions of their performance. Recognizing that physicians are constantly being monitored and evaluated "on stage" by patients, families, peers, and preceptors underscores the importance of developing strong communication and self-awareness skills. However, there is a critical part of communication individuals cannot completely control.

Meaning, understanding, and impression are based on the receiver's interpretation of communication events, and not on the intention of the actor.[28] Discussing or even debating intention is unproductive from a feedback standpoint because the communication behavior, and not the intention, is what the receiver must interpret to form his or her impression. Debating whether more significant weight should be attributed to "intention" over "impression" moves the feedback episode away from accepting that actions can have unintended consequences. To focus the feedback on the learner's behavior and its interpretation, the vice chair developed a feedback tool to help faculty and students in giving and receiving feedback in a way that deconstructs and distinguishes behaviors, impressions, and intentions.

DiCorcia's 4-Part Impression Management Feedback Statement

It is helpful to at least prime the educational pump by making learners aware that constructive feedback is an expected, natural, and necessary part of the process for skill acquisition, mastery, and professional identity formation. However, it was not uncommon at IUSM and elsewhere that learners did not recognize feedback when they received it. Part of the problem was that there was so much variability in feedback that without a consistent style, it was challenging to recognize it as feedback. Moreover, at times feedback pointed out a specific error but failed to broaden the learner's understanding concerning the greater implications of that error.

Therefore, the vice chair designed a theory-based feedback tool that would address the cognitive processes outlined above in order to facilitate learning in the clinical environment. The four main components needed are to identify (1) an observable behavior or error, (2) the effect the behavior or error has on an outcome, (3) the impression, if any, that the behavior or error could create in the mind of the audience, and (4) a specific remediation for correcting the observed behavior or error now and in the future.[22]

DiCorcia's 4-Part Impression Management Feedback Statement is structured to follow an important sequence and is illustrated below and in Table 18.2.

In the first part of the statement, it is important to simply identify the observable behavior (e.g., when you are late to clinic) or error, but without any

Table 18.2. DiCorcia's 4-Part Impression Management Feedback Statement

Suggested sequence

1. When you (identify the observable behavior or error),
2. The effects are (identify the effect the behavior or error has on an outcome),
3. The impression is/could be (identify, if any, the impression that the behavior or error can create in the mind of the audience),
4. I'd suggest (identify a specific remediation for correcting the observed behavior or error now and in the future).

EXAMPLE:

1. When you *are late to clinic,*
2. The effects are *that it inconveniences the patients who have to wait longer than they may have anticipated, which impacts their ability to return to their lives, and it potentially affects patient satisfaction and the clinic schedule for the rest of the day,*
3. The impression is/could be *that you don't care about your patients' time and that you aren't invested in this clinical rotation,*
4. I'd suggest *that you do whatever is necessary to get to clinic on time, whether that is set a second alarm clock or leave earlier for work in case there is traffic.*

interpretation or judgment (e.g., when you are inconsiderate and late to clinic). This can be harder than it appears, especially when training preceptors, who are accustomed to including interpretations in their feedback. However, the rationale is a simple one. Resistance to feedback is reduced when a behavior is observable, objective, and measurable. In contrast, people are more likely to feel defensive and close the lines of communication if they perceive the feedback to be an ad hominem attack or to assert a negative "intention" or drive behind the behavior or error.[29]

In the second part of the statement, it is important to create associations for the learner between behavior or error and potential effects or consequences. Resistance to persuasion is reduced when a person understands the "why" or "because" connection for a particular request.[30] These effects should relate directly to education, patient care, team dynamics, hospital policy, healthcare cost, professionalism, and professional identity. Therefore, in the example, "When you are late to clinic, the effects are that it inconveniences the patients, who have to wait longer than they may have anticipated, which impacts their ability to return to their lives and potentially affects patient satisfaction and the clinic schedule for the rest of the day."

The third part of the statement is where the preceptor has the opportunity to make the learner aware of the impression (not "intention") that the behavior or error either did or can create in the mind of the receiver or audience. Continuing with the current example, "When you are late to clinic … the impression could be that you don't care about your patients' time, and that you aren't invested in this clinical rotation."

Lastly, it is the fourth part of the statement that allows the preceptor to offer a potential solution that is often based on his or her own experience as a learner, preceptor, and/or clinician. As part of the mentoring process, the preceptor should offer what he or she would expect as a reasonable solution or response in order for the behavior or error to be corrected and considered remediated. Therefore, to bring the current example to conclusion, "…I'd suggest that you do whatever is necessary to get to clinic on time, whether that is set a second alarm clock or leave earlier for work in case there is traffic."

Utilizing DiCorcia's 4-Part Impression Management Feedback Statement provides preceptors with a consistent form and process for providing positive, reinforcing feedback and addressing problematic behaviors constructively, quickly, and succinctly. However, for a positive learning impact to follow, learners must first be trained in a process for accepting feedback.

DiCorcia's 4-Part Impression Management Response Statement

Giving feedback is only one-half of the process in fostering professional behavior and identity formation. Utilizing the same processes accounted for in the preceptor's feedback statement, it then became necessary to address them from the learner–receiver's perspective – to create a response for accepting feedback that would allow the learner an opportunity to recognize the behavior or error, express his or her thoughts and feelings, accept responsibility, and identify a plan for resolution. The four main components needed are to (1) apologize for the observable behavior or error, (2) recognize the lack of intentionality for the behavior or error, (3) identify an attribution but ultimately accept responsibility for the behavior or error, and (4) reinforce or identify the specific remediation for correcting the observed behavior or error now and in the future. DiCorcia's 4-Part Impression Management Response Statement is

Table 18.3. DiCorcia's 4-Part Impression Management Response Statement

Suggested sequence

1. I'm sorry I did/didn't (restate the observable behavior or error),
2. It wasn't my intention,
3. The reason was (identify and attribution), but I accept responsibility for it,
4. It won't happen again, as I will (reinforce a specific remediation for correcting the observed behavior or error now and in the future).

EXAMPLE:

1. I'm sorry I *was late to clinic,*
2. It wasn't my intention,
3. The reason was *there was an accident on Route 65 and traffic was backed up for miles,* but I accept responsibility for it,
4. It won't happen again as I will *leave for clinic a little earlier in case there is another accident, and if I get to work early I can use the time to read my textbook or review my patients' medical records for that day.*

structured to achieve these objectives and is illustrated above in Table 18.3.

In the first part of the statement, it is important for the learner to not only restate the behavior or error but also to apologize for it (e.g., "I'm sorry I was late to clinic."). The rationale is that the professional learner is responsible for ensuring the message was received, and in the process he or she learned an expectation that physicians will apologize for errors without fear of reprisal.

The second part of the statement is merely to neutralize any concerns that the learner has that his or her intentions could be called into question. It helps ensure that the recipient of the apology does not confound the act of apologizing with an admission of willful neglect or disregard for the person's well-being, emotions, or health.[22,31] It is therefore an expression of regret for an action that, although unfortunate and regrettable, was an accident. Continuing with the current example, "I'm sorry I was late to clinic, it wasn't my intention."

The third part of the statement is where the learner is allowed to assign a reason in an attempt to neutralize any doubt and suspicion regarding intention. It is necessary, and natural, to draw causal inferences between external factors and unintended actions, errors, or mistakes. However, regardless of the reason, the learner and future physician must be willing to accept responsibility for his or her actions. Therefore, furthering the example, "I'm sorry I was late to clinic, it wasn't my intention, the reason was there was an accident on Route 65 and traffic was backed up for miles but I accept responsibility for being late."

Lastly, the fourth part of the statement allows the learner to either recognize or amend the potential solution offered by the preceptor. This in essence becomes the acceptance of the remediation or learning contract between mentor and mentee, and holds the learner responsible for fulfilling the contract so that the issue can be "water under the bridge." Therefore, to conclude the current example, the learner's final statement would be, "It won't happen again as I will leave for clinic a little earlier in case there is another accident, and if I get to work early, I can use the time to read my textbook or review my patients' medical records for that day."

Utilizing DiCorcia's 4-Part Impression Management Response Statement provides learners with a consistent form and process for accepting feedback and creates a space for the learner to participate in the co-construction of feedback and identity formation. It also provides the learners with tools for fostering the mentor-mentee relationship in a gracious and collegial environment.

Tending the "garden of humanism"

Between 2008 and 2015, we set out to improve our departmental climate at IUSM, promote faculty vitality, and create an environment that would foster the professional formation of learners. With facilitation by local and national experts in appreciative inquiry and relationship-centered care, a vision and values statement was developed that expressed the aspirations of the faculty and implemented the faculty's proposals to move us closer to our vision. We better aligned faculty and resident recruitment practices with the professional attributes physicians most desire in their colleagues and themselves, and we developed strategies to recognize and celebrate those attributes. The "we" grew to comprise a community of faculty who have completed faculty development programs promoting humanism, who understand their roles in professional identity formation, and who work to create a positive departmental culture and learning climate. The success of the collective efforts is evident in a variety of qualitative and quantitative outcomes.

We compared medical student evaluations of the clerkship experience before and after implementing impression management and feedback training. There were significant improvements in the medical students' end-of-clerkship evaluations, including the specific items assessing how preceptors demonstrated respect for learners, listened to them, encouraged their participation in discussions, and encouraged them to bring up problems. The students noted that they received more frequent, constructive feedback, which included why the behavior was correct or incorrect, and suggestions for improvement. Preceptors were more likely to be viewed as models of professionalism and supportive of the team's emotions, to inspire the students' personal and professional growth, and to teach them communication and relationship-building skills. An increasing number of faculty and residents received the 4.0 Award based on student perception of teaching effectiveness and professionalism and humanism.

We witnessed an increase in medical student interest in our specialty as indicated by the number of internal residency program applicants rising from ten to twenty in the span of three academic years. In 2011, IUSM extended the Gold Humanism Honor Society to include six residents per year. Of the approximately 850 residents who were eligible, OBGYN residents, based on student nominations, have accounted for six of the eighteen inductees in 2011, 2012, and 2013 and one of six inductees in 2014. In the years following our initial efforts, we worked to consolidate our gains and prepare for new challenges.

The future of academic health centers is fraught with uncertainty and change.[32] During the past several years, the department has faced changes in the external environment caused by changes in affiliated health systems, the faculty practice plan, and the school of medicine. Uncertainty about the future provided an opportunity to test the resiliency of prior efforts and to develop new strategies for maintaining faculty vitality, protecting humanistic values, and maintaining focus on the patients and learners. In a time of rapid change it is essential to communicate frequently, distinguish facts from rumors, and demonstrate values of collaboration, respect, trust, and transparency. In addition to monthly faculty meetings, resident meetings, and new faculty mentoring lunches, the chair conducted separate meetings with each resident class on a rotating basis and invited the administrative chief resident to be present at every faculty meeting. When forming communications regarding externally imposed changes, we worked to model problem-solving communication, in contrast to pure expressions of frustration and concern, and to promote a more relationally coordinated culture.[33]

We also had access to focused faculty development opportunities. Two cohorts comprising eighteen faculty completed a twenty-eight-hour series of faculty development workshops to promote humanism through a grant from the Macy Foundation. The first cohort continues to meet monthly on a self-directed basis more than a year after completing the program. The workshops created dedicated time and space to deepen personal insights and mutual support as professional colleagues and role models, fostering greater resiliency.

Celebrating the impact we make keeps us centered on what matters most. No matter how the healthcare landscape may evolve, physicians hold enormous power to make enduring contributions to our patients, learners, and society. Patient care, teaching and learning, scholarship, and service are almost entirely under our direct control. Successes, small and large, provide opportunities to celebrate a job well done and value colleagues and team members. Truly appreciating the unique role of physicians in our society, and what we can accomplish in that role, creates a source of renewal on which we can perennially rely to recharge our humanism.

Additional initiatives are needed. More than half the current faculty joined the department after 2009 and did not have the opportunity to participate in the early retreats. Departmental leadership has a timely opportunity to refresh the vision and values statement, harvest new ideas, and form new initiatives for creating an aspirational environment in which to provide care and service, learn and educate, investigate, and support one another. Through these efforts the garden of humanism can continue to flourish – by pulling weeds, preparing the soil, planting seeds, and guiding the growth of what germinates.

References

1. Brater, DC. Viewpoint: infusing professionalism into a school of medicine: perspectives from the dean. *Acad Med*. 2007; **82**(11):1094–97.

2. Litzelman, DK, Cottingham, AH. The new formal competency-based curriculum and informal curriculum at Indiana University School of Medicine: overview and five-year analysis. *Acad Med*. 2007; **82**(4):410–21.

3. Cottingham, AH, Suchman, AL, Litzelman, DK, Frankel, RM, Mossbarger, DL, Williamson, PR, Baldwin, DC Jr, Inui, TS. Enhancing the informal curriculum of a medical school: a case study in organizational culture change. *J Gen Intern Med*. 2008; **23**(6):715–22.

4. Hafferty, FW. Beyond curriculum reform: confronting medicine's hidden curriculum. *Acad Med*. 1998; **73**(4):403–07.

5. Teherani, A, O'Sullivan, PS, Lovett, M, Hauer, KE. Categorization of unprofessional behaviours identified during administration of and remediation after a comprehensive clinical performance examination using a validated professionalism framework. *Med Teach*. 2009; **31**(11):1007–12.

6. Learman, LA, Autry, AM, O'Sullivan, P. Reliability and validity of reflection exercises for obstetrics and gynecology residents. *Am J Obstet Gynecol*. 2008; **198**(4):461.e1–e8, e8–e10.

7. Hickson, GB, Pichert, JW, Webb, LE, Gabbe, SG. A complementary approach to promoting professionalism: identifying, measuring, and addressing unprofessional behaviors. *Acad Med*. 2007; **82**(11):1040–48.

8. Janz, T. Initial comparison of patterned behaviour description interviews versus unstructured interviews. *J Appl Psychol*. 1982; **67**(5):577–80.

9. Lyon, D, Wiper, D. Finding our colleagues, finding ourselves: behavioral interviewing and critical assessment of how we identify and interview residency candidates. Unpublished paper. APGO/CREOG annual meeting: San Diego, CA; 2009.

10. Strand, EA, Moore, E, Laube, DW. Can a structured, behavior-based interview predict future resident success? *Am J Obstet Gynecol*. 2011; **204**(5):446.e1–e13.

11. Inui, TS, Cottingham, AH, Frankel, RM. Supporting teaching and learning of professionalism – changing the educational environment and students' "navigational skills." In Cruess, RL, Cruess, SR, Steinert, Y, eds. *Teaching Medical Professionalism*. New York, NY: Cambridge University Press; 2008;108–23.

12. Berger, PL, Luckmann, T. *The Social Construction of Reality: A Treatise in the Sociology of Knowledge*. New York, NY: Doubleday; 1966.

13. Huba, ME, Freed, JE. *Learner-Centered Assessment on College Campuses: Shifting the Focus from Teaching to Learning*. Boston, MA: Allyn & Bacon; 2000.

14. Fosnot, CT, Perry, RS. Constructivism: a psychological theory of learning. In Fosnot, CT, ed. *Constructivism: Theory, Perspectives, and Practice*. New York, NY: Teachers College Press; 2005:8–33.

15. Allen, MJ. *Assessing Academic Programs in Higher Education*. Boston, MA: Anker; 2004.

16. Cruess, RL, Cruess, SR, Boudreau, JD, Snell, L, Steinert, Y. Reframing medical education to support professionalism identity formation. *Acad Med*. 2014; **89**(11):1446–51.

17. Dornan, T, Boshuizen, H, King, N, Scherpbier, A. Experience-based learning: a model linking the processes and outcomes of medical students' workplace learning. *Med Educ*. 2007; **41**(1):84–91.

18. Amabile TM, Glazebrook, AH. A negativity bias in interpersonal evaluation. *J Exp Soc Psychol*. 1982; **18**(1):1–22.

19. Wong, BM, Levinson, W, Shojania, KG. Quality improvement in medical education: current state and future directions. *Med Educ*. 2012; **46**(1):107–19.

20. Goffman, E. *The Presentation of Self in Everyday Life*. New York, NY: Anchor Books; 1959.

21. Tseelon, E. Is the presenting self sincere? Goffman, impression management and the postmodern self. *Theory Cult Soc*. 1992; **9**(2):115–28.

22. DuBrin, AJ. *Impression Management in the Workplace: Research, Theory, and Practice*. New York, NY: Routledge; 2011.

23. Kelley, HH, Michela, JL. Attribution theory and research. *Annu Rev Psychol*. 1980; **31**:457–501.

24. Feldman, JM. Beyond attribution theory: cognitive processes in performance appraisal. *J Appl Psychol*. 1981; **66**(2):127–48.

25. Greene, K, Derlega, VJ, Yep, GA, Petronio, S. *Privacy and Disclosure of HIV in Interpersonal Relationships: A Sourcebook for Researchers and Practitioners*. Mahwah, NJ: Lawrence Erlbaum Associates; 2003.

26. Petronio, S, DiCorcia, MJ, Duggan, A. Navigating ethics of physician-patient confidentiality: a communication privacy management analysis. *Perm J*. 2012; **16**(4): 41–45.

27. Todorov, A, Chaiken, S, Henderson, MD. The heuristic-systematic model of social information processing. In Dillard, JP, Pfau, M, eds. *The Persuasion Handbook: Developments in Theory and Practice*. London, UK: Sage; 2002:195–211.

28. Andersen, PA. When one cannot not communicate: a challenge to Motley's traditional communication postulates. *Communication Studies*. 1991; **42**(4):309–25.

29. Knowles, ES, Linn, JA, eds. *Resistance and Persuasion*. Mahwah, NJ: Lawrence Erlbaum Associates; 2004.

30. Cialdini, RB. *Influence: Science and Practice*. Fifth edition. Boston, MA: Pearson Education; 2009.

31. Lazare, A. Apology in medical practice: an emerging clinical skill. *JAMA*. 2006; **296**(11):1401–04.

32. Dzau, VJ, Cho, A, Ellaissi, W, Yoediono, Z, Sangvai, D, Shah, B, Zaas, D, Udayakumar, K. Transforming academic health centers for an uncertain future. *N Engl J Med*. 2013; **369**(11):991–93.

33. Gittell, JH. Organizing work to support relational co-ordination. *International Journal of Human Resource Management*. 2000; **11**(3):517–39.

Chapter

19

Professional identities of the future: invisible and unconscious or deliberate and reflexive?

Brian D. Hodges

The philosophies of one age have become the absurdities of the next, and the foolishness of yesterday has become the wisdom of tomorrow.[1]

Introduction

In writing this chapter, I was given the task of pondering physician identities of the future. This deceptively complex challenge led me, by necessity, first into the past to see from whence we have come; then to scrutinize the present with the aim of finding clues to changes that might be in progress; and finally to project from the past and the present into a future – or more correctly, futures – that I can only half imagine.

Before launching into a consideration of those futures, it is important to do a little groundwork on what is meant by *future* and what gazing in that direction entails. I believe it is important to locate myself so as to make sense of my analysis. Briefly, I am a social constructionist, interested in history and discourse; a word about each follows.

Social constructionism

Some years ago I had the pleasure of chairing a group of international experts on the assessment of professionalism. The task assigned to us was to come up with a *consensus* on the assessment of medical professionalism. The most important contribution of this task force was to state that consensus was neither possible nor desirable. Indeed, the hard work of the committee was the identification of the wide range of beliefs about what we could say is known (epistemologies) about professionalism. We created a framework to help orient the many voices and perspectives on professionalism, a framework that was widely welcomed as helpful.[2]

The editors of this book have adopted the notion that *professionalism* is no longer, on its own, a sufficiently robust construct to capture the process that underpins becoming a physician; they would like to see a shift in the teaching of professionalism to support the development of professional identity. Had our task force, back in 2010, discussed identity rather than professionalism I am certain we would have encountered an equally diverse set of perspectives about what identity might be. Then, as now, my perspective is the one expressed as social constructionism: that professionalism and identity are social constructions arising from cultural contexts. Linked to this is my belief that there is no one, fixed universal definition of professionalism or of identity that can be said to be *true* in all places and in all periods of time. This means that in my mind there is no *one* future to predict; there are instead many possible *futures*.

Discourse

In order to consider possible futures, I am interested specifically in how language produces what it is possible to think, to say, and to be at different places and in different times. I am more interested in the social forces that shape who we are than I am in the inheritance of genes or the influence of an unseen developmental force. I have undertaken detailed studies of competence, incompetence, reflection, and assessment using this approach to understand how each of these has been constructed at different places and in different times and to understand more about what effects (including adverse or unintended) are achieved when each comes to be thought of in a particular way. By studying the traces of a society's language in text, speech, and graphic forms I get clues about how objects and roles are created by ways of thinking and

Teaching Medical Professionalism, 2nd Edition, ed. Richard L. Cruess, Sylvia R. Cruess and Yvonne Steinert.
Published by Cambridge University Press. © Cambridge University Press 2016.

speaking about them. Discourses are "practices that systematically form the objects of which they speak."[3] (p. 49)

The optimistic dimension of this perspective is that if we can see the constructive power of discourse, then we can, with some deliberate effort, shape it. However, it is not enough to simply think, talk, or write in a particular way to bring something into being. Culture, tradition, and power work to make particular ways of thinking, speaking, and being more viable, more legitimate, and thus more likely to dominate. It is this *more* that I am going to explore in this chapter. From an infinite number of ways we could think about professionalism and about professional identities, some are *much more likely* to shape the future than others.

A few definitions of identity

What better place to look for discourses about identity than the Oxford English Dictionary (OED) Historical Thesaurus?[4] This wonderful resource provides a snapshot of the way concepts and objects are defined in the present and how they have been defined in the past. For *identity*, OED gives a tripartite definition:

> Who or what a person or thing is;
>   a distinct impression of a single person or thing presented to or perceived by others;
>   a set of characteristics or a description that distinguishes a person or thing from others.[4]

There are three distinct concepts contained within the present definition; I will explore each of these below. But first let us also examine OED's historical examples of the use of the term *identity*:

> 1789 J. Morgan Ess. III. ii. 199 But, as to the proof of identity, whatever is sufficient to satisfy a jury, is good evidence.
> 1819 W. Irving Rip Van Winkle in Sketch Bk. i. 86 He doubted his own identity, and whether he was himself or another man.
> 1885 "E. Garrett" At Any Cost v. 89 Tom … had such a curious feeling of having lost his identity, that he wanted to reassure himself by the sight of his little belongings.
> 1926 People's Home Jrnl. Feb. 33/1 Everything indicated that he had been ready for flight and probably had some hiding place, either in town or out, where the rest of his loot was cached and where he had slipped into disguising clothes and a new identity.

> 2005 K. Harrison Starter Marriage 127 She has so many different identities, from trouble-shooting head teacher, to spiritual hippy chick, to glamorous property tycoon's wife, to country-bumpkin earth mother.[4]

Note how the 1789 usage suggests a *real* or *authentic* identity; one that can be proved or called into question. The 1819 and 1885 usages, on the other hand, bring into play the notions of *fluid* and *lost* identities. The 1926 selection adds the possibility of creating a *new* identity, while the 2005 example speaks to *multiple* identities.

These are not accidents of selection by the editors of the OED. During these epochs, there were many epistemological shifts. The 1789 citation comes from the classical era of positivism with its commitment to finding absolute and generalizable truths about the universe. The middle three citations were no doubt influenced by the notions of fluidity and the unconscious nature of phenomena introduced by psychoanalysis, surrealism, and existentialism in the late nineteenth and early twentieth centuries. Most recently, the last quote from 2005 illustrates the post-1950s concept of multiple identities and the constructed nature of reality associated with late twentieth century post-structuralism and post-modernism.

It is clear that what identity is, is shaped by dominant notions of what anything is or might be at a given period of history; identity is not a construction that one can understand by examining a single field as specific as medicine. Medicine and medical education do not exist on an epistemological island; the discourses that shape society in general shape medicine and medical education.

Gazing forward is not the same as science fiction

It is by now clear that I believe there are many possible formulations of identity and therefore hundreds of different futures could be written. What I describe below, however, are my speculations about what I think is *likely* based on what has already been (history of identity), what exists today (current dominant conceptions of identity), and what can reasonably be imagined to arise from these two.

All of this ignores the possibility of a convulsive paradigm shift. I do not deny that such a shift is possible. It could be, for example, that the role called *medical doctor* will disappear entirely in the future, replaced by one or more new professionals or by technologies. Although the role *doctor* has existed for about 2,000 years in the West, this is a rather short span compared with human existence. It also might be that the nature of disease and its treatment will change so drastically that the professional expertise required to treat disease will shift to another field, becoming a branch of engineering, for example. Modern surgery is an instructive example, having emerged as an outgrowth of barbering just a few hundred years ago. The use of medication, unknown to physicians for centuries, was appropriated from apothecaries during a relatively recent time frame. And consider that it has been just over a hundred years since we created the uneasy graft of the mind onto the biomedical body, uniting some of psychiatry's notions of psychodynamics and the unconscious very awkwardly with the rest of biomedicine. In the latter case there is perhaps a future to be imagined in which the care of the biomedical body is distinct from the care of the mind and of its consciousness, desires, and values. Finally, in many societies and cultures, the care and guidance of the spirit is not separate from the care of the body, and one could imagine a rapprochement between ministering to the mind, the spirit, and the body as a possible future for our field.

While these are all viable futures, imagining them takes us into the realm of science fiction. Tempting as it might be, I shall leave that exercise to individuals more gifted in the science fiction genre and instead project into a nearer, more graspable future. While we may not be able to completely predict the near future, we may be able to shape it, albeit such shaping will require a deliberate, concerted effort because calling for change is not the same as setting change in motion.

Calling for change is not the same as setting change in motion

Medical education is replete with calls for reform. Some have famously been associated with significant changes (e.g. the early twentieth-century Flexner reforms – see Flexner, 1910[5]) while others were completely forgotten.[6,7] Whitehead et al.[8] argue that there is an industry in medicine that thrives on publishing calls for change and that the content of these calls is remarkably repetitive. They argue that a sort of historical amnesia is brought about by attaching to these calls for reform a discourse of *newness* and sometimes of *crisis*.

Using this lens, we can look more critically at several contemporary calls for reform and wonder about the degree to which they will be heeded. For example, The Lancet's *Health Professionals for a New Century: Transforming Education to Strengthen Health Systems in an Interdependent World*[9] (p. 1951) calls for a shift from education that is *formative* to education that is *transformative* whereby health professional students and practitioners see it as part of their identity to advocate for and work toward systems change. Similarly, in the United States the Carnegie Foundation report *Educating Physicians: A Call for Reform of Medical School and Residency* calls for a greater emphasis on professional identity formation.[10] In Canada, the twin undergraduate and postgraduate reports on the *Future of Medical Education in Canada* call for renewed efforts at "ensuring that Canada's medical education system continues to meet the changing needs of Canadians, both now and into the future,"[11] giving major attention to professional identity formation as a strategy.

These are important and hopeful documents. As noted, however, history makes clear that much of what is called for in such reports never materializes. That is because to call for change is not the same as to accomplish the hard work of shifting the discourses and practices that make the desired change possible. Therefore, without significant faculty and institutional development, it is very possible that none of the change called for with respect to identity formation will occur. Indeed, continuation of the current state is my first predicted future. The second future I foresee is something of a return to the past, with its nostalgic focus on character. Finally, as will become apparent, my preference lies with a third possible future – one in which educators take a deliberate and reflexive approach to the formation of identities.

Here are the three futures I imagine:

(1) Future one: Identity continues to be thought of as a desirable competence or set of *characteristics*. Its formation takes places largely invisibly in the cracks and gaps of what is called a *hidden curriculum*.

(2) Future two: Identity reverts to a holistic notion of good *character*. Its formation is largely tacit, assumed to develop through unconscious identification and role modeling.

(3) Future three: Identity is reimagined, in the plural, as a form of self-construction. The formation of identities is deliberate and conscious through critical reflexivity.

Future 1: Identity continues to be thought of as a desirable competence or set of characteristics. Its formation takes places largely invisibly in cracks and gaps of what is called a hidden curriculum.

Identity: *a set of characteristics or a description that distinguishes a person or thing from others.*[4]

Let's begin with the possibility that very little will change at all. This is, in fact, the most likely future. Our present, at least in terms of notions of physician competence, is only about 50 years old, originating in the 1960s when a new discourse of medical competence as a set of definable *characteristics* took hold.[12] This development corresponded to the rising place of psychologists in medical education and the influence of their expertise on instrumentalization of personality and capacity.[13] In this period, admission and assessment models in medical education began to employ concepts from personality psychology and psychometrics. Most relevant for this chapter is the fact that the word *professionalism* came to be understood as a discrete competence or characteristic and was often treated as though it were separate from other competences. For example, in both the CanMEDS[14] and ACGME[15] competency frameworks, *professional* appears as a discrete role or competence that is to be defined and evaluated separately from other competencies. It is not surprising then that, when we look at the OED entry for identity, we also find it defined as a "set of characteristics."[4]

Our present is shaped significantly by the dominance of behaviorism: a way of understanding the world in which human motivation is conceptualized in terms of responding to stimuli in predictable and trainable ways. Behaviorist educational systems place value on response and reward. This explains medical education's assessment-heavy approach that rewards or punishes certain behaviors in order to shape medical students. The twentieth-century adoption of the notion of competence as a set of characteristics meant that more holistic concepts such as identity were either marginalized or understood as an assemblage of smaller pieces. The behaviorist impulse has meant that for half a century medical educators have spent a great deal of their time observing and recording individual behaviors in the hopes of reassembling them into a whole picture through processes of aggregation.[16]

Orienting medical schools around the codification, selection, and testing of specific characteristics of individuals did not seem problematic at first. In fact, competence frameworks advanced medical education in a number of positive ways.[17] However, toward the end of the twentieth century, scholars began to notice a problem. Something that was called the *hidden curriculum* appeared to exist in and around the formalized and codified teaching.[18] Indeed, it appeared that *most* of what we might call identity formation was a product of what happened when students were *not* focused on the formal curriculum. The experiences of being on-call with more senior residents, witnessing the way clinicians treated patients in the emergency department, overhearing the social conversation of senior trainees, and observing role models were all far more potent influences in shaping the emerging professional identities of medical students than anything that could be captured and packaged as a lecture, a textbook, or an e-learning module.

So while sequestering professionalism as a separate competence served in the beginning because it gave it a name and a place in curricula, as the twentieth century rolled into the twenty-first, educators became troubled that professional identity was developing more in the informal curriculum than the formal; more in the cracks between the roles and competencies than within them. Some began to suspect that dissociating professionalism and identity formation from other competencies might not be serving individual students or the profession well.

The above concern is expressed by the editors of this book as a call to link the concept of professionalism to identity formation and to re-center identity formation as the primary goal of medical education. In naming this book *Teaching Medical Professionalism: Supporting the Development of a Professional Identity*, the authors hope that by giving more attention to the concept of identity formation in medical schools, greater progress can be made to deal with what is perceived as an increasingly tenuous commitment to the "calling" and a rise in worrisome attitudes and behaviors.

The above position is a thoughtful direction. The notion of changing the premise of medical education and to anchor it in identity formation is one that I will explore in the next two futures. However, I want to emphasize that while identity formation is not the construct most often used to orient medical education today, the process of forming an identity certainly goes on nonetheless. In fact, it would be impossible *not* to form an identity during medical training. To reframe the problem slightly then, the concern appears to me to be that our current medical curricula, steeped as they are in the behaviorist tradition and oriented to help develop definable characteristics may not, in fact, be creating the identity educators *desire*. What then is it that medical schools are creating?

Frost and Regehr[19] have thoughtfully described a tension that runs through medical education today:

> The discourse of diversity emphasizes individuality, difference and plurality of possibilities and advances the notion that heterogeneity is beneficial to medical education and to patients. In contrast, the discourse of standardization strives for homogeneity, sameness, and a limited range of possibilities, and conveys that there is a single way to be a competent, professional physician.[19] (p. 1570)

My sense is that this tension arises, in part, because adoption of language from business creates a fertile ground for thinking about education in the way that we think about manufacturing. Schools are often compared (at least metaphorically) to *factories*, curricula to *conveyor belts*, students to *raw materials*, and graduates to *products*. Thus standardization and efficiency are positioned as key objectives in education and work, as Frost and Regehr[19] have described, at odds with diversification and multiplicity of perspectives. I have previously drawn parallels between the logic of manufacturing and use of these concepts in medical education by using the provocative name *i-Doc* to represent the notion that we can control the manufacturing of doctors with all of the right applications built in, creating a graduate who is *fit-for-purpose* and who will function with maximum efficiency.[20] Perhaps the ultimate extension of this way of thinking is The Doctor on *Star Trek: The Next Generation*. This doctor is a hologram, programmed to respond to medical situations, to diagnose, to treat, and sometimes, to manifest a form of programmed empathy. Perhaps he has a *professionalism app*. Thinking about education as a process of manufacturing doctors with the right built-in functionalities is powerfully aligned with assumptions about human behavior and the role of education that go well beyond medicine today. While there are important efforts to re-center medical education around humanism[21] and to balance caring and compassion with the technical aspects of healthcare,[22] the drive for standardization and efficiency is hard to resist. We may well, therefore, simply carry on thinking about identity as a producible set of *characteristics*, allowing identity formation to push up, here and there, through the cracks between our standardized roles and competencies.

Future 2: Identity reverts to a holistic notion of good character. Its formation is largely tacit, assumed to develop through unconscious identification and role modeling

Identity: *a distinct impression of a single person or thing presented to or perceived by others.*[4]

Whitehead et al.[12,23] have explored constructions of the "good doctor" across the twentieth century. They noted that in the early part of the century, before the rise of the discourse of characteristics discussed above, the emphasis was on *character*. Expressed as a holistic quality, character was thought essential to becoming a physician. Identifying the right character was a puzzle for medical schools and much debate raged about whether it was something inborn and therefore amenable to selection process or something that could be cultivated through education. In any case, the way character was discussed in this early literature makes it clear that it was something to be judged by *another person*. Such holistic constructions are also called *gestalt*. This way of thinking about identity corresponds better with the first part of the OED definition, which defines identity as "a distinct impression of a single person or thing presented to or perceived by others."[4]

As I have discussed, there is contemporary awareness of the limitations of thinking of identity as a set of separate roles or characteristics, and it would appear that a more holistic approach is once again gaining in appeal. Indeed, there are calls on many fronts to return to more holistic, integrated forms of curriculum and assessment in medicine and a seemingly renewed appreciation of teachers' assessments as holistic, social judgments.[24–26] Unlike 100 years ago, there are efforts today to extend judgment-based models to include the perspectives and evaluations of other health professionals and of patients and families. With holism and expert judgement models on the rise, it is possible that we are distancing ourselves from a rather reductionist era in the history of medical education. It is also possible that complex, integrated concepts such as identity formation will be given great prominence if this trend continues.

However, we should not dream of returning to a model of judging character exactly as was done in the early twentieth century. As Cruess et al. have written, "the early history of modern professionalism in the Anglo-American world reveals that it was more exclusionary than inclusive, with women, non-whites, and ethnic minorities having difficulty in finding a place."[27] Returning to an era in which the notion of good character meant being male, white, heterosexual and from the middle or upper classes would be regressive. And while we perhaps fancy ourselves in the twenty-first century to have risen above such exclusionary ways of thinking, current research illustrates quite clearly that the perils of entitlement and privilege continue to exist in the profession.[28] But assuming, for a moment, that a holistic approach to identity could be adopted without the discriminatory and exclusionary elements of its former twentieth-century form, what could a character-based sense of identity formation look like in the twenty-first century?

First of all, the shape of such a model would depend greatly on where medical educators fall on the nature-nurture debate about character. This debate has raged for decades and there is little reason to believe it has abated. Although the drive to find fixed and predictive traits and behaviors associated with professionalism has not been particularly successful[29,30], the belief that good doctors are born and not made is tenacious. A strong possibility, then, is that, were the behaviorist model to be less dominant in thinking, greater power might be conferred on ways of finding the right *characters*. The current fascination with mini-multiple interviews (a form of objective structured clinical examination adapted for admissions based on a behaviorist–characteristics model described earlier) can be seen holistically as a means of encouraging the right kind of thought, behavior, and perhaps identity.[31]

If, on the other hand, educators put less emphasis on admissions and more on processes of identity formation as curriculum, thinking about character holistically might foreground role modeling and the shaping effect of socialization. Concepts of extended mentorship, longitudinal learning, and working with authentic, contiguous teams might serve this agenda well. The editors of this book argue that "socialization, with its complex networks of social interaction, role models and mentors, experiential learning and implicit and tacit knowledge acquisition, influences each learner in medicine and causes them to gradually come to 'think, act and feel like a physician.'"[27] (p. 2) But perhaps most importantly, assessment systems that currently emphasize piecemeal bits and pieces of competence would have to give way to more integrated, holistic judgments. I have suggested elsewhere that posing simple questions such as "would you send a family member to see this clinician?" to a wide variety of professionals, patients, and family members might provide a more robust and better integrated picture of competence (and perhaps identity) than dozens of standardized written and performance tests.[17]

An interesting nuance, however, appears if we look again at this part of the OED definition of identity – identity is defined "as perceived by *others*."[4] This perspective brings to light what Canadian sociologist Erving Goffman[32] called a *dramaturgical* performance of roles in life. In his sense, good character is *performed* and the creation of a stable role is what Goffman called *impression management*. While attending to character, whether through admissions processes or through assessment that judges socialization, would be a gain in terms of holism, a possible weakness in such a model is the authenticity of role performance. Human beings are savvy and if the behaviorist model has taught us anything, it is that medical students will learn to respond as their teachers desire, at least while they are being watched. A second risk is the over-attribution of character to individuals. The influx of social scientists into medical education in the twentieth century helped make more visible the significant role that context and environment play in the attitudes and behaviors that individuals manifest. They helped show that competence, professionalism, and perhaps identities are transient, changeable, and shaped as much by circumstance as by any stable internal traits.[33]

Optimistically, medical education could this time incorporate into character multiple identities and address blind spots (gender, class, ethnicity, sexuality) that tarnished the early twentieth century. However, if the location for judging character remains external to the individual medical students, it seems more likely that teachers will continue to see what students think they are looking for – character as a performance. It is therefore possible that we might simply return to pre-Flexner times when educators simply *knew*, without having to unpack or critically examine their own knowing, who has the right character to be a doctor and who does not. And as we have seen, this unexamined knowing contained some problematic systematic biases. Returning to this form of identity as character in a *black box*, interpreted on the basis of unquestioned impressions, is what some call *nostalgic professionalism*. This future might give us back the doctor from a Norman Rockwell painting.

Future 3: Identity is reimagined, in the plural, as a form of self-construction. The formation of identities is deliberate and conscious through critical reflexivity.

Identity: *who or what a person or thing is.*[4]

By far the most philosophical part of the OED[4] definition is this one. Identity here is framed as an ontological puzzle – what is it possible to be? Though a more radical perspective, perhaps medical educators may come to see that there is no fixed state, no permanent identity to be achieved. Unlike characteristics or character that can be attained, defined, and perhaps selected or assessed at a particular point in time, the conception of identities as fluid and permanently changeable requires a paradigm shift.

Yet it is hard to deny that change is more characteristic of medical practice than is stability. There is no stable context in which physicians work. Taking a future orientation, today's graduates will be practicing after 2050 and what they will be doing is almost impossible to imagine. As the context of practice changes, identity must change with it. A solidified or even fossilized identity will work against adaptive competence in new contexts. Jarvis-Selinger et al.[34] have argued that identity formation is:

> ...an adaptive developmental process that happens simultaneously at two levels: (1) at the level of the individual, which involves the psychological development of the person and (2) at the collective level, which involves the socialization of the person into appropriate roles and forms of participation in the community's work. (p. 1186)

Unlike talking about identity as a way of judging character through external eyes in Future 2, this third future is one in which the primary driver of identity is internal to the student. As Cruess et al.[27] have written:

> It is important to realize that the development of a professional identity takes place within the context of individual identity formation, a process that begins at birth and results in a complex mix of identities (gender, nationality, race, religion, class, etc.) that represents how each individual is perceived and perceives themselves. (p. 1447)

It is this perception of *oneself* that is pivotal. Cruess et al. continue, "essentially individuals construct and situate themselves in 'progressively more complex systems for making sense of the world.'"[27] (p. 1447) This way of thinking stands in contrast to the positivist sense that identity formation is linear and auto-determined. Identity formation then is a windy road an individual travels along on which he or she meets challenges and crises that buffet and shape his or her (multiple) identities. The process is one of formation and reformation in social spaces much more than it is an unfolding of a master developmental plan. Formation of identities is often difficult or even painful. Thinking about identity formation in this way sheds light on the possible functions of medical training to foster *identity repression* and also *identity dissonance*.[27] (p. 1448) Frost and Regehr have pointed out the significant challenges a medical student faces in reconciling medicine's dominant discourse of standardization (discussed in Future 1) and the discourse of individual diversity.[19]

At the end of the twentieth century, the social sciences generally underwent a transformation, moving away from univocal *standpoints* in which the world was viewed (often critically) through one particular lens such as gender or sexuality, to a notion that all individuals embed multiple identities.[35] This perspective is called *intersectionality* and makes clear that identity is a fluid, changeable construct through which we engage multifaceted perspectives. For example, following on the work of sociologist bell hooks, a black female medical student may well know the corrosive forces of racism in a way that her white classmates do not – something that will not be addressed by taking a gender perspective alone.[36] Similarly, considering a religious student's perspective without also entertaining their sexual, cultural, and socioeconomic identities leaves much out. These dimensions of identity – some visible, some not – are the foundation on which students form their emerging professional identity. To choose to ignore them in medical education is to attend to only small parts of students' identity formation.

What students choose to reveal or suppress depends on the climate of training, and this observation is the key one in understanding the problems of external systems of assessment.[37] This latter point deserves emphasis, because it is not just any identity that will do for medical educators; the stakes are much higher for all concerned. The *modus operandi* of a medical school is a drive toward a *professional* identity. Indeed Cruess et al. (2014) take as a starting point that a physician's identity "is a representation of self, achieved in stages over time during which the characteristics, values, and norms of the medical profession are internalized, resulting in an individual thinking, acting, and feeling *like a physician*." (emphasis added)[27] (p. 1447) Educators must therefore be thoughtful about the ways in which they tacitly but strongly convey and enforce what is *acceptable*, or indeed *normal* to think, say, or be in medicine. Educators can never truly understand the life experiences or perspective of all of their students. Yet this does not mean that identities and their formation cannot be discussed. Indeed, the potential of this future is that it centers medical education precisely around such discussions. The notion of a hidden curriculum might no longer be needed because what was formerly hidden – the assumptions, discourses, and shaping contexts – are now thought of as *the* curriculum of identity formation.

There is a second element to a future in which identity formation is deliberate and conscious. Moving away from thinking about identity as something that takes place in interstitial spaces (in the characteristics model) or as a black box, tacit process (as in the character model), also means embracing *critical reflexivity* by students and their teachers. Central to this is acknowledging that there are other ways of knowing and being and that what we think of as appropriate or useful in medical practice today may be swept away as outmoded or inappropriate in the future. A good grasp of medical history and the sometimes amusing, sometimes-shocking, beliefs and practices of the past are an indispensable foundation for such reflection.[38] Indeed, it may be that one of the most important functions of a medical school is to teach students to see how strange some of our practices have been and to use lenses of history and cross-cultural studies to develop a healthy skepticism to any received wisdom. Today, the construction of medical practice and identity is largely anchored in western tradition. Yet it seems inevitable that what a doctor is, will shift through *hybridization* as non-Euro-American cultures continue to rise in dominance in world affairs and medical trainees and educators engage each other in a rapidly globalizing world. Ho is among a group of scholars who point out how shaky the foundation of ethics and practice can become when one crosses into medical education in a different culture.[39]

Martimianakis and Hafferty formulated some of the challenges medical teachers face when trying to reconcile, in the classroom, competing discourses of what a doctor is in a globalizing world.[40] For example, North American physicians (and students) have to navigate the commitment to serving the needs of individual patients in a relatively wealthy part of the world, while experiencing a greater and greater pull toward the enormous needs of those in underserved, deprived parts of the world that are increasingly made visible in media but also in the classroom. While social responsibility apparently underpins professionalism in that the responsibility of the medical profession to society is bound up in most of its definitions, how does an individual medical student create an identity as a socially responsible physician when he or she is torn between different and competing responsibilities that are local, national, and global? The burning questions for medical schools in the twenty-first century will be, social responsibility *to whom*? Tensions in identity formation are intrinsically woven into this question.

Finally, we must consider the individual versus the collective. To some degree, formation of identity in the reflexive way I have described will also require confronting the current overemphasis on a professional as an individual. If we were to relinquish, at least to some degree, our preoccupation with individuals as the sole source of professional competence and think about professional competence and identity as part of a collective, attention could shift (for admissions, assessment, quality, and maintenance of competence) to institutional contexts and collectives. Could we embrace a form of professional identity that has both collective and individual dimensions?

At a time of modularization of training, when boundaries between professions are constantly changing and scopes of practice overlap, some have argued that we cannot go on thinking about the identity of physicians without also thinking about the identity of all the other health professionals with whom they work.[41] To a large degree, taking a reflexive approach means examining how physician identity is defined in contradistinction to other health professions ("I am a doctor and not a nurse because...") and how the overlap in what each profession does and the boundaries between them are justified.

Taken together, this future hinges on a deep awareness of and responsibility for the self and a commitment by educational institutions and teachers to foster and promote fluid, changeable, and multifaceted identities. To a large degree, I think it also means abandoning much of the way we assess students today. Though I will not repeat the whole argument here, several recent papers have laid out clearly why critical reflection in the original sense of Dewey[42], Habermas[43] and to some degree Schön[44], is not compatible with external assessment. Too much instrumentalization of reflection (for example, through the marking or grading of reflection) works against the development of the self and the capacity for critical reflexivity.[45] The result, as I have argued, may be something more akin to *confession* than to personal growth. The overuse of external judgment may work against the formation of a robust, flexible, and critically insightful self.[46]

Another consequence of fostering identity formation as critical reflexivity is that students will, by definition, challenge the *status quo*. It is perhaps for this reason above all else that my personal hope is to see the dawn of this third future. Educators will need to embrace rather than shun attempts to shine light on the inconsistencies, problematic interpersonal and interprofessional dynamics, and even the frank power imbalances that riddle healthcare and its practice.[47] This might be a little painful at first, and I am not sure that the current professoriate is up to this challenge. Future 3, in which identity formation becomes a form of work on the self with the aim of developing the capacity for critical reflection, might require, to some degree, a differently constituted faculty. Just as at mid-century clinical teaching faculty began to displace basic scientists in medical schools, perhaps more of tomorrow's teachers should have as their primary strength, the capacity to model and foster critical reflection.

If we are to realize a future in which the formation of identities is deliberate and reflexive, watchwords for educators in the twenty-first century will need to be *adaptive expertise, metacognition, cognitive flexibility*, and *critical reflexivity*.[48] This will not occur without substantial investment in faculty and institutional development. Admissions policies, curricula, and assessment programs will need to be reconceptualized so that, at minimum, they do not work against identity formation and ideally so that they support the development of critical reflexivity. Curricula will have to evolve to promote healthy suspicion about any truth or practice that is prescriptive, dogmatic, or posited as universal, emphasizing that laws, practices, and professional codes of conduct are constructed and reconstructed across history and geography. Students will need to think of themselves as evolving, their competence as never finished, and each new context as a challenge requiring adaptation. If any common core can be identified for the physician of the future, it must surely revolve around compassion, caring, and healing. But the identification of a common set of values is not enough for this future to come into existence. Indeed, it is not the definition of commonalities that characterizes this form of identity formation; rather, the crucial dimension of this future is vigilance. The physician in this future will recognize the need to remain vigilant to beliefs, practices, and truths – including his or her own – that work against human freedom, dignity, health and well-being. This doctor will ask himself or herself, "Who am I?", "What am I?" and, "What are the effects of what I do and do not do?"

Because this future will not be compatible with strong external standardized testing, rigid rules, and prescriptive behavioral codes, there is a very good chance that it will not take root. To render identity formation the *point* of medical education will be strange and perhaps even disorienting for educators; to teach students to challenge assumptions and to think critically seems a daunting challenge. Nevertheless, to imagine a future in which becoming a physician is a process of forming multiple identities in a curriculum that is deliberate, critically reflexive, and never finished, is to imagine a medical profession that is highly adaptable, cognitively flexible, and oriented to the social and contextual as much as the individual and the personal.

References

1. Osler, W. Chauvinism in medicine. Montreal: M. J. 31:684, 1902. As cited in Bean, WB. Excerpts from Osler: a mosaic of bedside aphorisms and writings. *Arch Intern Med.* 1949; **84**(1):72–76.

2. Hodges, BD, Ginsburg, S, Cruess, R, Cruess, S, Delport, R, Hafferty, F, Ho, MJ, Holmboe, E, Holtman, M, Ohbu, S, Rees, C, Ten Cate, O, Tsugawa, Y, Van Mook, W, Wass, V, Wilkinson, T, Wade, W. Assessment of professionalism: recommendations from the Ottawa 2010 Conference. *Med Teach.* 2011; **33**(5):354–63.

3. Foucault, M. *The Archaeology of Knowledge.* New York, NY: Pantheon Books; 1972.

4. *Oxford English Dictionary.* Second edition. Oxford, UK: Oxford University Press; 1989. [Accessed Jan. 1, 2015]. Available from www.oed.com/view/Entry/91004?redirectedFrom=identity#eid.

5. Flexner, A. *Medical Education in the United States and Canada. A Report to the Carnegie Foundation for the Advancement of Teaching. Bulletin No. 4.* Boston, MA: Updike; 1910.

6. Bloom, SW. Structure and ideology in medical education: an analysis of resistance to change. *J Health Soc Behav.* 1988; **29**(4):294–306.

7. Christakis, NA. The similarity and frequency of proposals to reform US medical education. Constant concerns. *JAMA.* 1995; **274**(9):706–11.

8. Whitehead, CR, Hodges, BD, Austin, Z. Captive on a carousel: discourses of 'new' in medical education 1910–2010. *Adv Health Sci Educ Theory Pract.* 2013; **18**(4):755–68.

9. Frenk, J, Chen, L, Bhutta, ZA, Cohen, J, Crisp, N, Evans, T, Fineberg, H, Garcia, P, Ke, Y, Kelley, P, Kistnasamy, B, Meleis, A, Naylor, D, Pablos-Mendez, A, Reddy, S, Scrimshaw, S, Sepulveda, J, Serwadda, D, Zurayk, H. Health professionals for a new century: transforming education to strengthen health systems in an interdependent world. *Lancet.* 2010; **376**(9756):1923–58.

10. Cooke, M, Irby, DM, O'Brien, BC. *Educating Physicians: A Call for Reform of Medical School and Residency.* San Francisco, CA: Jossey-Bass; 2010.

11. Association of Faculties of Medicine of Canada. *The Future of Medical Education in Canada.* [Accessed Jan. 1, 2015.] Ottawa, ON; AFMC. Available from www.afmc.ca/future-of-medical-education-in-canada.

12. Whitehead, CR, Hodges, BD, Austin, Z. Dissecting the doctor: from character to characteristics in North American medical education. *Adv Health Sci Educ Theory Pract.* 2013; **18**(4):687–99.

13. Kuper, A, Albert, M, Hodges, BD. The origins of the field of medical education research. *Acad Med.* 2010; **85**(8):1347–53.

14. Frank, JR, Danoff, D. The CanMEDS initiative: implementing an outcomes-based framework of physician competencies. *Med Teach.* 2007; **29**(7):642–47.

15. Accreditation Council on Graduate Medical Education. *The ACGME Competency Framework.* Chicago, IL: ACGME. [Accessed Jan. 1, 2015.] Available from http://acgme.org/acgmeweb.

16. Hodges, BD. The shifting discourses of competence. In Hodges, BD, Lingard, L, eds. *The Question of Competence: Reconsidering Medical Education in the Twenty-first Century.* Ithaca, NY: Cornell University Press; 2012:14–41.

17. Hodges, B. Assessment in the post-psychometric era: learning to love the subjective and collective. *Med Teach.* 2013; **35**(7):564–68.

18. Hafferty, FW, O'Donnell, JF, eds. *The Hidden Curriculum in Health Professional Education.* Hanover, NH: Dartmouth College Press; 2015.

19. Frost, HD, Regehr, G. "I am a doctor": negotiating the discourses of standardization and diversity in professional identity construction. *Acad Med.* 2013; **88**(10):1570–77.

20. Hodges, BD. A tea-steeping or i-Doc model for medical education? *Acad Med.* 2010; **85**(9 Suppl): S34–S44.

21. The Arnold P. Gold Foundation. [Accessed Jan. 1, 2015.] Available from http://humanism-in-medicine.org.

22. AMS Phoenix Project. [Accessed Jan. 1, 2015.] Available from www.theamsphoenix.ca.

23. Whitehead, C. Recipes for medical education reform: will different ingredients create better doctors? A commentary on Sales and Schlaff. *Soc Sci Med.* 2010; **70**(11):1672–76.

24. Bogo, M, Regehr, C, Power, R, Hughes, J, Woodford M, Regehr, G. Toward new approaches for evaluating student field performance: tapping the implicit criteria used by experienced field instructors. *J Soc Work Educ.* 2004; **40**(3):417–26.

25. Gingerich, A, Regehr, G, Eva, KW. Rater-based assessments as social judgments: rethinking the etiology of rater errors. *Acad Med.* 2011; **86**(10 Suppl): S1–S7.

26. Ginsburg, S. Respecting the expertise of clinician assessors: construct alignment is one good answer. *Med Educ.* 2011; **45**(6):546–48.

27. Cruess, RL, Cruess, SR, Boudreau, JD, Snell, L, Steinert, Y. Reframing medical education to support professional identity formation. *Acad Med.* 2014; **89**(11):1446–51.

28. Razack, S, Lessard, D, Hodges, BD, Maguire, MH, Steinert, Y. The more it changes; the more it remains the same: a Foucauldian analysis of Canadian policy

documents relevant to student selection for medical school. *Adv Health Sci Educ Theory Pract*. 2014; **19**(2):161–81.

29. Colliver, JA, Markwell, SJ, Verhulst, SJ, Robbs, RS. The prognostic value of documented unprofessional behavior in medical school records for predicting and preventing subsequent medical board disciplinary action: the Papadakis studies revisited. *Teach Learn Med*. 2007; **19**(3):213–15.

30. Stern, DT, Frohna, AZ, Gruppen, LD. The prediction of professional behavior. *Med Educ*. 2005; **39**(1): 75–82.

31. Razack, S, Lessard, D, Hodges, B, McGuire, M, Steinert, Y. Representations of self in Multiple Mini interviews: a Goffman Performance Theory analysis. Unpublished manuscript.

32. Goffman, E. *The Presentation of Self in Everyday Life*. New York, NY: Doubleday; 1959.

33. Martimianakis, MA, Maniate, JM, Hodges, BD. Sociological interpretations of professionalism. *Med Educ*. 2009; **43**(9):829–37.

34. Jarvis-Selinger, S, Pratt, DD, Regehr, G. Competency is not enough: integrating identity formation into the medical education discourse. *Acad Med*. 2012; **87**(9):1185–90.

35. Kuper, A, Hodges, BD. Medical education in societies. In Dornan, T, Mann, KV, Scherpbier, AJJA, Spencer, JA, eds. *Medical Education: Theory and Practice*. London, UK: Elsevier; 2010:39–49.

36. hooks, b. Black women – shaping feminist theory. In *Feminist Theory – from Margin to Centre*. Boston, MA: South End Press; 1984.

37. Jaye, C, Egan, T, Parker, S. 'Do as I say, not as I do': medical education and Foucault's normalizing technologies of the self. *Anthropol Med*. 2006; **13**(2):141–55.

38. Hodges, B. The many and conflicting histories of medical education in Canada and the USA: an introduction to the paradigm wars. *Med Educ*. 2005; **39**(6):613–21.

39. Ho, MJ. Culturally sensitive medical professionalism. *Acad Med*. 2013; **88**(7):1014.

40. Martimianakis, MA, Hafferty, FW. The world as the new local clinic: a critical analysis of three discourses of global medical competency. *Soc Sci Med*. 2013; **87**:31–38.

41. Lingard, L. Rethinking competence in the context of teamwork. In Hodges, B, Lingard, L, eds. *The Question of Competence: Reconsidering Medical Education in the Twenty-First Century*. Ithaca, NY: Cornell University Press; 2012:42–69.

42. Dewey, J. *How We Think: A Restatement of the Relation of Reflective Thinking to the Educative Process*. New York, NY: DC Heath and Co; 1933.

43. Habermas, J. *Knowledge and Human Interests: A General Perspective*. Boston, MA: Beacon Press; 1971.

44. Schön, DA. *The Reflective Practitioner: How Professionals Think in Action*. New York, NY: Basic Books; 1983.

45. Ng, SL, Kinsella, EA, Friesen, F, Hodges, B. Reclaiming a theoretical orientation to reflection in medical education research: a critical narrative review. *Med Educ*. 2015; **49**(5):461–75.

46. Hodges, BD. Sea monsters & whirlpools: navigating between examination and reflection in medical education. *Med Teach*. 2015; **37**(3):261–66.

47. Hodges, BD. When I say … critical theory. *Med Educ*. 2014; **48**(11):1043–44.

48. Eichbaum, QG. Thinking about thinking and emotion: the metacognitive approach to the medical humanities that integrates humanities with the basic and clinical sciences. *Perm J*. 2014; **18**(4): 64–75.

Index

Printed in the United States
By Bookmasters